Radiographic Imaging and Exposure

TERRI L. FAUBER, EdD, RT(R)(M)

Professor Emeritus of Radiation Sciences
Department of Radiation Sciences
College of Health Professions
Virginia Commonwealth University
Richmond, Virginia

ELSEVIER

ELSEVIER

3251 Riverport Lane
St. Louis, Missouri 63043

Content Strategist: Sonya Seigafuse
Director, Content Development: Ellen M. Wurm-Cutter
Senior Content Development Specialist: Laura Klein
Publishing Services Manager: Shereen Jameel
Project Manager: Manikandan Chandrasekaran
Cover Design and Design Direction: Amy Buxton

Printed in India

Last digit is the print number: 9 8 7 6 5 4 3

CONTRIBUTOR

James N. Johnston, PhD, RT(R)(CV), FASRT
Professor Radiologic Sciences
Provost and Vice President for Academic Affairs
Midwestern State University
Wichita Falls, Texas

REVIEWERS

Sandra E. Moore, MA, RT(R)(M)(ARRT)
Director
Schools of Medical Imaging
Russell H. Morgan Department of Radiology and
    Radiologic Sciences
The Johns Hopkins Hospital
Baltimore, Maryland

Richard Sanders, MSRS, RT(R)(CT)
Clinical and Didactic Instructor
School of Radiologic Technology
Novant Health Presbyterian Medical Center
Charlotte, North Carolina

N. Tim Wilhelm, MEd, RT(R)
Associate Professor
Business and Allied Health
Central Virginia Community College
Lynchburg, Virginia

Ingrid Wright, MHSc, RT(R)
Program Director
Radiologic Technology Program
St. Johns River State College
St. Augustine, Florida

Radiographic Imaging and Exposure takes a unique and more effective approach to teaching imaging and exposure by focusing on the practical fundamentals. With a topic such as radiographic imaging, it is impossible to entirely depart from theoretic information, and we do not want to do so. A concerted effort was made to present the most important and relevant information on radiographic imaging and exposure. This book highlights the practical application of theoretical information to make it more immediately useful to students and practicing radiographers alike. Our ultimate goal is to provide the knowledge to effectively solve problems for consistently producing quality radiographic images in a clinical environment.

WHO WILL BENEFIT FROM THIS BOOK?

Radiographic Imaging and Exposure provides a fundamental presentation of topics that are vital for students to master to be competent radiographers. Moreover, radiographers will benefit from the practical approach to the topics of imaging and exposure presented here.

ORGANIZATION

Radiographic Imaging and Exposure begins with a description of Wilhelm Conrad Roentgen's discovery of x-rays in 1895 and the excitement it first caused among the members of the 19th-century society, who feared that private anatomy would be exposed for all to see! The introductory chapter moves into the realm of radiologic science with discussions of x-rays as energy, the unique characteristics of x-rays, and the fundamentals of radiation protection. Chapter 2 provides a more detailed discussion of the x-ray beam. The subsequent chapters describe image formation and radiographic quality (Chapter 3), digital image characteristics, receptors, and image acquisition (Chapter 4); digital image processing, display, and data management (Chapter 5); exposure technique factors (Chapter 6); and scatter control (Chapter 7). Chapter 8 focuses on the tools available to assist radiographers in selecting appropriate exposure techniques, such as automatic exposure control devices, anatomically programmed techniques, and exposure technique charts. Chapter 9 presents relevant content for those educators who still teach film-screen imaging. Chapter 10 discusses the components of fluoroscopic units, fluoroscopic features, and recording and viewing systems, with an expanded discussion on the digital fluoroscopic technology in use today.

Radiation exposure and imaging continues to be a complex subject even in the digital age. This text provides a thorough yet practical level of imaging and exposure to equip radiographers with the knowledge they need to produce high-quality images on the first attempt.

DISTINCTIVE FEATURES

Radiographic imaging and exposure is a complex topic, and a mastery of the fundamentals is necessary to become competent, whether you are a student or a practicing radiographer. Three special features have been integrated within each chapter to facilitate the understanding and retention of the concepts discussed and to underscore their applicability in a clinical setting. In addition, these special features give the practicing radiographer quick visual access to fundamental information that they need every day. Each feature is distinguished by its own icon for easy recognition.

Important Relationships summarize the relationships being discussed in the text, as each one occurs, for immediate summary and review. The topic of radiographic imaging and exposure is replete with fundamental, important relationships, and they are emphasized in short, meaningful ways at every opportunity.

 Mathematical Applications demonstrate the importance of mathematical formulas. Radiographic imaging also has a strong quantitative component, and this feature helps accustom readers to the necessity of mastering mathematical formulas. Because the formulas are presented with clinical scenarios, immediate applications and explanations of the formulas are provided.

 Radiation Protection Alerts emphasize the imaging and exposure variables that can have an impact on radiation exposure to patients and others. Because computer processing can mask exposure errors, it is even more important for radiographers to comprehend how their exposure technique choices can affect the patient.

NEW TO THIS EDITION

The digital imaging content has been expanded into two chapters for a more thorough coverage of current concepts. Data management has been added in Chapter 5 to provide the fundamentals of imaging informatics. Managing electronic health information and maintaining the safety and security of protected health information are responsibilities of all health care professionals, including radiographers. All discussion of film-screen imaging has been moved to Chapter 9. Educators who do not teach film-screen imaging can skip Chapter 9. As in previous editions, emphasis is placed on the responsibilities radiographers have in limiting the radiation exposure to their patients.

The sixth edition of *Radiographic Imaging and Exposure* includes the following:

1. Expanded and in-depth coverage of digital imaging and an increased coverage of digital fluoroscopy that meets the ARRT examination content specifications
2. Emphasis on radiographers' responsibilities in minimizing radiation exposure to patients and themselves

LEARNING AIDS

One of the primary goals of *Radiographic Imaging and Exposure* is to be a practical textbook that prepares student radiographers for the responsibilities of radiographic imaging in a clinical setting. Every effort has been made to make the material easily accessible and understandable while remaining thorough.

- The writing style is straightforward and concise, and the textbook includes numerous features to aid in the mastery of its content, including *Important Relationships, Mathematical Applications,* and *Radiation Protection Alerts.*
- All the *Important Relationships, Mathematical Applications,* and *Radiation Protection Alerts* are also collected in separate appendices for quick reference and review and are organized by chapter.
- *Radiographic Imaging and Exposure* also includes traditional learning aids. Each chapter begins with a list of objectives and key terms and concludes with a set of multiple-choice review questions, which help readers to evaluate whether they have achieved the chapter's objectives. An answer key is provided in the back of the book.

ANCILLARIES FOR INSTRUCTORS

Evolve Resources is an interactive learning environment designed to work in coordination with *Radiographic Imaging & Exposure,* 6th edition. It includes laboratory activities, PowerPoint slides, mathematical worksheets, an image collection of approximately 260 images, two practice tests with 60 questions each, and a Test Bank in Exam View with more than 620 questions.

The ancillary material on Evolve is useful for both practiced and novice educators. The laboratory exercises accommodate different available resources and instructor preferences for varying the recommended laboratory activities. Additional mathematical worksheets are included for educators to provide more practice for students if required.

Instructors may also use Evolve to provide an Internet-based course component that reinforces and expands the concepts presented in class. Evolve may be used to publish the class syllabus, outlines, and lecture notes; set up "virtual office hours" and e-mail communication; share important dates and information through the online class calendar; and encourage student participation through chat rooms and discussion boards. Evolve allows instructors to post exams and manage their grade books online. For more information, visit http://evolve.elsevier.com/Fauber/radiographic/ or contact an Elsevier sales representative.

ACKNOWLEDGMENTS

The study of digital imaging has expanded far beyond the fundamentals into the disciplines of data management and imaging informatics. As a result, radiographers have enormous responsibility to not only produce quality digital images but also protect patient health information.

It takes many dedicated and knowledgeable people to revise and improve a textbook on radiographic imaging and exposure. Sonya Seigafuse has been a steadfast supporter of me as an author and strong advocate for publishing a quality textbook. Laura Klein has been indispensable in managing the many challenges of a textbook revision, and it has been a pleasure to work with her. Manikandan Chandrasekaran has skillfully navigated the final stages of the textbook revision to ensure its accuracy and quality.

Comprehending the intricacies of digital imaging continues to be a challenge, and I am grateful for the knowledge and expertise of the reviewers who have challenged me to include more digital image processing and imaging informatics. Educators, students, and radiographers have inspired me to pursue excellence in producing an imaging textbook that is comprehensible, accurate, and relevant to radiographic imaging. I am truly humbled by the knowledge and skills required of radiographers in this digital age, and I applaud their determination to establish themselves in their unique health care role.

Terri L. Fauber

CONTENTS

Radiation and Its Discovery

CHAPTER OUTLINE

OBJECTIVES

After completing this chapter, the reader will be able to perform the following:

1. Define all the key terms in this chapter.
2. State all the important relationships in this chapter.
3. Describe the events surrounding the discovery of x-rays.
4. Describe the dual nature of x-ray energy.
5. State the characteristics of electromagnetic radiation.
6. Differentiate among the units of measurement for ionizing radiation.
7. List the properties of x-rays.
8. Recognize the fundamentals of radiation protection.

KEY TERMS

absorbed dose
air kerma
ALARA
dose equivalent
effective dose

electromagnetic radiation
exposure
fluorescence
frequency
photon

quantum
radioactivity
wavelength

X-rays were discovered in Europe in the late 19th century by German scientist Dr. Wilhelm Conrad Roentgen. Although Roentgen discovered x-rays by accident, he proceeded to study them so thoroughly that within a very short time, he identified all the properties of x-rays that are recognized today. Roentgen was more interested in the characteristics of x-rays as a form of energy than their practical application. X-rays are classified as a specific type of energy termed *electromagnetic radiation*, and like all other types of electromagnetic energy, x-rays act like both waves and particles.

DISCOVERY

X-rays were discovered on November 8, 1895, by Dr. Wilhelm Conrad Roentgen (Fig. 1-1), a German physicist and mathematician. Roentgen studied at the Polytechnic Institute in Zurich. He was appointed to the faculty of the University of Würzburg and was the director of the Physics

FIG. 1-1 Dr. Wilhelm Conrad Roentgen. (From Glasser O: *Wilhelm Conrad Roentgen and the early history of the roentgen rays,* 1933; Courtesy of Charles C Thomas, Springfield, IL.)

Institute at the time of his discovery. As a teacher and researcher, his academic interest was the conduction of high-voltage electricity through a low-vacuum tube. A low-vacuum tube is simply a glass tube from which a certain amount of air is evacuated. The specific type of tube that Roentgen was working with was called a *Crookes tube* (Fig. 1-2).

At the end of his workday on November 8, Roentgen prepared his research apparatus for the next experimental session to be conducted when he would return to his workplace. He darkened his laboratory to observe the electrical glow (cathode rays) that occurred when the tube was energized. This glow from the tube would indicate that the tube was receiving electricity and was ready for the next experiment. That day, Roentgen covered his tube with black cardboard and again electrified it. By chance, he noticed a faint glow coming from a certain material located several feet from his electrified tube. The source was a piece of paper coated with barium platinocyanide. Not believing that the cathode rays could reach that far from the tube, Roentgen repeated the experiment. Each time Roentgen energized his tube, he observed this glow coming from the barium platinocyanide–coated paper. He concluded that the energy emanating from his tube was causing this paper to produce light, or fluoresce. **Fluorescence** refers to the instantaneous production of light resulting from the interaction of some type of energy (in this case x-rays) and some element or compound (in this case barium platinocyanide).

Roentgen was understandably excited about this apparent discovery; however, at the same time, he was cautious not to make any early assumptions about what he had observed. Before

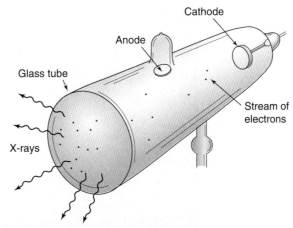

FIG. 1-2 A Crookes tube as used by Roentgen to discover x-rays.

sharing information about his discovery with colleagues, Roentgen spent time meticulously investigating the properties of this new type of energy. Of course, this new type of energy was not new at all; it had always existed and had likely been produced unknowingly by Roentgen and his contemporaries who were also involved in experiments with electricity and low-vacuum tubes. Knowing that others were doing similar research, Roentgen worked in earnest to exactly determine what this energy was.

Roentgen spent the next several weeks working feverishly in his laboratory to investigate as many properties of this energy as he could. He noticed that when he placed his hand between his energized tube and the barium platinocyanide–coated paper, he could see the bones of his hand glow on the paper, with this fluoroscopic image moving as he moved his hand. Curious about this, he produced a static (stationary) image of his wife Anna Bertha's hand using a 15-min exposure. This became the world's first radiograph (Fig. 1-3). Roentgen gathered other materials and interposed them between his energized tube and the fluorescent paper. Some materials, such as wood, allowed this energy to pass through and caused the paper to fluoresce, whereas some materials, such as platinum, did not.

In December 1895, Roentgen decided that his investigations of this energy were sufficient to inform his physicist colleagues of what he now believed to be a discovery of a new form of energy. He called this energy *x-rays*, with *x* representing the mathematical symbol for the unknown. On December 28, 1895, Roentgen submitted a scholarly paper on his research activities to his local professional society, the Würzburg Physico-Medical Society. Written in his native language, German, his article was titled "On a New Kind of Rays," and it caused a buzz of excitement in the medical and scientific communities. Within a short time, an English translation of this article appeared in the journal *Nature*, dated January 23, 1896.

Although Roentgen deemed his discovery important, he also considered it to have primarily academic value. His concern was in the x-ray itself as a form of energy and not in its possible practical applications. Others quickly began assembling their own x-ray–producing devices and exposed inanimate objects as well as tissue, both animal and human and both living and dead, to determine the range of use of these x-rays. Their efforts were driven largely by skepticism rather than belief that x-rays could do what had been claimed. Skepticism eventually gave way to productive curiosity as investigations concentrated on ways of imaging living human bodies for medical benefits.

As investigations into legitimate medical applications of the use of x-rays continued, the nonmedical and nonscientific communities began taking a different view of Roentgen's discovery. X-ray-proof underwear was offered as protection from these rays, which were known to penetrate

FIG. 1-3 The first radiograph that demonstrates the bones of the hand of Roentgen's wife, Anna Bertha, with a ring on one finger. (From Glasser O: *Wilhelm Conrad Roentgen and the early history of the roentgen rays*, 1933; Courtesy of Charles C Thomas, Springfield, IL.)

solid materials, and a New Jersey legislator attempted to enact legislation that would ban the use of x-ray–producing devices in opera glasses. Both these efforts were presumably aimed at protecting an individual's private anatomy from unscrupulous users of x-rays. The public furor reached such a height that a London newspaper, the *Pall Mall Gazette*, offered the following editorial in 1896: "We are sick of Roentgen rays. Perhaps the best thing would be for all civilized nations to combine to burn all the Roentgen rays, to execute all the discoverers, and to corner all the equipment in the world and to whelm it in the middle of the ocean. Let the fish contemplate each other's bones if they like, but not us."

In a similar vein but in a more creative fashion, another London periodical, *Photography*, in 1896 offered the following:

Roentgen Rays, Roentgen Rays?
What is this craze?
The town's ablaze
With this new phase
Of x-ray ways.
I'm full of daze, shock and amaze,
For nowadays
I hear they'll gaze
Through cloak and gown and even stays!
The naughty, naughty Roentgen rays!

Fortunately, despite these public distractions, the scientific applications of x-rays continued to be investigated for the benefit of society. Roentgen's discovery was lauded as one of great significance to science and medicine, and Roentgen received the first Nobel Prize presented for physics in 1901. The branch of medicine that was concerned with the use of x-rays was called *roentgenology*. A unit of radiation exposure was called the *roentgen*. X-rays were, at one time at least, called *roentgen rays*.

Excitement over this previously undiscovered type of energy was tempered by the realization in 1898 that x-rays could cause biological damage. This damage was first noticed as a reddening and burning of the skin (called *erythema*) of individuals who were exposed to large doses of x-rays required at that time. More serious effects, such as the growth of malignant tumors and chromosomal changes, were attributed in later decades to x-ray exposure. However, despite these disturbing findings, it was realized that x-rays could be used safely. When radiation-protection procedures to safeguard both the radiographer and the patient are followed, x-rays can assist medical diagnosis by imaging virtually every part of the human body.

X-RAYS AS ENERGY

Energy is the ability to do work, and it can exist in different forms, such as electrical energy, kinetic energy, thermal energy, and electromagnetic energy. Energy can also be transformed from one form to another, for instance, the electrical energy applied to a stove is changed into heat. Similarly, the electrical energy applied to an x-ray tube is transformed into heat and x-rays.

X-radiations, or x-rays, are a type of electromagnetic radiation. **Electromagnetic radiation** refers to radiation that has both electrical and magnetic properties. All radiations that are electromagnetic make up a spectrum (Fig. 1-4).

In the academic discipline of physics, energy can generally be described as behaving according to the wave or the particle concept of physics. X-rays have a dual nature: they behave like both waves and particles. Higher-energy electromagnetic radiation, such as x-rays, tends to exhibit more particle-like characteristics, and lower-energy electromagnetic radiation, such as radiowaves, tend to exhibit more wave-like characteristics.

 IMPORTANT RELATIONSHIP

The Dual Nature of X-ray Energy

X-rays act like both waves and particles.

X-rays can be described as waves because they move in waves that have wavelength and frequency. Looking at a sine wave (Fig. 1-5), one can see that the **wavelength** represents the distance between two successive crests or troughs. Wavelength is represented by the Greek letter lambda (λ), and its values are given in units of angstroms (Å). An angstrom is a metric unit of length equal to one ten-billionth of a meter, or 10^{-10} m. X-rays used in radiography range in wavelength from approximately 0.1 to 1.0 Å. Another unit of measurement for wavelength is nanometer (nm); 1 Å equals 0.1 nm, which equals 10^{-9} m.

The sine wave (Fig. 1-5) also demonstrates that **frequency** represents the number of waves (cycles) passing a given point per given unit of time (second). Frequency is represented by a lowercase *f* or by the Greek letter nu (ν), and its values are given in units of Hertz (Hz). One Hertz is equal to one cycle per second. X-rays used in radiography range in frequency from approximately 3×10^{19} to 3×10^{18} Hz. Wavelength and frequency are inversely related—that is, as one increases, the other decreases. Higher-energy electromagnetic radiation has high frequencies and low wavelengths.

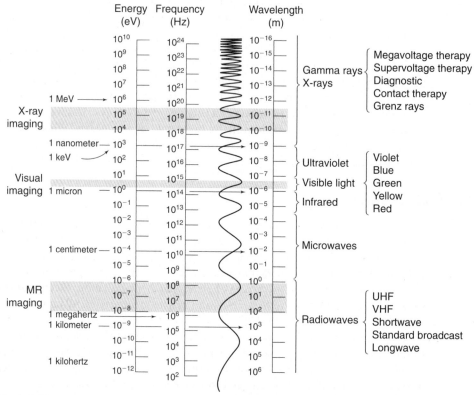

FIG. 1-4 Electromagnetic spectrum. Radiowaves are the least energetic on the spectrum, and gamma rays are the most energetic. *MR,* Magnetic resonance; *UHF,* ultra high frequency; *VHF,* very high frequency.

IMPORTANT RELATIONSHIP

Wavelength and Frequency

Wavelength and frequency are inversely related. Higher-energy x-rays have decreased wavelength and increased frequency. Lower-energy x-rays have increased wavelength and decreased frequency.

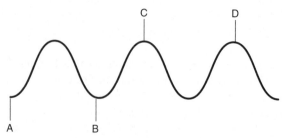

FIG. 1-5 Sine wave demonstrating wavelength and frequency. One wavelength is equal to the distance between two successive troughs (points *A* to *B*) or the distance between two successive crests (points *C* to *D*).

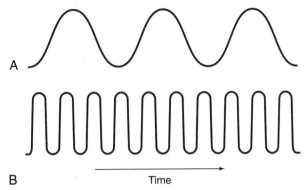

FIG. 1-6 A, Sine wave demonstrating long wavelength and low frequency. **B,** Sine wave demonstrating short wavelength and high frequency; comparison of sine waves. **A** and **B** demonstrate the inverse relationship between wavelength and frequency.

This relationship can be observed in Fig. 1-6 and is demonstrated by the expression $c = \lambda v$, in which c represents the speed of light. In this expression, if wavelength increases, frequency must decrease because the speed of light is a constant velocity (3×10^8 m/s or 186,000 miles/s). Conversely, if wavelength decreases, frequency must increase, again because the speed of light is constant. Mathematically, the formulas are $\lambda = c/v$ to solve for wavelength and $v = c/\lambda$ to solve for frequency. These formulas illustrate the inverse relationship between wavelength and frequency.

X-rays also behave like particles and move as photons or quanta (plural). A **photon** or **quantum** (singular) is a small, discrete bundle of energy. For most applications in radiography, x-rays are referred to as *photons*. When x-rays interact with matter, they behave more like particles than waves. The energy of an individual photon is measured in units of electron volts (eV) and the energy of diagnostic x-rays is approximately between 10^4 and 10^5 eV. Decreasing the wavelength and/or increasing the frequency of the x-ray will increase its energy.

Radiation Units of Measurement

It is important to recognize the units of radiation quantity to obtain an accurate understanding of radiation exposure, dose, and biologic effect. There are two systems for quantifying radiation exposure: the Standard (British) System and the International System (SI). SI has become the more widely adopted of the two. Radiation exposure can be measured in the following units:

Unit of Measure	Standard	International System (SI)
Exposure in air (a)	roentgen (R)	coulomb/kilogram air kerma (Gy_a)
Absorbed dose in tissue (t)	radiation absorbed dose (rad)	gray (Gy_t)
Dose equivalent	radiation equivalent in man (rem)	sievert (Sv)
Radioactivity	curie (Ci)	becquerel (Bq)

Exposure

The quantity of radiation **exposure** expressed in roentgens (R) measures the amount of ionization or electrical charge in a specified amount of air; this is a measure of the *intensity* of radiation exposure. The coulomb/kilogram is equivalent to the roentgen. The coulomb/kilogram is a measure of the number of electrons liberated by ionization per kilogram of air. Ionization is the removal of electrons from atoms. The roentgen or coulomb/kilogram is generally used as a unit of measure for such phenomena as the output intensity of x-ray equipment or intensity in air. The relationship between the two is:

$$1 \, C/kg = 3876 \, R$$

or

$$1 \, R = 2.58 \times 10^{-4} \, C/kg$$

Another radiation quantity used to express exposure or intensity is **air kerma** (**k**inetic **en**ergy **r**eleased per unit **ma**ss). Air kerma is used to describe the quantity of radiation energy delivered to a given point. The quantity of energy released by 1 R of exposure in air is equal to approximately 0.01 air kerma. Air kerma is the amount of energy deposited in a unit mass of air (kg) and expressed in units of joules (J) or J/kg, which is also the radiation unit, the gray (Gy). 1 R of exposure in air is equal to approximately 0.01 (Gy_a) air kerma; however, radiation exposure is typically expressed in smaller units by adding the prefix "milli," in which 1 R = 1000 mR and 1 Gy = 1000 mGy.

Absorbed Dose

The rad and gray are units measuring the transfer of radiation energy into matter (e.g., tissue), known as the **absorbed dose**. One rad is equal to an energy transfer of 100 ergs per gram of any absorbing matter. One gray (Gy_t) is defined as 1 joule of energy absorbed in each kilogram of absorbing material. The joule is the SI unit for the transfer of energy into matter and more commonly used today; 100 ergs per gram is equal to 0.01 joule per kilogram of irradiated matter. One rad is equal to 0.01 gray, and a conversion factor of 0.01 is used to convert a rad into a gray. For example, an absorbed dose of 5 rad = 0.05 Gy_t.

Absorbed dose is typically used in referring to patient low-dose medical radiation absorbed exposure and the potential biologic effects and is expressed as millirad or mGy_t. The amount of absorbed dose is dependent on the energy of the ionizing radiation and the type of interacting tissues.

Dose Equivalent

The units used in measuring occupational radiation exposure (**dose equivalent** [similarly known as equivalent dose]) are radiation equivalents in man (rem) and sieverts (Sv). One sievert equals 100 rem or 0.01 Sv equals 1 rem. These units are derived by multiplying a quality factor for dose equivalent and a radiation weighting factor (W_r) for equivalent dose by the units of absorbed exposure, rads or grays. The quality factor or W_r takes into consideration the biological effects of different types of ionizing radiation (Table 1-1). Although dose equivalent and equivalent dose may be used interchangeably, the quality factor and W_r are not equal for all ionizing radiations. However, x- and gamma rays have the same quality factor or W_r of 1 and therefore are equal in their biological effect on tissues. Consequently, 1 rad or 0.01 Gy is equal to 1 rem or 0.01 Sv.

TABLE 1-1 **International Commission of Radiologic Protection (ICRP) Radiation Weighting Factors**	
Type of Radiation	**Weighting Factor (W_r)**
X-rays, gamma rays, beta particles, and electrons	1
Protons	2
Fast neutrons and alpha particles	20

TABLE 1-2 International Commission of Radiologic Protection (ICRP)–Recommended Tissue Weighting Factors (ICRP 103)

Tissue	Weighting Factor (W_t)
Breast, adrenals, bone marrow, colon, extrathoracic region, gallbladder, heart, kidneys, lung, lymph nodes, muscle, oral mucosa, pancreas, prostate, small intestine, spleen, stomach, thymus, uterus, cervix	0.12
Gonads	0.08
Bladder, esophagus, liver, thyroid	0.04
Bone surface, brain, salivary glands, skin	0.01

Differing particulate radiations, such as alpha particles, have differing associated quality factors and W_r, resulting in changes in the biologic effects following exposure.

Effective dose is an expression of the *relative risk to humans* (whole-body exposure) of exposure to ionizing radiation. It is a calculated measure and concept most useful in radiation protection applications. However, effective dose does not consider patient variability such as age, gender, or weight and therefore should be used for populations and not individual patients. It is measured in Sv but is calculated by multiplying the absorbed dose (in Gy [but equal to Sv for x- and gamma rays]), the W_r and the tissue weighting factor (W_t). W_t is used as a correction factor because not all tissues, organs, or systems have the same level of sensitivity to radiation (radiosensitivity). If more than one tissue, organ, or system is exposed, the effective doses are added together (summed). Table 1-2 is the International Commission of Radiologic Protection (ICRP)–recommended tissue weighting factors.

It is important to note that our knowledge about tissue radiosensitivity and low-dose radiation risk has uncertainties and continues to evolve. There have been variations over the years regarding tissue radiosensitivity because of these inherent uncertainties, and therefore the W_t has varied. Nevertheless, ionizing radiation has the potential to produce biologic harm and should be administered wisely.

Radioactivity

Unstable atoms spontaneously emit particles and energy from the nucleus in an effort to reach stability (**radioactivity**). This process is called radioactive disintegration or decay. Radioisotopes are the radioactive elements used in nuclear medicine and radiation therapy.

The curie (Ci) and the becquerel (Bq) measure the rate of nuclear disintegration or decay of a material. Radioactive disintegration or decay refers to the decrease in the activity of a radiation source. Half-life is a term that describes the time it takes for the radiation activity to reduce to 50% of its original activity. For example, radioisotopes used in nuclear medicine typically have half-lives in a number of hours or days.

PROPERTIES OF X-RAYS

X-rays are known to have several characteristics or properties. These characteristics are briefly explained here and presented in Box 1-1.

- *X-rays are invisible.* In addition to being unable to see x-rays, one cannot feel, smell, or hear them.
- *X-rays are electrically neutral.* X-rays have neither a positive nor a negative charge; they cannot be accelerated or made to change direction by a magnet or electrical field.

BOX 1-1   Characteristics of X-rays

Are invisible
Are electrically neutral
Have no mass
Travel at the speed of light in a vacuum
Cannot be optically focused
Form a polyenergetic (heterogeneous) beam
Can be produced in a range of energies
Travel in straight lines
Can cause some substances to fluoresce
Can penetrate the human body
Can be absorbed or scattered in the human body
Can produce secondary radiation
Can cause damage to living tissue

- *X-rays have no mass.* X-rays create no resistance to being put into motion and cannot produce force.
- *X-rays travel at the speed of light in a vacuum.* X-rays move at a constant velocity of 3×10^8 m/s or 186,000 miles/s in a vacuum.
- *X-rays cannot be optically focused.* Optical lenses have no ability to focus or refract x-ray photons.
- *X-rays form polyenergetic (heterogeneous) beams.* The x-ray beam that is used in diagnostic radiography is composed of photons that have many different energies. The maximum energy that a photon in any beam may have is expressed by the kilovoltage peak (kVp), which is set on the control panel of the radiographic unit by the radiographer.
- *X-rays can be produced in a range of energies.* These are useful for different purposes in diagnostic routine radiography. The medically useful diagnostic range of x-ray energies is 30 to 150 KeV.
- *X-rays travel in straight lines.* X-rays used in diagnostic radiography form a divergent beam in which each individual photon travels in a straight line.
- *X-rays can cause certain substances to fluoresce.* When x-rays strike certain substances, the substances produce light. These substances are used in some types of radiographic image receptors.
- *X-rays can penetrate the human body.* X-rays have the ability to pass through the body based on the energy of the x-rays and on the compositions and thicknesses of the tissues being exposed.
- *X-rays can be absorbed or scattered by tissues in the human body.* Depending on the energy of an individual x-ray photon, that photon may be absorbed in the body or made to scatter, moving in another direction.
- *X-rays can produce secondary radiation.* When x-rays are absorbed as a result of a specific type of interaction with matter (photoelectric effect), a secondary or characteristic photon is produced.
- *X-rays can cause chemical and biologic damage to living tissue.* Through excitation and ionization (removal of electrons) of atoms comprising cells, damage to the cells (mainly through ionization of water in the body) can occur.

THE FUNDAMENTALS OF RADIATION PROTECTION

A central message throughout this textbook is that it is the radiographer's responsibility to minimize the radiation dose to the patient, to themselves, and to others in accordance with the **as low as reasonably achievable** (**ALARA**) principle. Although the ALARA principle is primarily intended for occupational exposures to imaging professionals, it has also been applied to patient radiation exposure. The concept of *dose optimization* is currently advocated, meaning the radiation exposure should be appropriate to the imaging procedure and avoid unnecessary exposure to the patient.

> ### ! RADIATION PROTECTION ALERT
> #### *ALARA Principle*
>
> It is the radiographer's responsibility to minimize the radiation dose to the patient, to themselves, and to others in accordance with the **a**s **l**ow **a**s **r**easonably **a**chievable (ALARA) principle.

Central to minimizing the radiation dose to oneself and to others are the cardinal principles of shielding, time, and distance. Shielding broadly refers to the use of radiopaque materials (i.e., materials through which x-rays do *not* pass easily) to greatly reduce radiation exposure to areas of the patient not essential for the exam being performed, to radiographers during exams, and to others. Lead-impregnated materials are a common example. Leaded and rubber sheets of varying sizes may be directly laid on the patient to shield radiosensitive areas. One example of this is gonadal shielding; these are specifically shaped lead materials that are placed directly over the gonadal area to minimize radiation dose to these radiosensitive areas. They must be carefully and precisely placed to prevent interference with the image and the anatomic area of interest. They should be used on all patients within reproductive age, all children, and when it will not interfere with the primary imaging objective of the examination being performed. Although the effectiveness of gonadal shielding is unresolved, it is recommended by many regulatory and professional organizations. Lead aprons must be worn by the radiographer and other health care workers when it is necessary to be in close proximity to the patient during an exposure. In addition, thyroid shields are commonly used in conjunction with lead aprons, especially during fluoroscopic exams by personnel who remain in the room. This collar wraps around the neck and fastens in the back to shield the entire front portion of the neck. Leaded curtains may be draped from the fluoroscopy tower to provide a barrier between the fluoroscopist (one operating the fluoroscope) and the x-ray beam during fluoroscopic exams. The walls of the radiographic suite are permeated with lead or lead equivalent (thicknesses of other materials that provide equivalent radiopaque properties as lead) to limit exposure beyond that intended for the radiological exam. The primary barriers are those to which the x-ray beam is routinely directed, such as the floor beneath the x-ray table and the wall behind the upright Bucky. Secondary barriers are the others, such as the wall separating the control panel from the room and the ceiling to protect those outside the room from scatter radiation. The general rule of thumb is to always maximize shielding (use as much as possible).

Time broadly refers to the duration of exposure to ionizing radiation and the time spent in a health care environment where exposure to ionizing radiation is accumulated. This may include the length of the exposure and number of times the patient is exposed for a radiological exam or the time a radiographer spends in a fluoroscopy suite (or any procedure involving fluoroscopy). Whether one is referring to the patient, to the radiographer, or to other health care workers, the general rule of thumb is to always minimize time (limit duration of exposure to ionizing radiation).

Distance refers to the space between oneself and the source of ionizing radiation. This is an effective means of limiting exposure simply because the intensity (quantity) of radiation diminishes over distance. This is an application of the inverse-square law discussed in detail in Chapter 6. Suffice it to say here that as one increases the distance from an ionizing radiation source, the radiation intensity from that source significantly decreases. This principle is applied mostly to radiographers and others to maintain a safe distance from the source of radiation during exposure. The general rule of thumb is always to maximize distance (maintain a safe distance from the radiation source during exposure).

❗ RADIATION PROTECTION ALERT

Cardinal Principles for Minimizing Radiation Dose

Time: Limit the amount of time exposed to ionizing radiation.
Distance: Maintain a safe distance from the source of ionizing radiation exposure.
Shielding: Maximize the use of shielding from ionizing radiation exposure.

Another important *tool* in radiation protection is the limiting of the field of x-ray exposure, essentially beam restriction, through the use of a collimator. By limiting the area of exposure, this device limits the radiation dose to the patient; that is, the smaller the area of x-ray exposure, the lower the total dose to the patient. When we discuss radiation interactions in the body, we are talking about x-ray photons interacting with atoms of tissue. The greater the volume of tissue we expose, the greater is the opportunity for such interactions to occur. With these interactions, the photon's energy will either be totally absorbed (which contributes to patient dose) or scattered (which may contribute to the dose to radiographers or others if in the immediate area). See Chapter 3 for a full discussion of x-ray interactions with matter.

❗ RADIATION PROTECTION ALERT

Beam Restriction

Limiting the size of the x-ray exposure field reduces the volume of tissue irradiated and reduces the radiation dose to the patient.

Next among our *tools* of radiation protection are the primary controls of the x-ray beam's kVp, milliamperage (mA), and duration (s), mAs = mA × s. These are the factors selected by the radiographer to produce an x-ray beam of a given quality (penetrating power) controlled by kVp and quantity (number of photons) ultimately controlled by mAs. The combination of kVp and mAs is selected on the basis of a number of considerations, including the anatomic part being examined, patient age, condition, pathology, and so on, and should be ideally suited to the circumstance to minimize radiation dose while producing optimum exposure to the image receptor. See Chapter 6 for a complete discussion of these factors.

❗ RADIATION PROTECTION ALERT

Primary Exposure Factors

The combination of kVp and mAs is selected based on a number of considerations, including the anatomic part being examined, patient age, condition, and pathology, and should be ideally suited to the circumstance to minimize radiation dose while producing optimum exposure to the image receptor.

Finally, there are a number of daily *workflow* tasks and processes that address radiation protection. A major one, for which the radiographer serves as a frontline advocate for the patient, is the avoidance of unnecessary duplication of exams. This means preventing the patient from having the same exam performed twice owing to an error. With so much computerization, automation, and team approach to patient care, it is easy to duplicate an order (accidentally order the same radiographic exam more than once) or for two different physicians involved in a patient's care who unknowingly order the same thing. There are instances when a patient's condition rapidly changes, and it is necessary to perform the same exam a number of times in succession, but it is appropriate to double-check an order or to stop and question. The radiographer must recognize and accept his or her role as a patient advocate and do what is necessary to avoid unnecessary duplication of exams. Think of each duplicate exam as a doubling of the radiation dose that is otherwise needed (the first exam was a normal dose, and the unnecessary one doubles that dose). Thus, this radiation protection measure alone significantly impacts the radiation dose administered to the patient and to others.

! RADIATION PROTECTION ALERT

Avoid Unnecessary Duplicate Exams

The radiographer must recognize and accept his or her role as a patient advocate and do what is necessary to avoid unnecessary duplication of exams.

Screening for pregnancy is another important task for minimizing unnecessary exposure to a developing fetus. Departmental protocols for pregnancy screening may vary and should be consistently used. When it is necessary to perform a radiographic exam on a pregnant patient, shielding materials and precise collimation, as discussed previously, should be used to minimize radiation dose administered to the fetus. Be sure to follow the clinical site policy for pregnancy screening.

! RADIATION PROTECTION ALERT

Screening for Pregnancy

Screening for pregnancy is another important task for minimizing unnecessary exposure to a developing fetus. When it is necessary to perform a radiographic exam on a pregnant patient, shielding materials and precise collimation should be used to minimize the radiation dose administered to the fetus.

Last, as a developing radiographer, good work habits and skills have not yet been developed. Use sufficient time and concentration to *get it right the first time.* Develop a mental checklist for radiographic procedures and perform them the same way every time. By doing so, mistakes involving the details of a task can be minimized along with unnecessary radiation dose administered to the patient and to others. See Box 1-2 for a summary of radiation protection fundamentals.

Since the publication of Roentgen's scientific paper, no other properties of x-rays have been discovered. However, the discussion of x-rays has expanded far beyond the early concerns about modesty or even danger. Today, x-rays are accepted as an important diagnostic tool in medicine, and the radiographer is an important member of the health care team. The radiographic imaging professional is responsible for the care of the patient in the radiology department, the production and control of x-rays, and the formation of a quality radiographic image. Fig. 1-7 shows a standard radiographic room that includes an x-ray table, an overhead x-ray tube and collimator, and a control panel for the selection of exposure technique factors. The subsequent chapters of this book uncover the intricate and fascinating details of the art and science of medical radiography.

BOX 1-2   Summary of Radiation Protection Fundamentals

- Minimize the radiation dose to the patient, to themselves, and to others in accordance with the **a**s **l**ow **a**s **r**easonably **a**chievable (**ALARA**) principle.
- Limit the amount of *time* exposed to ionizing radiation.
- Maintain a safe *distance* from source of ionizing radiation exposure.
- Maximize the use of *shielding* from ionizing radiation exposure.
- Limit the size of the x-ray exposure field to the area of interest.
- Select a combination of kVp and mAs to produce a diagnostic image while minimizing patient radiation exposure.
- Avoid unnecessary duplicate exams.
- Screen for pregnancy.
- Develop a mental checklist for radiographic procedures and perform consistently.

FIG. 1-7 A, Typical radiographic unit showing the x-ray table, overhead x-ray tube, and collimator. (From Ehrlich RA: *Patient Care in Radiography: With an Introduction to Medical Imaging*, ed 9, St. Louis Elsevier Inc.) **B,** Control panel. (From Johnston JN, Fauber TL: *Essentials of Radiographic Physics and Imaging*, ed 3, St. Louis, 2020, Elsevier.)

CHAPTER SUMMARY

- X-rays were discovered on November 8, 1895, by Dr. Wilhelm Conrad Roentgen, a German physicist, mathematician, and recipient of the first Nobel Prize for physics.
- The discovery of x-rays was met with skepticism and curiosity and subsequently by acceptance of its medical benefit.
- X-rays are a type of electromagnetic radiation with both electrical and magnetic properties.
- Electromagnetic radiation is a form of energy that moves in waves with wavelength and frequency.
- Wavelength and frequency are inversely related. Higher-energy x-rays have decreased wavelength and increased frequency.
- X-rays act like both waves and particles and have a higher energy than other types of electromagnetic radiation, such as visible light.
- There are two systems of quantifying radiation exposure: the standard system and the International System (SI). Exposure in air: coulomb/kilogram, roentgen (R), and air kerma (Gy$_a$);

absorbed dose: radiation absorbed dose (rad) and gray (Gy_t); equivalent dose: radiation equivalent in man (rem) and sievert (Sv); effective dose: an expression of the relative risk to humans of exposure to ionizing radiation; radioactivity: curie (Ci) and becquerel (Bq).

- X-rays have several important characteristics. They are invisible and electrically neutral, have no mass, travel at the speed of light, penetrate matter, and can cause chemical and biologic changes.
- The fundamentals of radiation protection include adhering to the ALARA principle, dose optimization, time, distance, shielding, beam restriction, careful selection of exposure technique factors, avoidance of duplicate exams, and screening for pregnancy.

REVIEW QUESTIONS

1. In what year were x-rays discovered?
   A. 1892
   B. 1895
   C. 1898
   D. 1901
2. In what year were some of the biologically damaging effects of x-rays discovered?
   A. 1892
   B. 1895
   C. 1898
   D. 1901
3. X-rays were discovered in experiments dealing with electricity and _____.
   A. ionization
   B. magnetism
   C. atomic structure
   D. vacuum tubes
4. X-rays were discovered when they caused a barium platinocyanide-coated plate to _____.
   A. fluoresce
   B. phosphoresce
   C. vibrate
   D. burn and redden
5. X-radiation is classified in which spectrum?
   A. Radiation
   B. Energy
   C. Atomic
   D. Electromagnetic
6. X-rays have a dual nature, which means that they behave like both _____.
   A. atoms and molecules
   B. photons and quanta
   C. waves and particles
   D. charged and uncharged particles
7. The wavelength and frequency of x-rays are _____ related.
   A. directly
   B. inversely
   C. partially
   D. not

8. X-rays have _____ electrical charge.
   A. a positive
   B. a negative
   C. an alternately positive and negative
   D. no

9. X-rays have _____.
   A. no mass
   B. the same mass as electrons
   C. the same mass as protons
   D. the same mass as neutrons

10. The x-ray beam used in diagnostic radiography can be described as being _____.
    A. homogeneous
    B. monoenergetic
    C. polyenergetic
    D. scattered

11. The unit that measures the transfer of radiation energy into tissues is known as the _____.
    A. roentgen
    B. kerma
    C. gray
    D. sievert

12. What is defined as the measure of the intensity of radiation exposure?
    A. Absorbed dose
    B. Exposure
    C. Equivalent Dose
    D. Effective dose

13. What is the radiation weighting factor (W_r) for x- and gamma rays?
    A. 1
    B. 2
    C. 10
    D. 20

14. Which of the following will minimize radiation exposure to the patient?
    A. Beam restriction
    B. Gonadal shielding
    C. Avoid unnecessary duplicate exams
    D. All of the above

The X-ray Beam

OBJECTIVES

After completing this chapter, the reader will be able to perform the following:

1. Define all the key terms in this chapter.
2. State all the important relationships in this chapter.
3. Describe the construction of an x-ray tube.
4. State the function of each component of an x-ray tube.
5. Describe how x-rays are produced.
6. Explain the role of the primary exposure factors in determining the quality and quantity of x-rays.
7. Explain the line-focus principle.
8. State how the anode heel effect can be used in radiography.
9. Differentiate among the types of filtration and explain their purpose.
10. Calculate heat units.
11. Recognize how changing generator output, kVp, mA, and filtration affect the x-ray emission spectrum.
12. List the guidelines followed to extend the life of an x-ray tube.

KEY TERMS

actual focal spot size
added filtration
anode
anode heel effect
bremsstrahlung interactions
cathode
characteristic interactions
compensating filters
dosimeter
effective focal spot size
exposure time
filament

filament current
focusing cup
half-value layer (HVL)
heat unit (HU)
inherent filtration
kilovoltage
leakage radiation
line-focus principle
milliamperage (mA)
off-focus radiation
rotor
space charge

space charge effect
stator
target
thermionic emission
total filtration
trough filter
tube current
voltage ripple
wedge filter
x-ray emission spectrum

The x-ray tube is the most important part of the x-ray machine because the tube is where the x-rays are produced. Radiographers must understand the construction and operation of an x-ray tube. The radiographer controls many actions that occur within the tube. Kilovoltage peak (kVp), milliamperage (mA), and exposure time all are factors that the radiographer adjusts on the control panel to produce a quality image. The radiographer also needs to be aware of the amount of heat produced during x-ray production because excessive heat can damage the tube.

X-RAY PRODUCTION

The production of x-rays requires a rapidly moving stream of electrons that are suddenly decelerated or stopped. The source of electrons is a cathode, or negative electrode. The negative electrode is heated, and electrons are emitted. The electrons are attracted to the positively charged anode (positive electrode) and move rapidly toward the anode, where they are stopped or decelerated. When the kinetic energy (energy of motion) of the electrons is transferred to the anode, x-rays and heat are produced (Fig. 2-1).

Cathode

The **cathode** of an x-ray tube is a negatively charged electrode. It comprises a filament and a focusing cup. Fig. 2-2 shows a double-filament cathode surrounded by a focusing cup. The **filament** is a coiled tungsten wire, which is the source of electrons during x-ray production.

FIG. 2-1 X-ray tube inside protective housing. (Modified From Johnston JN, Fauber TL: *Essentials of Radiographic Physics and Imaging*, ed 2, St. Louis, 2016, Mosby.)

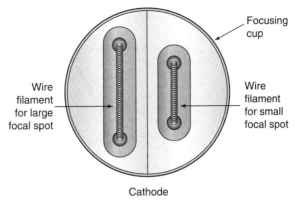

FIG. 2-2 Most x-ray tubes use a small filament and a large filament, corresponding to a small focal spot size and a large focal spot size.

 IMPORTANT RELATIONSHIP

Filament

The filament is the source of electrons during x-ray production.

Most x-ray tubes are referred to as *dual-focus tubes* because they have two filaments: one large and one small. Only one filament is energized at any one time during x-ray production. If the radiographer selects a large focal spot when setting the control panel, the large filament is energized. If a small focal spot is chosen, the small filament is energized. The **focusing cup** is made of nickel and nearly surrounds the filament. It is open at one end to allow electrons to flow freely across the tube from the cathode to the anode. It has a negative charge, which keeps the cloud of electrons emitted from the filament from spreading apart. The purpose of the focusing cup is to focus the stream of electrons from the filament toward the anode target.

Anode

The **anode** of an x-ray tube is a positively charged electrode composed of molybdenum, copper, tungsten, and graphite. These materials are used for their thermal and electrical conductive properties. The anode consists of a target and, in rotating anode tubes, a stator and rotor. The **target** is made of a metal that abruptly decelerates and stops electrons in the tube current, allowing the production of x-rays. The target can be either rotating or stationary. Tubes with rotating targets are more common than tubes with stationary ones. Rotating anodes are manufactured to rotate at a set speed ranging from 3000 to 10,000 revolutions per minute (rpm). Fig. 2-3 shows how a rotating anode and stationary anode differ in appearance.

 IMPORTANT RELATIONSHIP

Target

The target is the part of the anode that is struck by the focused stream of electrons coming from the cathode. The target stops the electrons and creates the opportunity for the production of x-rays.

FIG. 2-3 Side views of a stationary anode (**A**) and a rotating anode (**B**).

Tungsten–
rhenium
alloy

Molybdenum

Graphite

FIG. 2-4 Typical construction of a rotating anode.

The target of the rotating anode tubes is made of a tungsten and rhenium alloy. This layer, or focal track, is embedded in a base of molybdenum and graphite (Fig. 2-4). Tungsten generally constitutes 90% of the composition of the rotating target, with rhenium constituting the other 10%. The face of the anode is angled to help the x-ray photons exit the tube. Rotating targets generally have a target angle ranging from 5 to 20 degrees. Tungsten is used for both rotating and stationary targets because it has a high atomic number of 74 for efficient x-ray production and a high melting point of 3400°C (6152°F). Most of the energy produced by an x-ray tube is heat; thus, melting of the target can sometimes become a problem, especially with high exposures.

IMPORTANT RELATIONSHIP

Tungsten

Because tungsten has a high atomic number (74) and a high melting point (3400°C [6,152°F]), it efficiently produces x-rays.

To turn the anode during x-ray production, a rotating anode tube requires a stator and rotor (Fig. 2-5). The **stator** is an electric motor that turns the rotor at very high speed. The **rotor** (made of copper) is rigidly connected to the target through the anode stem (made of molybdenum), causing the target to rapidly rotate during x-ray production. High-strength ball bearings in the rotor allow it to smoothly rotate at high speeds.

During x-ray production, most of the energy produced at the anode is heat, with a very small percentage being x-ray energy. Heat can pose a problem if allowed to build up; hence, it is transferred to the envelope and then to the insulating oil surrounding the tube. Moreover, many tube assemblies have a fan that blows air over the tube to help dissipate heat.

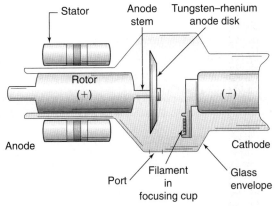

FIG. 2-5 Structure of a typical x-ray tube, including the major operational parts.

Dissipating Heat

The heat produced when the x-ray exposure is activated is transferred to the insulating oil that surrounds the x-ray tube.

Rotating anodes can withstand high heat loads; this ability relates to the actual focal spot, which is the physical area of the target that is bombarded by electrons during x-ray production. With stationary targets, the focal spot is a fixed area on the surface of the target. With rotating targets, this area is represented by a focal track. Fig. 2-6 shows the stationary anode's focal spot and the rotating anode with its focal track. The size of the focal spot is not altered with a rotating anode, but the actual physical area of the target bombarded by electrons is constantly

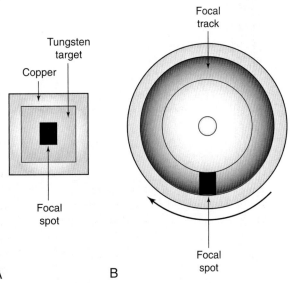

FIG. 2-6 A, Front view of a stationary anode. **B,** The target area of the rotating anode turns during exposure along with an increased physical area—a focal track—that is exposed to electrons.

moving, causing a greater area of the *focal track* to be exposed to electrons. Because of the larger area of the target being bombarded during an exposure, the rotating anode is able to withstand higher heat loads produced by greater exposure factors. Rotating anode x-ray tubes are used in all applications in radiography, whereas stationary anode tubes are limited to studies of small anatomic structures such as teeth.

IMPORTANT RELATIONSHIP

Rotating Anodes

> Rotating anodes can withstand higher heat loads than stationary anodes because the rotation causes a greater physical area, or focal track, to be exposed to electrons.

X-ray Tube Housing

The components necessary for x-ray production are housed in a glass or metal envelope. Fig. 2-7 shows the appearance of a glass x-ray tube. Metal envelopes are more commonly used because of their superior electrical properties.

A disadvantage of a glass envelope x-ray tube is that tungsten evaporated from the filament during exposure can be deposited upon the inside of the glass, especially in the middle portion of the envelope. This evaporation can affect the flow of electrons and cause the tube to fail. Replacing this section of glass with metal prevents these problems and extends the tube life. An additional advantage of a metal envelope is the reduction of **off-focus radiation.** Off-focus radiation occurs when projectile electrons are reflected and x-rays are produced from outside the focal spot. The metal tube envelope can collect these electrons and conduct them away from the anode.

The envelope allows air to be completely evacuated from the x-ray tube, which in turn allows an efficient flow of electrons from cathode to anode. The envelope serves two additional functions: it provides some insulation from electrical shock that may occur because the cathode and anode contain electrical charges, and it dissipates heat in the tube by conducting it to the insulating oil surrounding the envelope. The purpose of insulating oil is to provide more insulation from electrical shock and to help dissipate heat away from the tube. All of these components are surrounded by metal tube housing on all sides except for a port, or window, which allows the primary beam to exit the tube. It is the metal tube housing that the radiographer observes and handles when moving the x-ray tube. The tube housing is lined with lead to provide additional shielding from **leakage radiation**. Leakage radiation refers to any x-rays, other than the primary

FIG. 2-7 A glass envelope x-ray tube as it appears before installation in a tube housing.

beam, that escape the tube housing. The tube housing is required to allow a leakage radiation of no more than 100 mR/h (1 mGy$_a$/h) to escape when measured at a distance of 1 m from the source while the tube operates at maximum output. Electrical current is supplied to the x-ray tube using two high-voltage cables that enter the top of the tube assembly.

TARGET INTERACTIONS

The electrons that move from the cathode to the anode travel extremely fast, approximately at half the speed of light. The moving electrons, which have kinetic energy, strike the target and interact with the tungsten atoms in the anode to produce x-rays.

 IMPORTANT RELATIONSHIP

Production of X-rays

As electrons strike the target, their kinetic energy is transferred to the tungsten atoms in the anode to produce x-rays.

These interactions occur within the top 0.5 mm of the anode surface. Two types of interactions produce x-ray photons: bremsstrahlung interactions and characteristic interactions.

 IMPORTANT RELATIONSHIP

Interactions that Produce X-ray Photons

Bremsstrahlung interactions and characteristic interactions both produce x-ray photons.

Bremsstrahlung Interactions

Bremsstrahlung is a German word meaning *braking* or *slowing down radiation*. **Bremsstrahlung interactions** occur when a projectile (incident) electron completely avoids the orbital electrons of a tungsten atom and travels very close to its nucleus. The very strong electrostatic force of the positively charged nucleus causes the negatively charged electron to suddenly *slow down*. As the electron loses energy, it suddenly changes its direction, and the energy loss then reappears as an x-ray photon (Fig. 2-8). The closer the projectile electron travels to the nucleus, the stronger the attraction. The stronger this attraction, the more energy the projectile electron loses and the stronger the resultant x-ray photon (higher energy). Projectile electrons that travel farther from the nucleus create x-ray photons with less energy.

X-ray energy is measured in kiloelectron volts (keV [1 keV = 1000 electron volts]). The energy of a bremsstrahlung x-ray photon can be found by subtracting the energy that the projectile electron exits the atom with from the energy it had upon entering. For example, a projectile electron enters an atom with 120 keV of energy, passes very close to the nucleus, and exits with 40 keV of energy. The x-ray photon produced is 80 keV (120 keV – 40 keV = 80 keV). If that same projectile electron traveled farther from the nucleus and exited with 90 keV of energy, the x-ray photon produced would be 30 keV (120 keV – 90 keV = 30 keV).

In the diagnostic energy range from 30 to 150 keV, most x-ray interactions are bremsstrahlung. Below 70 kVp (with a tungsten target), 100% of the x-ray beam results from bremsstrahlung interactions. Above 70 kVp, approximately 85% of the beam results from bremsstrahlung interactions.

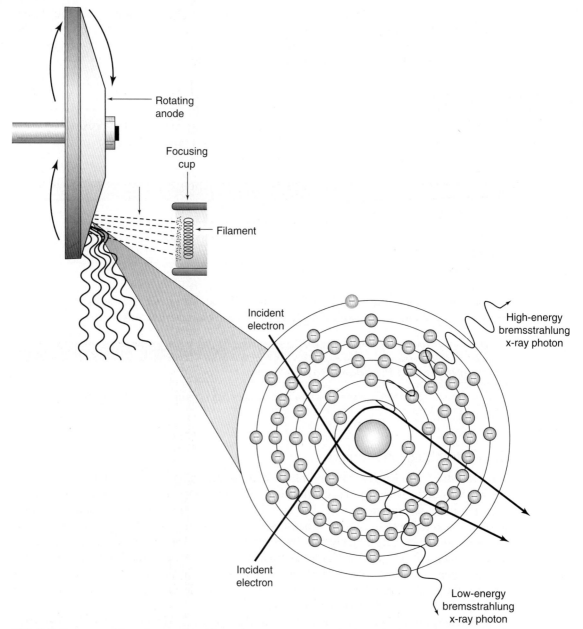

Rotating anode

Focusing cup

Filament

Incident electron

High-energy bremsstrahlung x-ray photon

Incident electron

Low-energy bremsstrahlung x-ray photon

FIG. 2-8 Bremsstrahlung interaction. X-ray photons are created when the incident electrons travel close to the atom's nucleus of the rotating tungsten anode.

IMPORTANT RELATIONSHIP

Bremsstrahlung Interactions

Bremsstrahlung interactions occur when a projectile (incident) electron completely avoids the orbital electrons of a tungsten atom and travels very close to its nucleus. The closer the projectile electron travels to the nucleus, the stronger the attraction. The stronger this attraction, the more energy the projectile electron loses and the stronger the resultant x-ray photon (higher energy). Projectile electrons that travel farther from the nucleus create x-ray photons with less energy. Most x-ray interactions in the diagnostic energy range are bremsstrahlung.

Characteristic Interactions

Characteristic interactions are produced when a projectile (incident) electron interacts with an electron from the inner shell (K-shell) of a tungsten atom. The electron must have enough energy to eject the K-shell electron from its orbit. The electron shells of each element have specific binding energies (Table 2-1). K-shell electrons in tungsten have the strongest binding energy at 69.5 keV. For a projectile electron to remove this orbital electron, it must possess energy equal to or greater than 69.5 keV (a 70-kVp setting on the control panel). When the K-shell electron is ejected from its orbit, an outer-shell electron drops into the open position and creates an energy difference. The energy difference is emitted as an x-ray photon (Fig. 2-9). Electrons from the L-, M-, O-, and P-shells of the tungsten atom are also ejected from their orbits, as they are attracted to the open positions nearer to the nucleus. However, the photons created from these interactions have very low energy and, depending on filtration, may not even reach the patient. K-shell characteristic x-rays in the x-ray beam have an energy range of approximately 57 to 69 keV; therefore, they contribute a small percentage to the useful x-ray beams. Below 70 kVp (with a tungsten target), no characteristic x-rays are present in the beam; above 70 kVp, approximately 15% of the beam consists of characteristic x-rays. X-rays produced through these interactions are termed *characteristic x-rays* because their energies are characteristic of the tungsten target element.

 IMPORTANT RELATIONSHIP

Characteristic Interactions

Characteristic interactions are produced when a projectile (incident) electron interacts with an electron from the inner shell (K-shell) of a tungsten atom. Characteristic x-rays can be produced in a tungsten target only when the kVp is set at 70 or greater because the binding energy of the K-shell electron is 69.5 keV.

TABLE 2-1 **Binding Energies for Tungsten**	
Electron Shell	**Binding Energy (keV)**
K-shell	69.5
L-shell	12.1
M-shell	2.82
N-shell	0.6
O-shell	0.08
P-shell	0.008

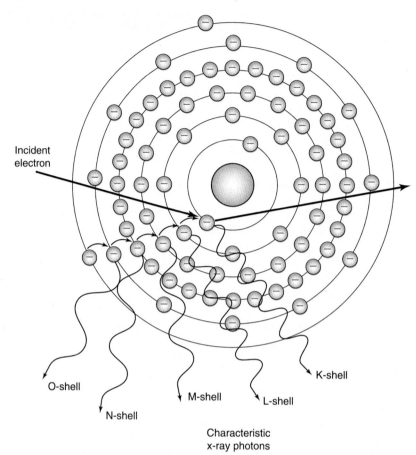

Incident electron

O-shell

N-shell

M-shell

L-shell

K-shell

Characteristic
x-ray photons

FIG. 2-9 Characteristic interaction. X-ray photons are created when the incident electrons interact with inner-shell electrons within the atoms of the rotating tungsten anode.

▶▶ MATHEMATICAL APPLICATION

Characteristic X-ray Photons

To find the energy of a characteristic x-ray photon, one must know the shell-binding energies of the element and the shells involved. The projectile electron must possess kinetic energy equal to or greater than the shell-binding energy to remove it from orbit. The photon energy is then equal to the difference in the binding energy of the shells involved.

Example:

A projectile electron removes a K-shell electron, and an L-shell electron fills the vacancy:

K-shell binding energy = 69.5 keV

L-shell binding energy = 12.1 keV

$69.5 - 12.1 = 57.4$ keV

The energy of the K-shell characteristic x-ray photon produced is 57.4 keV.

To summarize, when comparing bremsstrahlung and characteristic interactions, most x-ray interactions produced in diagnostic radiology result from bremsstrahlung interactions. There is no difference between a bremsstrahlung x-ray and a characteristic x-ray at the same energy level; they are simply produced by different processes.

X-RAY EMISSION SPECTRUM

The x-ray beam is polyenergetic (has many energies) and consists of a wide range of energies known as the **x-ray emission spectrum**. The lowest energies are always approximately 15 to 20 keV, and the highest energies cannot exceed the kVp set on the control panel. For example, an 80-kVp x-ray exposure technique produces x-ray energies ranging from 15 to 80 keV (Fig. 2-10). The smallest number of x-rays occurs at the extreme low and high ends of the spectrum. The greatest number of x-ray energies (peak of the curve) occurs between 30 and 40 keV for an 80 kVp exposure (about one third of the kVp selected). The x-ray emission spectrum, or the range and intensity of x-rays emitted, changes with different exposure technique settings on the control panel.

X-RAY EXPOSURE

A radiographic exposure is produced by a radiographer using two switches located on the control panel of the x-ray unit. These are sometimes combined into a single switching device that has two levels of operation corresponding to rotor preparation and x-ray exposure. In either case, the switches that are used to make an x-ray exposure are called *deadman switches*. Deadman switches require positive pressure to be applied during the entire x-ray exposure process. If the radiographer lets off either switch, thus releasing positive pressure, the exposure process is immediately terminated.

The first switch is usually called the *rotor*, or *prep button*, and the second switch is usually called the *exposure*, or *x-ray button*. The activation of the exposure switch by the radiographer produces specific reactions inside the x-ray tube. The rotor must be activated before the x-ray exposure to properly produce an x-ray exposure.

Pushing the rotor, or prep button, causes an electrical current to be induced across the filament in the cathode. This **filament current** is approximately 3 to 5 A and operates at approximately 10 V. The amount of current flowing through the filament depends on the mA set at the control panel. The filament current heats the tungsten filament. This heating of the filament causes thermionic emission to occur. **Thermionic emission** refers to the boiling off of electrons from the filament.

FIG. 2-10 An 80-kVp x-ray emission spectrum from a tungsten target. Most x-rays occur between 30 and 40 keV. Characteristic x-ray energies are discrete and are represented by the line at 69 keV. (From Johnston JN, Fauber TL: *Essentials of Radiographic Physics and Imaging*, ed 2, St. Louis, 2016, Mosby.)

IMPORTANT RELATIONSHIP

Thermionic Emission

> When the tungsten filament gains enough heat (therm), the outer-shell electrons (ions) of the filament atoms are boiled off, or emitted, from the filament.

The electrons liberated from the filament during thermionic emission form a cloud around the filament called **space charge**. This term is descriptive because there is an actual negative charge from these electrons that exists in the space around the filament. The **space charge effect** refers to the tendency of the space charge to prevent more electrons to be boiled off of the filament. The focusing cup, with its own negative charge, forces the electrons in the space charge to remain together.

By pushing the rotor, or prep button, the radiographer also activates the stator that drives the rotor and rotating target (Box 2-1). While thermionic emission is occurring and the space charge is forming, the stator starts to turn the anode, accelerating it to top speed in preparation for x-ray production. If an exposure were to be made before the target was up to speed, the heat produced would be too great for the slowly rotating target, causing serious damage. The machine therefore does not allow such an exposure to occur until the target is up to full speed, even when the exposure switch is activated. The radiographer can press the rotor and exposure switches one after the other, and the machine makes the exposure as soon as it is ready, with no damage to the tube. It takes only a few seconds for the space charge to be produced and for the rotating target to reach its top speed (Fig. 2-11).

When the radiographer pushes the exposure, or x-ray button, the x-ray exposure begins (Box 2-2). The kVp level, which depends on the actual kVp value set on the control panel by the radiographer, is applied across the tube from cathode to anode. This creates potential difference and the cathode becomes highly negatively charged, strongly repelling the thus created negatively charged electrons. The anode becomes positively charged, strongly attracting the electrons.

Electrons that comprised the space charge now flow quickly from the cathode to the anode in a current. **Tube current** refers to the flow of electrons from cathode to anode and is measured in units called *milliamperes*. It is important to note that electrons flow only in one direction in the x-ray tube—from cathode to anode.

BOX 2-1   Preparing the Tube for Exposure

When the rotor, or prep button, is activated:

On the Cathode Side of the X-ray Tube
1. The filament current heats up the filament.
2. This heat boils electrons off the filament (thermionic emission).
3. These electrons gather in a cloud around the filament (space charge).
4. The negatively charged focusing cup keeps the electron cloud focused together.
5. The number of electrons in the space charge is limited (space charge effect).

On the Anode Side of the X-ray Tube
1. The rotating target begins to turn rapidly, quickly reaching top speed.

Rotating anode

Space charge of electrons

Filament

Focusing cup

FIG. 2-11 When the radiographer activates the rotor, or prep button, a filament current is induced across the filament, causing electrons to be burned off and gather in a cloud around the filament. Simultaneously, the rotating anode begins to turn.

BOX 2-2   Making an X-ray Exposure

After activation of the rotor and the exposure is initiated:

On the Cathode Side of the X-ray Tube
1. High negative charge strongly repels electrons.
2. These electrons stream away from the cathode and toward the anode (tube current).

On the Anode Side of the X-ray Tube
1. High positive charge strongly attracts electrons in the tube current.
2. These electrons strike the anode.
3. X-rays and heat are produced.

IMPORTANT RELATIONSHIP

Tube Current

Electrons flow only in one direction in the x-ray tube—from cathode to anode. This flow of electrons is called the *tube current* and is measured in mA.

As these electrons strike the anode target, their kinetic energy is converted into either electromagnetic energy (x-rays) or thermal energy (heat); in other words, an energy conversion occurs. Most of the electron kinetic energy in the tube current (greater than 99%) is converted to heat, whereas less than 1% of it is converted to x-rays. These events are illustrated in Fig. 2-12.

IMPORTANT RELATIONSHIP

Energy Conversion in the X-ray Tube

As electrons strike the anode target, more than 99% of their kinetic energy is converted to heat, whereas less than 1% of their energy is converted to x-rays.

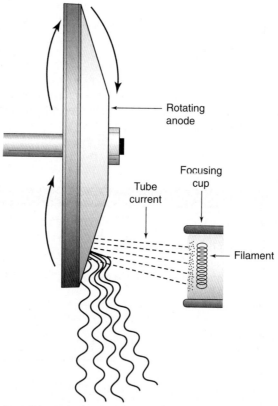

FIG. 2-12 After activation of the rotor and initiation of the exposure, a high voltage, or kilovoltage, is applied across the tube, making the cathode highly negative and the anode highly positive. Electrons are repelled from the cathode side and attracted to the anode side. The negatively charged focusing cup focuses the electrons into a stream, and they quickly cross the tube gap in a tube current. The kinetic energy of electrons interacting with the target is converted into x-rays and heat.

X-RAY QUALITY AND QUANTITY

The radiographer initiates and controls the production of x-rays. Manipulating the prime exposure factors on the control panel (kVp, mA, and exposure time) allows both the quantity and the quality of the x-ray beam to be altered. The quantity of the x-ray beam indicates the number of x-ray photons in the primary beam, and the quality of the x-ray beam indicates its penetrating power. Knowledge of the prime exposure factors and their effect on the production of x-rays assists the radiographer in producing quality radiographic images.

Kilovoltage

The **kilovoltage** that is set by the radiographer and applied across the x-ray tube at the time the exposure is initiated determines the speed at which the electrons in the tube current move.

 IMPORTANT RELATIONSHIP

Kilovoltage and the Speed of Electrons

The speed of the electrons traveling from the cathode to the anode increases as the kilovoltage applied across the x-ray tube increases.

Selecting a higher voltage results in greater repulsion of electrons from the cathode and greater attraction of electrons toward the anode. The speed at which the electrons in the tube current move determines the quality or energy of the x-rays that are produced. The higher the energy of the x-ray photons, the greater their penetrability, or ease with which they move through tissue. Whether addressing the x-ray photons themselves or the primary beam, *quality* refers to the energy level of the radiation produced (Box 2-3).

 IMPORTANT RELATIONSHIP

Speed of Electrons and Quality of X-rays

The speed of the electrons in the tube current determines the quality or energy of the x-rays that are produced. The quality or energy of the x-rays in turn determines the penetrability of the primary beam (ease with which it moves through tissue).

 IMPORTANT RELATIONSHIP

kVp and Beam Penetrability

As kVp increases, beam penetrability increases; as kVp decreases, beam penetrability decreases.

BOX 2-3   kVp and X-ray Quality

1. Higher kVp results in electrons that move faster in the tube current from the cathode to the anode.
2. The faster the movement of the electrons in the tube current, the greater the energy of the x-rays produced.
3. The greater the energy of the x-rays produced, the greater the penetrability of the primary beam.
4. The quality of the x-ray beam refers to its energy level; hence, adjusting kVp affects the quality of the x-ray beam.

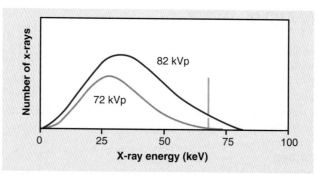

FIG. 2-13 Increasing the kVp from 72 to 82 shows an increase in the quantity of x-rays (amplitude), and the x-ray emission shifts toward the right, indicating an increase in the energy or quality of the beam. (From Johnston JN, Fauber TL: *Essentials of Radiographic Physics and Imaging*, ed 2, St. Louis, 2016, Mosby.)

In addition to kVp affecting the quality of x-ray photons produced, it affects the quantity or number of x-ray photons produced (Fig. 2-13). Increased kVp results in more x-rays being produced because it increases the efficiency of x-ray production. (Box 2-4 describes quality-control methods for evaluating kilovoltage accuracy.)

To provide a sufficient potential difference (kVp) to allow x-ray production, a generator is required to convert low voltage (volts) to high voltage (kilovolts), 1 kilovolt = 1000 volts. Three basic types of x-ray generators are available: single phase, three phase, and high frequency. Each generator produces a different voltage waveform (Fig. 2-14). These waveforms are a reflection of the consistency of the voltage supplied to the x-ray tube during an x-ray exposure. The term **voltage ripple** describes voltage waveforms in terms of how much the voltage varies during x-ray production. Fig. 2-14 shows that for single-phase generation, voltage varies from the peak to a value of zero. The voltage ripple for single-phase generators is said to be 100% because there is total variation in the voltage waveform, from peak voltage to zero voltage. For three-phase generators, the voltage ripple is 13% for the 6-pulse mode and 4% for the 12-pulse mode. High-frequency generators produce a voltage ripple of less than 1%. Voltage used in the x-ray tube is most consistent with high-frequency generators. The more consistent the voltage applied to the x-ray tube throughout the exposure, the greater the quantity and energy level (quality) of the x-ray beam. Fig. 2-15 shows x-ray emissions for different types of generators.

Milliamperage

Milliamperage (mA) is selected on the x-ray control panel to operate the tube current. Tube current is the number of electrons flowing per unit time between the cathode and the anode. For example, at 200 mA, there is a specific amount of current applied to the filament, causing a certain amount of thermionic emission. Based on the amount of thermionic emission, there

---

BOX 2-4   Quality-Control Check: Kilovoltage Accuracy

- X-ray quality can be affected if the actual kilovoltage used is inaccurate.
- A digital kVp meter measures the actual kilovoltage. An older method is a Wisconsin Test Cassette, which estimates the kilovoltage by measuring densities (blackness) produced on a film.
- The maximum variability of the kilovoltage is ±5%.

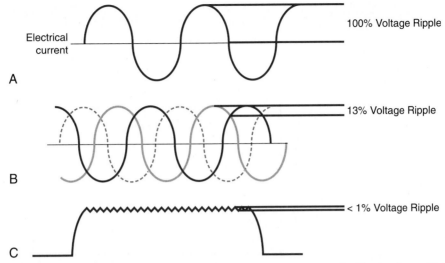

FIG. 2-14 Voltage waveforms produced by various x-ray generators. **A,** Single phase. **B,** Three phase. **C,** High frequency.

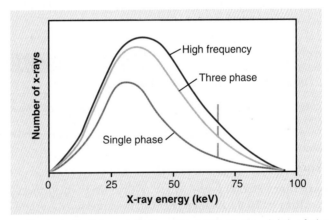

FIG. 2-15 The quantity (amplitude) and the quality (shift to the right) of the x-ray beam are increased when using high-frequency and three-phase generators because they are more efficient in x-ray production. (From Johnston JN, Fauber TL: *Essentials of Radiographic Physics and Imaging*, ed 2, St. Louis, 2016, Mosby.)

is a space charge consisting of a certain number of electrons; 200 mA indicates the number of electrons (based on the space charge) flowing in the tube per second. Generally, changing to the 400-mA station on the control panel causes twice as much thermionic emission, twice as big a space charge, and twice as many electrons to flow per second. The mA set by the radiographer determines the number of electrons flowing in the tube and the quantity of x-rays produced (Box 2-5). The quantity of electrons in the tube current is directly proportional to the mA. If the mA increases, the quantity of electrons and x-rays proportionally increases, and if it decreases, the quantity of electrons and x-rays proportionally decreases. The mA does not affect the quality or energy of the x-rays produced (Fig. 2-16).

BOX 2-5   mA and X-ray Quantity

1. Higher mA results in more electrons moving in the tube current from the cathode to the anode.
2. The more electrons in the tube current, the more x-rays produced.
3. The number of x-rays produced is directly proportional to mA.

FIG. 2-16 Changing the mA results in a proportional change in the quantity (amplitude) of x-rays produced. (From Johnston JN, Fauber TL: *Essentials of Radiographic Physics and Imaging*, ed 2, St. Louis, 2016, Mosby.)

 IMPORTANT RELATIONSHIP

mA, Tube Current, and X-ray Quantity

The quantity of electrons in the tube current and quantity of x-rays produced are directly proportional to the mA.

Exposure Time

Exposure time determines the length of time over which the x-ray tube produces x-rays. The exposure time set by the radiographer can be expressed in seconds or milliseconds (ms) as either a fraction (older units) or a decimal (0.001 s = 1000 ms). This exposure time determines the length of time for which the tube current is allowed to flow from cathode to anode. The longer the exposure time, the greater the quantity of electrons that flow from the cathode to the anode and the greater the quantity of x-rays produced (Box 2-6). For example, if an exposure time of 0.25 s at 400 mA produces 5000 x-rays, then doubling the exposure time to 0.50 s at 400 mA would produce 10,000 x-rays. Changes in exposure time produce the same effect on the number of x-rays produced as do changes in mA. (Box 2-7 describes quality-control methods for evaluating exposure timer accuracy.)

BOX 2-6   Exposure Time and X-ray Quantity

1. A longer exposure time results in more electrons moving in the tube current from the cathode to the anode.
2. The more electrons in the tube current, the more x-rays produced.
3. The number of x-rays produced is directly proportional to the exposure time.

BOX 2-7 Quality-Control Check: Exposure Timer Accuracy

- X-ray quantity can be affected if the actual exposure time used is inaccurate. A digital timer device measures the actual exposure time. An older method uses a synchronous spinning top test device to estimate the actual time by measuring the density (blackness) arc produced on film with a timer protractor or by counting the number of black dots expected for the type of x-ray generator.
- The maximum variability of the exposure timer is ±5% for times >10 ms and ±10% for times <10 ms.

 IMPORTANT RELATIONSHIP

Exposure Time, Tube Current, and X-ray Quantity

The quantity of electrons flowing from the cathode to the anode and the quantity of x-rays produced are directly proportional to the exposure time.

Milliamperage and Time

When mA is multiplied by exposure time, the result is known as mAs (milliamperage-seconds), which the radiographer can set at the control panel. Mathematically, mAs is simply expressed as follows: $mA \times s = mAs$, where s represents the exposure time in fractions of a second (as actual fractions or in decimal form) or in seconds.

 MATHEMATICAL APPLICATION

Calculating mAs

$$mAs = mA \times seconds$$

Examples:

$$200\,mA \times 0.25\,s = 50\,mAs$$

$$500\,mA \times 2/5\,s = 200\,mAs$$

$$800\,mA \times 100\,ms\,(milliseconds\ or\ 0.1\,s) = 80\,mAs$$

The quantity of electrons flowing from the cathode to the anode is directly proportional to mAs (Box 2-8). The quantity of x-ray photons produced is directly proportional to this quantity of electrons. An increase or decrease in mA, exposure time, or mAs directly affects the quantity of x-rays produced; mAs has no effect on the quality of the x-rays produced. (Box 2-9 describes quality-control methods for evaluating radiation output.)

BOX 2-8 mAs and X-ray Quantity

1. Higher mAs results in more electrons moving within the tube current from the cathode to the anode.
2. The more electrons in the tube current, the more x-rays produced.
3. The number of x-rays produced is directly proportional to the mAs.
4. mAs affects only the quantity of x-rays produced; it has no effect on the quality of the x-rays.

BOX 2-9   Quality-Control Check: Radiation Output

- Variations in the generator or x-ray tube performance may cause inconsistent exposures and affect the x-ray quantity. Three quality-control tests are typically performed with a **dosimeter** (a device that measures x-ray exposure) to evaluate the radiation output by measuring the radiation intensity: reproducibility of exposure, mAs reciprocity, and mA and exposure time linearity.
- **Reproducibility of exposure** verifies the consistency of the radiation output for a given set of exposure factors. The maximum variability of the reproducibility of radiation exposures is ±5%.
- **mAs reciprocity** verifies the consistency of radiation intensity for changes in mA and exposure time with constant mAs. The maximum variability of reciprocity is ±10%.
- **mA and exposure time linearity** verifies that proportional changes in mA or exposure time or both likewise change the radiation intensity. Doubling the mA or exposure time should double the radiation intensity. The maximum variability of linearity is ±10%.

 IMPORTANT RELATIONSHIP

Quantity of Electrons, X-rays, and mAs

The quantity of electrons flowing from the cathode to the anode and the quantity of x-rays produced are directly proportional to mAs.

LINE-FOCUS PRINCIPLE

The **line-focus principle** describes the relationship between the actual and the effective focal spots in an x-ray tube.

 IMPORTANT RELATIONSHIP

Line-Focus Principle

The line-focus principle describes the relationship between the actual focal spot, where the electrons in the tube current bombard the target, and the effective focal spot, which is the same area as seen from directly below the tube.

The **actual focal spot size** refers to the size of the area on the anode target that is exposed to electrons from the tube current. It depends on the size of the filament producing the electron stream. The **effective focal spot size** refers to focal spot size as measured directly under the anode target (Fig. 2-17).

A tube's focal spot is an important factor because a large focal spot can withstand the heat produced by large exposures, whereas a small one produces better image quality. The line-focus principle demonstrates how, by angling the face of the anode target, the actual focal spot can remain relatively large while the effective focal spot is reduced in size. Greater heat capacity can be achieved while maintaining good image quality.

When manufactured, every tube has a specific anode target angle, typically ranging from 5 to 20 degrees. Based on the line-focus principle, the amount of the target angle determines the size of the effective focal spot. It should be noted that the anode target angle is determined on the basis of the intended use of the tube and is not something the radiographer *selects* at the operating console.

A larger target angle produces a larger effective focal spot, and a smaller target angle produces a smaller one. The relationship among target angle, effective focal spot size, and actual focal spot size is illustrated in Fig. 2-18.

FIG. 2-17 The line-focus principle addresses the relationship between the size of the actual focal spot (where the electrons actually bombard the target) and the effective focal spot (the same area as viewed and measured directly below the target).

FIG. 2-18 Based on the line-focus principle, a large target angle produces a large effective focal spot size (**A**), and a small target angle produces a small one (**B**). Both actual focal spot sizes are the same, meaning that they can withstand the same heat loading. The smaller effective focal spot results in improved image quality.

IMPORTANT RELATIONSHIP

Anode Angle and Effective Focal Spot Size

Based on the line-focus principle, the smaller the anode target angle, the smaller the effective focal spot size.

ANODE HEEL EFFECT

A phenomenon known as the **anode heel effect** occurs because of the angle of the target. The heel effect describes how the x-ray beam has greater intensity (number of x-rays) on the cathode side of the tube but a lower intensity toward the anode side (Fig. 2-19).

 IMPORTANT RELATIONSHIP

Anode Heel Effect

X-rays are more intense on the cathode side of the tube; their intensity decreases toward the anode side.

As x-rays are produced, they leave the anode in all directions. The x-rays that are emitted toward the anode side of the tube have farther to travel, and some are absorbed by the anode itself (anode heel), reducing them in number compared with the photons that are emitted in the direction of the cathode. The difference in the intensities between the two ends can be as

FIG. 2-19 Anode heel effect.

much as 45%. The heel effect can be used to advantage in radiography because the cathode end of the tube can be placed over a thicker body part, resulting in a more even exposure to the image receptor.

The anode heel effect can be used in imaging the thoracic spine, which has small vertebrae at the top and large vertebrae at the bottom. By placing the patient's head under the anode end of the tube, more intense radiation is directed toward the lower, larger portion of the spine, and the upper, smaller vertebrae are exposed to less intense radiation exposure.

BEAM FILTRATION

The x-ray beam produced at the anode exits the tube housing to become the primary beam. The remnant (exit) beam is the x-ray beam that eventually records the body part onto the image receptor. The x-rays that exit the tube are polyenergetic; they consist of low-energy, medium-energy, and high-energy photons. The low-energy photons cannot penetrate parts of the anatomy and do not contribute to image formation. They contribute only to patient dose.

 IMPORTANT RELATIONSHIP

Low-Energy Photons, Patient Dose, and Image Formation

Low-energy photons serve only to increase patient dose and do not contribute to image formation.

Reduction of the low-energy photons requires that filtration be added to the x-ray beam to attenuate or absorb these photons. **Added filtration** describes the filtration that is added to the port of the x-ray tube. Aluminum is the material primarily used for this purpose because it absorbs more low-energy photons while the useful higher-energy photons can exit (Fig. 2-20).

Various components within the x-ray tube assembly also contribute to the attenuation of low-energy x-rays. **Inherent filtration** refers to the filtration that is permanently in the path of the x-ray beam. Three components contribute to inherent filtration: (1) the envelope of the tube, (2) the oil that surrounds the tube, and (3) the window in the tube housing. The mirror inside the collimator (beam restrictor located just below the x-ray tube) adds additional filtration (see Fig. 2-20). The **total filtration** in the x-ray beam is the sum of the added and inherent filtration. The US government sets standards for total filtration to ensure that patients receive minimal doses of radiation. The current guidelines state that x-ray tubes operating at above 70 kVp must have a minimum total filtration of 2.5 mm of aluminum or its equivalent. Increasing the amount of tube filtration increases the x-ray beam quality because there is a greater percentage of x-rays that have high energy rather than low energy. In addition, increasing tube filtration decreases the quantity of x-rays or x-ray emission (Fig. 2-21). (Box 2-10 describes quality-control methods for evaluating filtration.)

! RADIATION PROTECTION ALERT

Beam Filtration

Low-energy photons, created during x-ray production, are unable to penetrate the patient. Patients are protected from unnecessary exposure to this low-energy radiation by the placement of inherent and added filtration in the path of the x-ray beam.

FIG. 2-20 Aluminum (Al)-added filtration is shown at the port, or window, of the x-ray tube and the collimator mirror. The inherent filtration of the envelope and the oil are shown.

FIG. 2-21 Increasing beam filtration decreases the quantity (amplitude) and increases the quality (shift to the right) of the x-ray beam. (From Johnston JN, Fauber TL: *Essentials of Radiographic Physics and Imaging*, ed 2, St. Louis, 2016, Mosby.)

BOX 2-10   Quality-Control Check: Beam Filtration

- **Half-value layer (HVL)**, the amount of filtration that reduces the intensity of the x-ray beam to half of its original value, is considered the best method for describing x-ray quality.
- The HVL can be used as an indirect measure of the total filtration in the path of the x-ray beam. It is expressed in millimeters of aluminum (mm-Al).
- During the HVL test, a radiation-measuring device, such as a dosimeter, is used to measure both the radiation intensity of the original exposure and that following the addition of increasing mm-Al filtration in the path of the primary beam. The radiation intensity can be graphed for the increasing levels of aluminum filtration to determine the HVL.
- According to the NCRP Report #102, for equipment operated at or above 70 kVp, the required minimum total filtration should be at least 2.5 mm, which indicates the total filtration in the x-ray tube is adequate to protect patients from unnecessary low-energy radiation.
- Normal HVL of general diagnostic beams is 3–5 mm-Al.

COMPENSATING FILTERS

Compensating filters can be added to the primary beam to alter its intensity. These types of filters are used to image anatomic areas that are non-uniform in makeup and assist in producing more consistent exposure to the image receptor.

The most common type of compensating filter is a simple **wedge filter** (Fig. 2-22A). The thicker part of the wedge filter is lined up with the thinner portion of the anatomic part being imaged, allowing fewer x-ray photons to reach that end of the part. A wedge filter may be used for an anteroposterior (AP) projection of the femur, where the hip end is considerably larger than the knee end. A **trough filter** performs a function similar to a wedge filter; however, it is differently designed (Fig. 2-22B). In particular, the trough filter has a double wedge. A trough filter may be used for an AP projection of the thorax to compensate for the easily penetrated air-filled lungs.

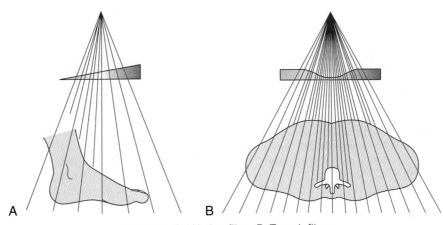

FIG. 2-22 A, Wedge filter. **B,** Trough filter.

HEAT UNITS

During x-ray production, most of the kinetic energy of the electrons is converted to heat. This heat can damage the x-ray tube and the anode target. The amount of heat produced from any given exposure is expressed by the **heat unit (HU)**. The number of HUs produced depends on the type of x-ray generator being used and the exposure factors selected for a particular exposure and can be mathematically expressed as follows:

$$HU = mA \times Time \times kVp \times Generator\ factor$$

The generator factor (Table 2-2) accounts for the fact that the use of more consistent x-ray generators results in more heat.

▶ MATHEMATICAL APPLICATION
Calculating Heat Units

An exposure is made with a three-phase x-ray unit at 600 mA and 75 kVp over 0.05 s. How many heat units are produced from this exposure?

$$HU = mA \times time \times kVp \times generator\ factor$$
$$HU = 600 \times 0.05 \times 75 \times 1.35$$
$$3037.5\ HU$$

Different models of x-ray tubes vary in their ability to withstand the heat produced by x-ray exposures. Prior to modern x-ray tubes, radiographers were responsible for evaluating their exposure technique selection to avoid excessive heat load. Box 2-11 explains the use of tube-rating charts to avoid heat damage. Manufacturers of current x-ray units build their equipment so that tube-damaging exposures cannot be made. In general, if an inappropriate technique is set, the radiographer sees a message such as *Technique Overload*, or the machine may simply not expose after the button is activated. The routine use of high-exposure techniques, although within the x-ray tube's limit, can potentially damage the x-ray tube.

TABLE 2-2 Generator Factor	
Generator Type	**Factor**
Single phase	1.00
Three phase	1.35
High frequency	1.40

BOX 2-11   Tube-Rating Charts

Before the development of today's x-ray tubes, manufacturers used instantaneous-load tube-rating charts, also called *single-exposure rating charts*, to describe the exposure limits of x-ray tubes. An instantaneous-load tube-rating chart is used to determine whether a particular exposure would be safe to make and to determine what limits on kVp, mA, and exposure time must be made for safe exposure. Violation of these limits, as indicated by the tube-rating chart, would almost certainly result in permanent and irreparable damage to the x-ray tube. Fig. 2-23 shows a typical instantaneous-load tube-rating chart. For example, the maximum kVp that can be used with 700 mA and 0.3-s exposure time is 90 kVp. The maximum mA that can be used with 105 kVp and 0.2-s exposure time is 600 mA. The maximum exposure time that can be used with 85 kVp and 900 mA is 0.05 s. Although 130 kVp, 500 mA, and 0.1 s would produce a safe exposure, 130 kVp, 500 mA, and 0.2 s would not.

In addition to tube-rating charts, manufacturers provided anode and housing cooling charts. Based on the quantity of heat units, these charts provided radiographers with information regarding the amount of time that must elapse before initiating another exposure.

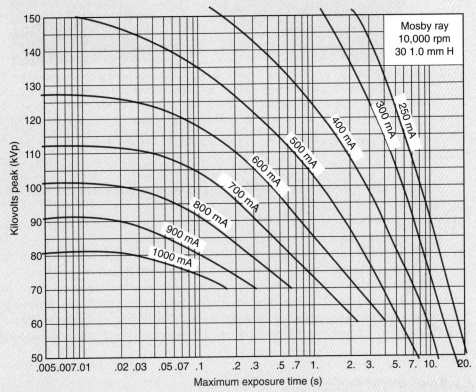

FIG. 2-23 Typical instantaneous-load tube-rating chart that can be used to determine safe and unsafe exposures.

EXTENDING X-RAY TUBE LIFE

X-ray tubes are expensive devices that can fail because of radiographer errors or carelessness. Not only do failed tubes result in an expense for purchasing a new tube, but there is also a downtime for a radiographic room when a failed tube is being replaced, thus decreasing the room's productivity. A few simple but important guidelines for x-ray tube operation should be consistently adhered to by the radiographer to extend tube life:

- If applicable, warm up the tube according to the manufacturer's specifications, especially if it has not been energized for 2 hours or more.
- Avoid excessive heat unit generation. Repeatedly using exposure techniques near an x-ray tube's limit increases the total number of heat units. Fig. 2-24 shows anode targets that have been damaged as a result of excessive heat loading.
- Do not hold down the rotor button without making an exposure. Unnecessarily holding down the rotor button causes excessive wear on both the filament and the rotor.

FIG. 2-24 Two heat-damaged anode targets. **A,** Target shows pitting of the anode track caused by consistent overloading of exposure factors. **B,** Target shows melting of the focal track caused by failure of the rotor to rotate the anode. This failure is usually due to heat damage to the rotor bearings from overloading the exposure factors. (Courtesy of Varian Medical Systems, North Charleston, SC.)

- Use lower tube currents with longer exposure times when possible to minimize wear on the filament.
- Do not move the tube while it is energized. This movement can cause damage to the anode and anode stem as a result of torque (a twisting or rotation force).
- If the rotor makes noticeable noise, stop using the tube until it has been inspected by a qualified service personnel. Noises can be indicative of a potentially serious problem.

Radiographers create diagnostic images by producing an x-ray beam to visualize anatomic structures. The x-rays produced by the radiographer affect not only the quality of the image but also the life of the x-ray tube. Understanding the prime exposure factors and their effect on the x-ray beam and knowing what happens inside the x-ray tube are important considerations in radiography.

CHAPTER SUMMARY

- X-rays are produced when electrons are boiled off (thermionic emission) the cathode filament, accelerated across to the anode target, and suddenly stopped. Heat is also produced.
- The anode, containing a tungsten–rhenium alloy target, typically rotates, allowing for larger exposures.
- X-rays are produced by bremsstrahlung (primarily) and characteristic interactions that occur as the electrons interact with the tungsten atoms in the target.
- Manipulation of the primary factors affects the quality and quantity of radiation. kVp affects both the quality (energy and penetrability) and the quantity of x-rays, whereas mA and exposure time (or mAs when combined) affect only quantity.
- The line-focus principle describes the relationship between the anode angle and the effective focal spot. The anode heel effect results in more intense radiation exiting the tube toward the cathode side.
- Added and inherent beam filtration ensures that a minimal amount of low-energy x-ray photons reach the patient. The half-value layer (HVL) is an indirect measure of total filtration and is used to describe x-ray quality.
- There are numerous methods for extending tube life, including attending to the amount of heat produced during x-ray production. Heat units are the measure of the amount of heat produced using specific exposure factors.

REVIEW QUESTIONS

1. Which x-ray tube component serves as a source of electrons for x-ray production?
   A. Focusing cup
   B. Filament
   C. Stator
   D. Target

2. Electrons interact with the _____ to produce x-rays and heat.
   A. focusing cup
   B. filament
   C. stator
   D. target

3. The cloud of electrons that forms before x-ray production is referred to as _____.
   A. thermionic emission
   B. space charge
   C. space charge effect
   D. tube current

4. The burning or boiling-off of electrons at the cathode is referred to as _____.
   A. thermionic emission
   B. space charge
   C. space charge effect
   D. tube current

5. Which primary exposure factor influences both the quantity and the quality of x-ray photons?
   A. mA
   B. mAs
   C. kVp
   D. Exposure time

6. The unit used to express tube current is _____.
   A. mA
   B. mAs
   C. kVp
   D. s

7. What percentage of the kinetic energy is converted to heat when moving electrons strike the anode target?
   A. 1%
   B. 25%
   C. 59%
   D. 99%

8. The intensity of the x-ray beam is greater on the _____.
   A. cathode side of the tube
   B. anode side of the tube
   C. short axis of the beam
   D. long axis of the beam

9. According to the line-focus principle, as the target angle decreases, the _____.
   A. actual focal spot size decreases
   B. actual focal spot size increases
   C. effective focal spot size decreases
   D. effective focal spot size increases

10. _____ extends x-ray tube life.
    A. Selecting higher tube currents
    B. Using small focal spots when possible
    C. Producing exposures with a wide range of kVp values
    D. Warming up the tube after 2 hours of non-use

11. Which type of target interaction is responsible for most of the x-rays in the diagnostic beam?
    A. Characteristic interaction
    B. Thermionic emission
    C. Bremsstrahlung interaction
    D. None of the above

12. What value of mAs is produced when the radiographer sets a kVp of 70, an mA of 600, and an exposure time of 50 ms?
    A. 3.5 mAs
    B. 30 mAs
    C. 300 mAs
    D. 350 mAs

13. Increasing the kVp results in _____.
    A. x-rays with higher energy
    B. x-rays with lower energy
    C. more x-rays
    D. A and C
    E. B and C

14. Total filtration in the x-ray beam includes _____.
    A. compensating filters
    B. inherent filtration
    C. added filtration
    D. B and C
    E. all of the above

15. How many heat units result from an exposure made on a single-phase x-ray unit using a beam current of 400 mA, an exposure time of 0.2 s, and a kVp of 70?
    A. 5600 HU
    B. 7560 HU
    C. 7896 HU
    D. 8120 HU

Image Formation and Radiographic Quality

OBJECTIVES

After completing this chapter, the reader will be able to perform the following:

1. Define all the key terms in this chapter.
2. State all the important relationships in this chapter.
3. Describe the process of radiographic image formation.
4. Explain the process of beam attenuation.
5. Identify the factors that affect beam attenuation.
6. Describe the x-ray interactions termed *photoelectric effect* and *Compton effect*.
7. Define the term *ionization*.
8. State the composition of exit radiation.
9. Explain the process of creating the various shades of image brightness.
10. Describe the necessary components of radiographic quality.
11. Explain the importance of brightness and contrast to image quality.
12. Differentiate between high-contrast and low-contrast images.
13. Explain the importance of spatial resolution and both size and shape distortion to image quality.
14. State the effects of quantum noise, scatter, and image artifacts on image quality.
15. Recognize the advantages of digital imaging and the limitations of film-screen imaging.
16. Differentiate radiographic imaging from dynamic imaging.

KEY TERMS

absorption
artifact
attenuation
brightness
coherent scattering
Compton effect
Compton electron
contrast resolution
differential absorption
distortion

dynamic range
elongation
exit radiation
fluoroscopy
fog
foreshortening
grayscale
high-contrast images
image receptor (IR)
invisible image

ionization
latent image
low-contrast images
magnification
manifest image
photoelectric effect
photoelectron
quantum noise
remnant radiation
saturation

To produce a radiographic image, x-ray photons must pass through tissue and interact with an **image receptor (IR)**, a device that receives the radiation leaving the patient. Both the quantity and the quality of the primary x-ray beam affect its interactions within the various tissues that make up anatomic parts. In addition, the composition of the anatomic tissues affects the x-ray beam interaction. The absorption characteristics of the anatomic part are determined by its thickness, atomic number of the atoms contained within it, and tissue density or compactness of the cellular structures. Finally, the radiation that exits the patient is composed of varying energies and interacts with the IR to form a latent or invisible image and must be processed.

A visible radiographic image is produced following the processing of the latent or invisible image. Depending on the type of imaging system, the acquiring, processing, and displaying of images can vary significantly. However, the attributes of a quality radiographic image are similar regardless of the type of imaging system. This chapter focuses on how images are formed and their quality after processing.

IMAGE FORMATION

Differential Absorption

The process of image formation is a result of **differential absorption** of the x-ray beam as it interacts with anatomic tissue. Differential absorption is a process whereby some amount of the x-ray beam is absorbed in the tissue, and some passes through (transmits) the anatomic part. The term *differential* is used because varying anatomic parts do not *absorb* the primary beam to the same degree. Anatomic parts composed of bone absorb more x-ray photons than parts filled with air. Differential absorption of the primary x-ray beam creates an image that structurally represents the anatomic area of interest (Fig. 3-1).

 IMPORTANT RELATIONSHIP

Differential Absorption and Image Formation

A radiographic image is created when an x-ray beam passes through a patient and then interacts with an IR, such as a digital imaging system. The variations in the absorption and transmission of the exiting x-ray beam structurally represent the anatomic area of interest.

Creating a radiographic image by differential absorption requires several processes to occur: beam attenuation, absorption, and transmission.

Beam Attenuation

As the primary x-ray beam passes through anatomic tissue, it loses some of its energy (intensity). Fewer x-ray photons remain in the beam after it interacts with anatomic tissue. This reduction in the intensity or number of photons in the primary x-ray beam is known as **attenuation**. Beam attenuation occurs as a result of the photon interactions with the atomic structures that comprise the tissues. Two distinct processes occur during beam attenuation: absorption and scattering.

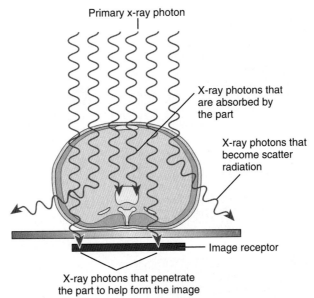

Primary x-ray photon

X-ray photons that
are absorbed by
the part

X-ray photons that
become scatter
radiation

Image receptor

X-ray photons that penetrate
the part to help form the image

FIG. 3-1 As the primary x-ray beam interacts with an anatomic part, photons are absorbed, scattered, and transmitted. The differences in the absorption characteristics of the anatomic part create an image that structurally represents the part. (From Johnston JN, Fauber TL: *Essentials of Radiographic Physics and Imaging*, ed 2, St. Louis, 2016, Mosby.)

Absorption. As the energy of the primary x-ray beam is deposited within the atoms comprising the tissue, some x-ray photons are completely absorbed. Complete **absorption** of the incoming x-ray photon occurs when it has enough energy to remove (eject) an inner-shell electron. The ejected electron is called a **photoelectron**, and it quickly loses energy by interacting with nearby tissues. The ability to remove (eject) electrons, known as **ionization**, is a characteristic of x-rays. In the diagnostic range, this x-ray interaction with matter is known as the **photoelectric effect**.

With the photoelectric effect, an ionized atom has a vacancy, or electron hole, in its inner shell. An electron from an outer shell drops down to fill this vacancy. Because of the difference in binding energies between the two electron shells, a secondary x-ray photon is emitted (Fig. 3-2). This secondary x-ray photon typically has a very low energy and is unlikely to exit the patient.

IMPORTANT RELATIONSHIP

X-ray Photon Absorption

During attenuation of the x-ray beam, the photoelectric effect is responsible for the total absorption of the incoming x-ray photon.

The probability of total photon absorption by the photoelectric effect depends on the energy of the incoming x-ray photon and the atomic number of the anatomic tissue. The energy of the incoming x-ray photon must be at least equal to the binding energy of the inner-shell electron. After absorption of a portion of x-ray photons, the overall quantity of the primary beam decreases as it passes through the anatomic part.

Scattering. Some incoming photons are not absorbed but lose energy and change direction during interactions with the atoms comprising the tissue. This process is called **scattering**.

Photoelectric effect

1 Incident photon interacts with an inner orbital, K or L, electron, giving all of its energy to the electron, ejecting it from orbit. The photon is "absorbed."

2 The ejected electron (photo-electron) imparts the atom with energy equal to the excess of the electron's binding energy.

3 There is a vacancy in the inner orbital shell, K or L, which must be filled. One of the electrons from the outer orbital shell, usually the next orbit out, drops to the void.

4 As the electron drops to the void, it may shed its excess energy as a secondary photon.

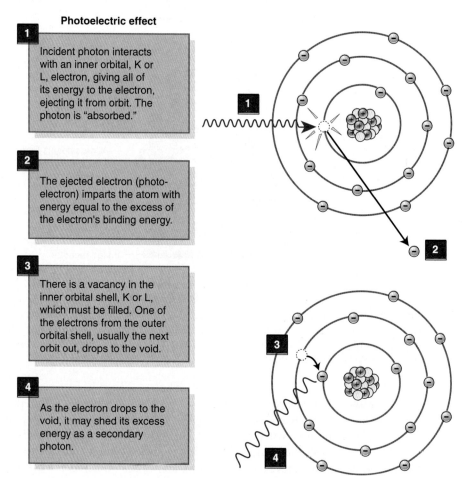

FIG. 3-2 The photoelectric effect is responsible for total absorption of the incoming x-ray photon. (From Johnston JN, Fauber TL: *Essentials of Radiographic Physics and Imaging*, ed 2, St. Louis, 2016, Mosby.)

It results from an interaction between diagnostic x-rays and matter, known as the **Compton effect**. The loss of energy of the incoming photon occurs when it ejects an outer-shell electron from a tissue atom. The ejected electron is called a **Compton electron** or **secondary electron**. The remaining lower-energy x-ray photon changes direction and may leave the anatomic part and interact with the IR (Fig. 3-3).

IMPORTANT RELATIONSHIP

X-ray Beam Scattering

During attenuation of the x-ray beam, the incoming x-ray photon may lose energy and change direction as a result of the Compton effect.

Compton interactions can occur at any diagnostic x-ray energy and are an important interaction in radiography. The probability of a Compton interaction occurring depends on the energy of the incoming photon. It does not depend on the atomic number of the anatomic tissue. For example, a Compton interaction is just as likely to occur in soft tissue as in tissue composed of bone;

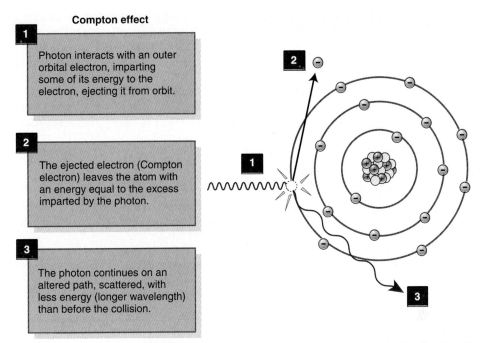

Compton effect

1 | Photon interacts with an outer orbital electron, imparting some of its energy to the electron, ejecting it from orbit.

2 | The ejected electron (Compton electron) leaves the atom with an energy equal to the excess imparted by the photon.

3 | The photon continues on an altered path, scattered, with less energy (longer wavelength) than before the collision.

FIG. 3-3 During the Compton effect, the incoming photon loses energy and changes its direction. (From Johnston JN, Fauber TL: *Essentials of Radiographic Physics and Imaging*, ed 2, St. Louis, 2016, Mosby.)

however, if the tissue has more complex atoms, there are more opportunities for interaction. With higher atomic number particles, such as bone, if the energy of the incoming photon is sufficiently high, more scatter will occur; otherwise, more absorption will occur. For Compton interactions to occur, the energy of the photon is more important, whereas the atomic number of elements in the tissue is only related to the opportunity for x-ray interactions. When a higher kilovoltage peak (kVp) within the diagnostic range is used, the overall number of x-ray interactions within matter decrease because of increased photon transmission; however, the percentage of photoelectric interactions generally decreases at higher kilovoltages within the diagnostic range, whereas the percentage of Compton interactions is likely to increase at higher kilovoltages within the diagnostic range. Box 3-1 compares photoelectric and Compton interactions. Scattered and secondary radiations provide no useful information and must be controlled during radiographic imaging.

Coherent scattering is an interaction that occurs with low-energy x-rays, typically below the diagnostic range, also known as classical scattering. The incoming photon interacts with the atom, causing it to become excited. The x-ray does not lose energy, but it changes direction (Fig. 3-4). Coherent scattering could occur within the diagnostic range of the x-rays and may interact with the IR, but it is not considered an important interaction in radiography.

If a scattered photon strikes the IR, it does not contribute any useful information about the anatomic area of interest. If scattered photons are absorbed within the anatomic tissue, they contribute to radiation exposure to the patient. In addition, if the scattered photon leaves the patient and does not strike the IR, it could contribute to radiation exposure of anyone near the patient.

The preceding discussion focused on photon interactions that occur in radiography when using x-ray energies within the moderate range. X-rays with energies above the diagnostic range result in other interactions, namely, pair production and photodisintegration. X-ray interactions above the diagnostic range are important in positron emission tomography (PET) and radiation therapy.

BOX 3-1 Comparing the Photoelectric and Compton Effects

Photoelectric Effect
- An incoming photon has sufficient energy to eject an inner-shell electron and be completely absorbed.
- An electron from an upper-level shell fills the electron hole or vacancy.
- A secondary photon is created because of the difference in the electrons' binding energies.
- The probability of this effect depends on the energy of the incoming x-ray photon and the composition of the anatomic tissue.
- Fewer photon interactions occur at a higher kVp, but of those interactions, a smaller percentage are photoelectric interactions.

Compton Effect
- An incoming photon loses energy when it ejects an outer-shell electron and changes direction.
- The scattered photon may be absorbed within the patient tissues leave the anatomic part, interact with the IR, or expose anyone near the patient.
- Scattered photons that strike the IR provide no useful information.
- The probability of this effect depends on the energy of the incoming x-ray photon but not on the composition of the anatomic tissue.
- Fewer photon interactions occur at a higher kVp, but a greater percentage of those interactions are Compton interactions.

Classical scattering

FIG. 3-4 Coherent (classical) scattering. The incoming photon interacts with the atom, causing it to become excited. The x-ray does not lose energy, but it changes direction. (From Johnston JN, Fauber TL: *Essentials of Radiographic Physics and Imaging*, ed 2, St. Louis, 2016, Mosby.)

Factors Affecting Beam Attenuation

The amount of x-ray beam attenuation is affected by the thickness of the anatomic part, the atomic number of the atoms contained within it, its tissue density, and the energy of the x-ray beam.

Tissue Thickness. Increasing the thickness of a given anatomic tissue increases beam attenuation by either absorption or scattering (Fig. 3-5). X-rays are exponentially attenuated and are generally reduced by approximately 50% for each 4 to 5 cm (1.6–2 inches) of tissue thickness (Fig. 3-6). More x-rays are needed to produce a radiographic image for a thicker anatomic part. Fewer x-rays are needed to produce a radiographic image for a thinner anatomic part.

Type of Tissue. Tissues composed of elements with a higher atomic number, such as bone (which has an effective atomic number of 13.8), attenuate the x-ray beam more than tissue

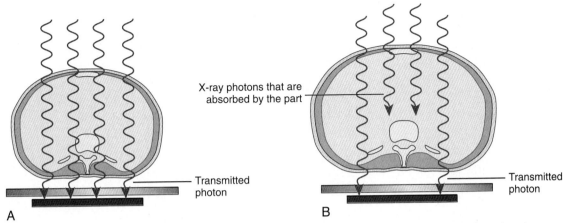

X-ray photons that are
absorbed by the part

Transmitted
photon

Transmitted
photon

A

B

FIG. 3-5 A, A thinner patient transmits more radiation than a thicker patient. **B,** A thicker patient absorbs more radiation than a thinner patient. (From Johnston JN, Fauber TL: *Essentials of Radiographic Physics and Imaging*, ed 2, St. Louis, 2016, Mosby.)

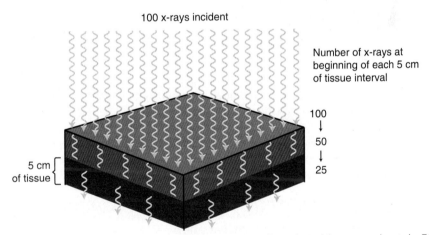

100 x-rays incident

Number of x-rays at
beginning of each 5 cm
of tissue interval

100
↓
50
↓
25

5 cm
of tissue

FIG. 3-6 X-rays are exponentially attenuated and generally reduced by approximately 50% for each 4 to 5 cm (1.6–2 inches) of tissue thickness. (From Johnston JN, Fauber TL: *Essentials of Radiographic Physics and Imaging,* ed 2, St. Louis, 2016, Mosby.)

composed of elements with a lower atomic number, such as fat (which has an effective atomic number of 6.3). The higher atomic number indicates there are more atomic particles for interactions with x-ray photons. X-ray absorption is more likely to occur in tissues with a higher effective atomic number than in those with a lower effective atomic number (Fig. 3-7).

Tissue density (matter per unit volume), or the compactness of atomic particles composing the anatomic part, also affects the amount of beam attenuation. For example, muscle (effective atomic number 7.4) and fat (effective atomic number 6.3) tissue are similar in effective atomic number; however, their atomic particles differ in compactness, and their tissue densities vary. Muscle tissue has atomic particles that are more densely packed or compact and therefore attenuate the x-ray beam more than fat cells. Bone is composed of tissue with a higher atomic number, and the atomic particles are more compacted or densely packed. Anatomic tissues are typically ranked on the basis of their attenuation properties. Four substances account for most of the beam attenuation in the

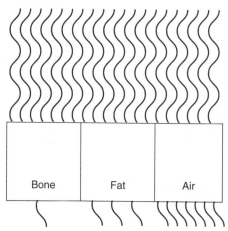

FIG. 3-7 Bone absorbs more radiation than fat and air. Air transmits more radiation than fat and bone. (From Johnston JN, Fauber TL: *Essentials of Radiographic Physics and Imaging,* ed 2, St. Louis, 2016, Mosby.)

human body: bone, muscle, fat, and air. Bone attenuates the x-ray beam more than muscle, muscle attenuates the x-ray beam more than fat, and fat attenuates the x-ray beam more than air. The effective atomic number of the anatomic part and its tissue density affect x-ray beam attenuation.

X-ray Beam Quality. The quality of the x-ray beam or its penetrating ability affects its interaction with anatomic tissue. Higher-penetrating x-rays (shorter wavelength with higher frequency) are more likely to be transmitted through anatomic tissue without interacting with the tissues' atomic structures. Lower-penetrating x-rays (longer wavelength with lower frequency) are more likely to interact with the atomic structures and be absorbed. The kilovoltage selected during x-ray production determines the energy or penetrability of the x-ray photon, and this affects its attenuation in anatomic tissue (Fig. 3-8). Beam attenuation decreases with a higher-energy x-ray beam and increases with a lower-energy x-ray beam. See Table 3-1 for factors affecting beam attenuation.

> ### ✦ IMPORTANT RELATIONSHIP
> #### *Factors Affecting Beam Attenuation*
> Increasing tissue thickness, atomic number, and tissue density increases x-ray beam attenuation because more x-rays are absorbed by the tissue. Increasing the quality of the x-ray beam decreases beam attenuation because the higher-energy x-rays penetrate the tissue.

Transmission. If the incoming x-ray photon passes through the anatomic part without any interaction with the atomic structures, it is called **transmission** (Fig. 3-9). The combination of absorption and transmission of the x-ray beam provides an image that structurally represents the anatomic part. Because scatter radiation is also a process that occurs during interaction of the x-ray beam and the anatomic part, the quality of the image created is compromised if scattered photons strike the IR.

Exit Radiation

When the attenuated x-ray beam leaves the patient, the remaining x-ray beam, referred to as **exit radiation** or **remnant radiation**, is composed of both transmitted and scattered radiation (Fig. 3-10). The varying amounts of transmitted and absorbed radiation (differential absorption) create an image that structurally represents the anatomic area of interest. Scatter exit radiation

Low-energy (kVp) beam

High-energy (kVp) beam

Most x-ray photons are absorbed. Few emerge to strike the image receptor.

Photons have more energy to penetrate the part.

FIG. 3-8 The energy of the x-ray beam affects its interaction within anatomic tissues. Lower kVp results in more absorption in the tissue; higher kVp results in more transmission through the tissue. (From Johnston JN, Fauber TL: *Essentials of Radiographic Physics and Imaging*, ed 2, St. Louis, 2016, Mosby.)

TABLE 3-1 Factors Affecting Beam Attenuation			
Factor	**Beam Attenuation**	**Absorption**	**Transmission**
Tissue Thickness			
• Increasing thickness	↑	↑	↓
• Decreasing thickness	↓	↓	↑
Tissue Atomic Number			
• Increasing atomic number	↑	↑	↓
• Decreasing atomic number	↓	↓	↑
Tissue Density			
• Increasing tissue density	↑	↑	↓
• Decreasing tissue density	↓	↓	↑
X-ray Beam Quality			
• Increasing beam quality	↓	↓	↑
• Decreasing beam quality	↑	↑	↓

(Compton interactions) that reach the IR do not provide any diagnostic information about the anatomic area. Scatter radiation creates unwanted exposure on the image called **fog**. Methods used to decrease the amount of scatter radiation reaching the IR are discussed in Chapter 7.

IMPORTANT RELATIONSHIP

X-ray Interaction with Matter

When the diagnostic primary x-ray beam interacts with anatomic tissues, three processes occur: absorption, scattering, and transmission.

The areas within the anatomic tissue that absorb incoming x-ray photons (photoelectric effect) create the light areas (increased brightness) on the displayed image. The incoming x-ray photons

FIG. 3-9 Some incoming x-ray photons pass through the anatomic part without any interactions. (From Johnston JN, Fauber TL: *Essentials of Radiographic Physics and Imaging*, ed 2, St. Louis, 2016, Mosby.)

FIG. 3-10 Radiation that exits the anatomic part comprises transmitted and scattered radiation. (From Johnston JN, Fauber TL: *Essentials of Radiographic Physics and Imaging*, ed 2, St. Louis, 2016, Mosby.)

that are transmitted create dark areas (decreased brightness) on the displayed image. Anatomic tissues that vary in absorption and transmission create a range of dark and light areas (shades of gray) (Fig. 3-11). The various shades of gray recorded in the radiographic image make anatomic tissues visible. Skeletal bones are differentiated from the air-filled lungs because of their differences in absorption and transmission.

Less than 5% of the primary x-ray beam interacting with the anatomic part actually reaches the IR, and an even lower percentage is used to create the radiographic image. The exit radiation interacting with an IR creates the **latent image**, or **invisible image**. This latent image is not visible until it is processed to produce the **manifest image**, or **visible image**. IRs, acquisition, processing, and display are discussed in Chapters 4 and 5.

— Increased brightness

— Shades of gray

— Decreased brightness

FIG. 3-11 Anatomic tissues vary in their absorption and transmission of x-ray photons to create the range of brightness or gray levels that structurally represent the anatomic area of interest. Increased brightness represents absorbed radiation, whereas decreased brightness represents transmitted radiation. (From Johnston JN, Fauber TL: *Essentials of Radiographic Physics and Imaging*, ed 2, St. Louis, 2016, Mosby.)

IMPORTANT RELATIONSHIP

Image Brightness

The range of image brightness levels visible after processing is a result of the variation in x-ray absorption and transmission as the x-ray beam passes through anatomic tissues.

RADIOGRAPHIC QUALITY

A quality radiographic image accurately represents the anatomic area of interest, and information is well visualized for diagnosis. It is important to identify the attributes of a quality radiographic image before comprehending all the factors that affect its quality.

The *visibility* of the anatomic structures and the *accuracy* of their recorded structural lines (sharpness) determine the overall quality of the radiographic image. The visibility of the anatomic detail refers to the *brightness* and *contrast* of the image, and the accuracy of the structural lines is achieved by maximizing the amount of *spatial resolution* and minimizing the amount of *distortion* (Fig. 3-12). Visibility of the anatomic structures is achieved by the proper balance of image brightness and contrast.

Image Brightness

Because the digital image is composed of numerical data, the brightness level displayed on the computer monitor can be easily altered to visualize the range of anatomic structures recorded. **Brightness** is the amount of luminance (light emission) of a display monitor.

Radiographic Quality

FIG. 3-12 Factors affecting radiographic image quality. **A,** Visibility factors. **B,** Sharpness factors. (From Johnston JN, Fauber TL: *Essentials of Radiographic Physics and Imaging*, ed 2, St. Louis, 2016, Mosby.)

FIG. 3-13 Brightness. Radiographic image with sufficient brightness. (From Johnston JN, Fauber TL: *Essentials of Radiographic Physics and Imaging*, ed 3, St. Louis, 2020, Mosby.)

FIG. 3-14 Brightness. Radiographic image with excessive brightness. Brightness altered with postprocessing. (From Johnston JN, Fauber TL: *Essentials of Radiographic Physics and Imaging*, ed 3, St. Louis, 2020, Mosby.)

A radiographic image must have sufficient brightness to visualize the anatomic structures of interest (Fig. 3-13). A radiographic image that is too light has too much brightness to visualize the structures of the anatomic part (Fig. 3-14). Conversely, a radiographic image that is too dark has insufficient brightness, and the anatomic part cannot be well visualized (Fig. 3-15). The radiographer must evaluate the overall brightness in the image to determine whether it is sufficient to

FIG. 3-15 Brightness. Radiographic image with insufficient brightness. Brightness altered with postprocessing. (From Johnston JN, Fauber TL: *Essentials of Radiographic Physics and Imaging,* ed 3, St. Louis, 2020, Mosby.)

visualize the anatomic area of interest. He or she then decides whether the radiographic image is diagnostic or unacceptable.

 IMPORTANT RELATIONSHIP
Brightness and Radiographic Quality

A radiographic image must have sufficient brightness to visualize the anatomic structures of interest.

The x-ray beam that exits the patient contains a wide range of x-ray intensities (often varying by more than 1000-fold). To adequately capture these intensity extremes, a receptor with a wide dynamic range is required. Because digital imaging provides a wide dynamic range and the computer can adjust for exposure errors, a greater margin of error exists for exposure techniques to yield acceptable brightness levels.

Because digital image processing can compensate for exposure errors, the image may display the appropriate level of brightness yet also have been over- or underexposed. As a result, the radiographer may be unaware of the exposure error. However, extreme exposure errors can affect image quality and be visible to the radiographer. When exposure to the digital IR is too low for

FIG. 3-16 Saturation. **A,** Radiographic image with sufficient exposure. **B,** Radiographic image with extreme overexposure; the quality is severely degraded. (From Johnston JN, Fauber TL: *Essentials of Radiographic Physics and Imaging*, ed 3, St. Louis, 2020, Mosby.

the anatomic area, excessive quantum noise (discussed later in this chapter) may be visible. When the IR is extremely overexposed, **saturation** may occur where the image cannot be properly processed, and the quality is severely degraded (Fig. 3-16).

Image Contrast

In addition to sufficient brightness, the radiographic image must exhibit differences in the brightness levels (image contrast) to differentiate among anatomic tissues. The range of brightness levels is a result of the tissues' differential absorption of the x-ray photons. An image that has sufficient brightness but no differences appears as a homogeneous object (Fig. 3-17). This appearance indicates that the absorption characteristics of the object are equal. When the absorption characteristics of an object differ, the image has varying levels of brightness (Fig. 3-18). The anatomic tissues are easily differentiated because of these differences in brightness levels (i.e., contrast). Tissues that attenuate the x-ray beam equally are more difficult to visualize because the brightness levels are too similar to differentiate.

Radiographic contrast is the combined result of multiple factors associated with the anatomic structure, radiation quality, image-receptor capabilities, computer processing, and display. **Subject contrast** refers to the absorption characteristics of the anatomic tissue imaged and the quality of the x-ray beam. Differences in tissue thickness, density, and effective atomic number contribute to subject contrast (Fig. 3-19). For example, the chest is composed of tissues that vary greatly in x-ray lucency, such as the air-filled lungs, the heart, and the bony thorax. This anatomic region creates high subject contrast because the tissues attenuate the x-ray beam very differently compared with the abdomen for the same beam quality. When the thorax is imaged, great differences in brightness levels are recorded for the varying tissues (Fig. 3-20). The abdomen is composed of tissues that attenuate the x-ray beam similarly and is considered to be a region of low subject contrast. The brightness levels representing the organs

FIG. 3-17 Radiograph of a homogeneous object having no differences in brightness levels.

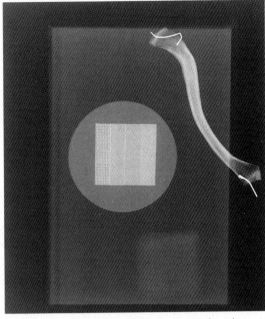

FIG. 3-18 An object with different absorption characteristics produces an image with varying brightness levels.

in the abdomen are more similar (Fig. 3-21). Therefore, it is difficult to distinguish the stomach from the kidneys. As previously discussed, the quality of the x-ray beam also affects its attenuation in tissues, which alters subject contrast. Increasing the penetrating power of the x-ray beam decreases attenuation, reduces absorption, and increases x-ray transmission, resulting in fewer differences in the brightness levels recorded in the radiographic image.

IMPORTANT RELATIONSHIP

Differentiating Among Anatomic Tissues

The ability to distinguish among types of tissues is determined by the differences in brightness levels in the image, or contrast. Anatomic tissues that attenuate the beam similarly have low subject contrast. Anatomic tissues that attenuate the beam very differently have high subject contrast.

Brightness is easily measurable; however, contrast is a more complex attribute. Evaluating radiographic quality in terms of contrast is more subjective. (It is affected by individual preferences.) The level of radiographic contrast desired in an image is determined by the composition of the anatomic tissue to be imaged and the amount of information needed to visualize the tissue for an accurate diagnosis. For example, the level of contrast desired in a chest image is different from that required in an extremity image.

Radiographic or *image contrast* is a term used to describe variations in brightness levels. In digital imaging, the number of different shades of gray that can be stored and displayed by a computer system is termed **grayscale**. Because the digital image is processed and reconstructed in the computer as digital data, its grayscale or contrast can be altered. Digital images can be displayed

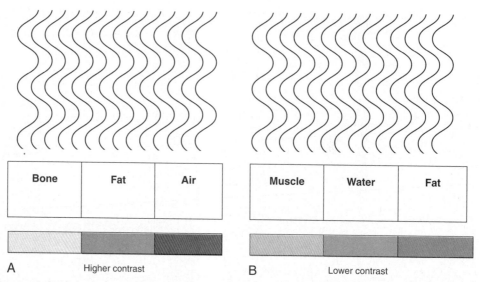

Bone	Fat	Air

A   Higher contrast

Muscle	Water	Fat

B   Lower contrast

FIG. 3-19 A, Higher contrast resulting from great differences in radiation absorption between tissues that vary greatly in composition. **B,** Lower contrast resulting from fewer differences in the radiation absorption for tissues that are more similarly composed.

FIG. 3-20 The thorax is an anatomic area of high subject contrast because there is great variation in tissue composition.

FIG. 3-21 The abdomen is an anatomic area of low subject contrast because it is composed of similar tissue types.

to show a range of gray levels from high to low contrast. **High-contrast images** display fewer shades of gray but greater differences among them (Fig. 3-22). **Low-contrast images** display a greater number of gray shades but smaller differences among them (Fig. 3-23).

FIG. 3-22 High-contrast image showing fewer gray levels and greater differences among them.

FIG. 3-23 Low-contrast image showing many gray levels and few differences among them.

Contrast resolution is a term associated with digital imaging and is used to describe the ability of the imaging system to distinguish between small objects that attenuate the x-ray beam similarly. The contrast resolution of the imaging system determines the level of visibility of small objects having similar brightness levels or shades of gray. Increasing the number of shades of gray increases the contrast resolution within the image. An image with increased contrast resolution increases the visibility of anatomic structures and the ability to distinguish among small anatomic areas of interest.

Spatial Resolution

The quality of a radiographic image depends on both the visibility and the accuracy of the anatomic structural lines (sharpness) displayed. Adequate visualization of the anatomic area of interest (brightness and contrast) is just one component of radiographic quality. To produce a quality radiographic image, the anatomic structures must be accurately recorded and with the greatest amount of sharpness. **Spatial resolution** is a term used to evaluate the accuracy of the anatomic structural lines displayed. Spatial resolution refers to the smallest object that can be detected in an image.

The ability of a radiographic image to demonstrate sharp lines determines the quality of the spatial resolution. The imaging process makes it impossible to produce a radiographic image without a certain degree of unsharpness. A radiographic image that has greater spatial resolution minimizes the unsharpness of the anatomic structural lines.

IMPORTANT RELATIONSHIP
Sharpness of Anatomic Detail

The accuracy of the anatomic structural lines displayed in the radiographic image is determined by its spatial resolution.

A radiographic image cannot be an exact reconstruction of the anatomic structure. Some information is always lost during the process of image formation. In addition, factors such as patient motion increase the amount of unsharpness recorded in the image (Fig. 3-24). Eliminating motion unsharpness is an important skill required of the radiographer. Voluntary motion, under the control of the patient, is best alleviated by effective communication. However, in some situations such as with children and older adults, patients may have difficulty controlling voluntary motion. Reducing the exposure time and using immobilization devices may be needed in addition to effective communication. Reducing the exposure time is the best method to eliminate motion unsharpness for involuntary motion, not under the control of the patient. A less common type of motion unsharpness is a result of equipment malfunction and is more difficult to identify.

It is the radiographer's responsibility to minimize the amount of information lost by manipulating the factors that affect the sharpness of the displayed image. Diagnostic quality is achieved by maximizing the amount of spatial resolution and minimizing the amount of image distortion.

FIG. 3-24 Image showing motion unsharpness. (From *Mosby's Instructional Radiographic Series: Radiographic Imaging*, St. Louis, 1998, Mosby.)

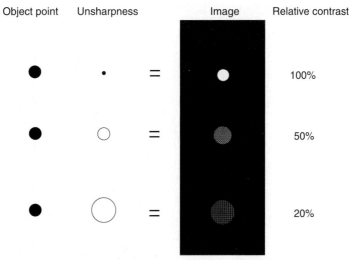

| Object point | Unsharpness | | Image | Relative contrast |

FIG. 3-25 Unsharpness and image contrast. Increasing the amount of unsharpness decreases the brightness between the area of interest and its surrounding background. (Modified from Sprawls P: *Physical Principles of Medical Imaging Online*, ed 2, http://www.sprawls.org/ppmi2.)

The sharpness and visibility of recorded detail have typically been discussed as two separate qualities of a radiographic image. Generally, this separation remains true except when imaging small anatomic structures. A small anatomic structure is best visualized when its brightness varies significantly from the background. If unsharpness is increased, the visibility of small anatomic details is compromised. An increase in the amount of unsharpness displayed in the image decreases the contrast of small anatomic structures, reducing the overall visibility of the structural lines. The spreading of the structural lines with increased unsharpness decreases the differences in brightness levels between the structural lines of the area of interest and the background. As a result, the difference in brightness levels between the area of interest and the background lessens (low contrast) and the visibility of the anatomic structure is reduced (Fig. 3-25).

Distortion

Distortion results from the radiographic misrepresentation of either the size (magnification) or the shape of the anatomic part. When an image is distorted, spatial resolution is also reduced.

Size Distortion (Magnification)

The term **size distortion** (or **magnification**) refers to an increase in the image size of an object compared with its true or actual size. Radiographic images of objects are always magnified in terms of the true object size. The source-to-image receptor distance (SID) and object-to-image receptor distance (OID) have a geometric relationship and play an important role in minimizing the amount of size distortion of the radiographic image.

Because radiographers produce radiographs of three-dimensional objects, some size distortion always occurs as a result of OID. The parts of the object that are farther away from the IR are radiographically represented with greater size distortion than the parts of the object that are closer to the IR. Even if the object is in close contact with the IR, some part of the object is farther away than other parts of the object. SID also influences the total amount of magnification of the image. As SID increases, size distortion (magnification) decreases; as SID decreases, size distortion (magnification) increases.

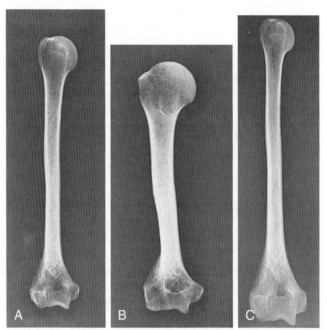

FIG. 3-26 A, No distortion. **B,** Foreshortened. **C,** Elongated. (From *Mosby's Instructional Radiographic Series: Radiographic Imaging*, St. Louis, 1998, Mosby.)

 IMPORTANT RELATIONSHIP

Size Distortion

> Radiographic images of objects are always magnified in terms of the true object size. The SID and OID have a geometric relationship and play an important role in minimizing the amount of size distortion of the radiographic image.

Shape Distortion

In addition to size distortion, objects that are being imaged can be radiographically misrepresented by distortion of their shape. **Shape distortion** can radiographically appear in two different ways: elongation or foreshortening. **Elongation** refers to images of objects that appear longer than the true objects. **Foreshortening** refers to images that appear shorter than the true objects. Examples of elongation and foreshortening can be seen in Fig. 3-26.

Shape distortion can arise from inaccurate central ray (CR) alignment of the tube, the part being radiographed, or the IR. Any misalignment of the CR among these three factors—tube, part, or IR—alters the shape of the part recorded in the image.

 IMPORTANT RELATIONSHIP

Shape Distortion

> Shape distortion can occur from inaccurate CR alignment of the tube, the part being radiographed, or the IR. Elongation refers to images of objects that appear longer than the true objects. Foreshortening refers to images that appear shorter than the true objects.

FIG. 3-27 Scatter and fog.

Sometimes shape distortion is advantageous in particular projections or positions. For example, CR angulation is sometimes required to elongate a part so that a particular anatomic structure can be visualized better. Also, rotating the part (and therefore creating shape distortion) is sometimes required to eliminate superimposition of objects that normally obstruct visualization of the area of interest. In general, shape distortion is not a necessary or desirable characteristic of radiographic images.

Both SID and OID determine the amount of magnification of the anatomic structures on the image. In addition, improper alignment of the CR, anatomic part, IR, or a combination of these components distorts the shape of the image.

Scatter

Scatter radiation, as previously described, can add unwanted exposure to the radiographic image as a result of Compton interactions. Unwanted exposure or fog on the image does not provide information about the anatomic area of interest. Scatter degrades or decreases the visibility of the anatomic structures. The scatter or unwanted exposure displayed in the image has the effect of decreasing the contrast by masking the desired brightness of the image and changing the degree of difference (Fig. 3-27).

Fog produced because of scatter reaching the IR can be visualized on a digital image. Even though the computer can change the contrast or gray levels displayed in a digital image, scatter radiation reaching the IR does not provide any information about the area of interest. Because digital IRs can detect low levels of radiation intensity, they are more sensitive to scatter radiation.

Quantum Noise

Image noise contributes no useful diagnostic information and serves only to detract from the quality of an image. **Quantum noise** (mottle) is a concern in digital imaging and is photon

FIG. 3-28 A, Image created using an appropriate x-ray exposure technique. **B,** Image shows increased quantum noise as a result of insufficient x-ray exposure to the image receptor. (From Johnston JN, Fauber TL: *Essentials of Radiographic Physics and Imaging*, ed 2, St. Louis, 2016, Mosby.)

dependent. Quantum noise is visible as brightness fluctuations in the image. The fewer the photons reaching the IR to form the image, the greater the visibility of quantum noise on the digital image.

> ### IMPORTANT RELATIONSHIP
> #### Number of Photons and Quantum Noise
>
> Decreasing the number of photons reaching the IR may increase the amount of quantum noise within the radiographic image; increasing the number of photons reaching the IR may decrease the amount of quantum noise within the radiographic image.

As previously mentioned, the digital computer system can adjust for low or high x-ray exposures during image acquisition. When the x-ray exposure to the IR is too low (i.e., when there is a decreased number of photons), computer processing alters the appearance of the digital image to make the brightness acceptable, but the image displays increased quantum noise (Fig. 3-28). Certain postprocessing options may render quantum noise more or less noticeable.

The exposure technique should be selected on the basis of the requirements of the type of radiographic procedure being performed. Although the computer can adjust for both low- and high-exposure technique errors, the radiographer is still responsible for selecting exposure techniques that produce diagnostic quality images while avoiding unnecessary exposure to the patient. Exposures that are too low adversely affect the quantum noise of an image even though the computer can adjust the brightness. Exposures that are too high result in excessive radiation exposure to the patient.

Image Artifacts

An **artifact** is any unwanted brightness level on a radiographic image. Artifacts are detrimental to images because they can impede visibility of anatomy, pathologic conditions, or patient-identification information. They decrease the overall quality of the radiographic image.

FIG. 3-29 Image artifact. (From Long B, Rollins J, Smith B: *Merrill's Atlas of Radiographic Positioning and Procedures*, ed 13, St. Louis, 2016, Mosby.)

Errors such as double-exposing an IR or the improper use of equipment can result in image artifacts and must be avoided. Foreign bodies are a class of artifacts imaged within a patient's body. Variation in exposure techniques may be necessary when imaging for a suspected foreign body.

Artifacts from patient clothing and items imaged that are not a part of the area of interest are the same regardless of the type of imaging systems. The radiographer must be diligent in removing clothing or items that could obstruct visibility of the anatomic area of interest (Fig. 3-29). Scatter radiation or fog and image noise have also been classified as radiographic artifacts because they add unwanted information on the displayed image.

Digital image artifacts can be a result of errors during extraction of the latent image from the IR, inadequate CR imaging plate erasure, or performance of the electronic detectors and will be discussed in subsequent chapters.

Digital versus Film-Screen Imaging

Although film-screen imaging served as a good medium for radiographic imaging for many decades, it has many limitations that can be overcome with digital imaging. One major deficiency is the limited **dynamic range** (the range of exposure intensities an IR can accurately detect). This limitation renders a film-screen IR very sensitive to underexposure or overexposure, which may necessitate image retakes. A limited dynamic range also restricts the visibility of structures that differ greatly in x-ray attenuation. An example is the difficulty of optimally visualizing both soft tissue and bony structures within a given film image.

> **IMPORTANT RELATIONSHIP**
>
> *Dynamic Range and Film-Screen Imaging*
>
> The range of exposure intensities that film can accurately detect is limited (limited dynamic range). This renders film more susceptible to overexposure and underexposure and restricts its ability to display tissues that vary greatly in x-ray attenuation.

Other drawbacks of film-screen imaging involve the cost of film itself, the necessity of developing the latent image into a manifest image via chemical processing, and potential artifacts related to film handling and chemical processing. The time required to process the film before viewing the radiograph can delay the progress of an examination or diagnosis. Automatic film processors incur considerable equipment and maintenance costs and demand frequent quality-control procedures.

Another restriction associated with a film image is that after the film has been processed, the image is permanent, and further adjustments cannot be made. There is no option to alter the brightness (for film, density, the amount of blackness after processing) or contrast of the manifest image. Therefore, the anatomic area that is to be optimally imaged must be selected at the time of exposure. For example, when an image is taken in the thoracic region, the exposure technique must be selected depending on whether the area of interest is the lungs or the ribs. A related issue is the limited contrast resolution, which is the ability to distinguish tissues of similar subject contrast, of film-screen receptors. Even if technique factors are chosen to optimize soft tissue contrast, the differential absorption among various soft tissues is slight and not well differentiated using film-screen imaging.

In addition, film images cannot be electronically stored or duplicated, displayed on computer monitors, or transmitted over computer networks unless they are digitized after processing. Traditional film archives consume significant space and are frequently prone to loss of films. In addition, personnel costs associated with maintaining the archive and the expense of storing radiographs and then retrieving them when needed for comparison is prohibitive. Film-screen imaging is discussed more thoroughly in Chapter 9.

Digital imaging overcomes many limitations of film-screen radiography. Digital radiographic images can be quickly acquired and displayed and can be efficiently transmitted, processed, interpreted on a display monitor, stored, and retrieved via electronic means.

Radiography creates a static (stationary) image of the anatomic area of interest whereas dynamic imaging, or fluoroscopy, provides imaging of the movement of internal structures.

DYNAMIC IMAGING: FLUOROSCOPY

Fluoroscopy (Fig. 3-30) differs from static imaging by its use of a continuous beam of x-rays to create images of moving internal anatomic structures that can be viewed on a display monitor. Internal structures, such as the vascular or gastrointestinal systems, can be visualized in their normal state of motion with the aid of special liquid or gas substances (contrast media) that are either injected or instilled (i.e., ingested). The equipment used in fluoroscopy has undergone major changes over the past few years. Image-intensified fluoroscopy is rapidly being replaced with flat-panel detector fluoroscopy. Regardless of the type of fluoroscopic equipment, the x-ray tube is usually positioned underneath the table, and the x-rays pass through the patient to interact with a device that converts the x-rays into either light intensities (image-intensified) or digital data (flat-panel detector).

FIG. 3-30 Digital fluoroscopy using flat-panel detector technology. (Courtesy of Siemens Healthcare, Malvern, PA.)

 IMPORTANT RELATIONSHIP

Fluoroscopy

Dynamic imaging of internal anatomic structures can be visualized with the use of a flat-panel detector or image intensifier. The exit radiation interacts with the acquisition device, is processed or converted, and is then transmitted to the display monitor for viewing.

Fluoroscopy is discussed in detail in Chapter 10.

Regardless of the type of imaging system (digital, film, or fluoroscopic), the process of differential absorption for image formation remains the same. The varying x-ray intensities exiting the anatomic area of interest form the image.

 IMPORTANT RELATIONSHIP

Image Formation

The process of differential absorption for image formation remains the same regardless of the type of imaging system, digital, film, or fluoroscopic. The varying x-ray intensities exiting the anatomic area of interest form the image which is displayed on a monitor or film.

CHAPTER SUMMARY

- A radiographic image is a result of the differential absorption of the primary x-rays that interact with tissues of varying composition within the anatomic area of interest.
- Beam attenuation occurs when the primary x-ray beam loses energy as it interacts with anatomic tissues.

- X-rays have the ability to eject electrons (ionization) from atoms within anatomic tissue.
- Three primary processes occur during x-ray interaction with anatomic tissues: absorption, transmission, and scattering.
- Total absorption of the incoming x-ray photon is a result of the photoelectric effect.
- Scattering of the incoming x-ray photon is a result of the Compton effect.
- Scatter radiation reaching the IR provides no useful information and creates unwanted exposure or fog on the radiographic image.
- The process of differential absorption remains the same for image formation regardless of the type of IR.
- A radiographic image is composed of varying brightness levels that structurally represent the anatomic area of interest.
- The visibility and accuracy of the recorded anatomic structural lines determine thwe overall quality of the radiographic image.
- Visibility of the anatomic structures is achieved by the proper balance of image brightness and contrast.
- Image contrast provides the ability to distinguish among the types of irradiated tissues.
- Grayscale is the number of different shades of gray that can be stored and displayed in a digital image.
- Spatial resolution refers to the accuracy of the anatomic structural lines displayed.
- Distortion describes the magnification or misrepresentation in shape of the anatomic structures.
- Scatter radiation produces unwanted exposure on the image, known as fog.
- Quantum noise is a result of too few photons reaching the IR and is a concern in digital imaging.
- An artifact is any unwanted brightness level on a radiographic image.
- Digital IRs have a wider dynamic range compared with film-screen IRs.
- Fluoroscopy differs from static imaging by its use of a continuous beam of x-rays to create images of moving internal structures (dynamic imaging) that can be viewed on a display monitor.

REVIEW QUESTIONS

1. The process whereby a radiographic image is created by variations in absorption and transmission of the exiting x-ray beam is known as _____.
   - **A.** attenuation
   - **B.** the photoelectric effect
   - **C.** the Compton effect
   - **D.** differential absorption

2. Which of the following processes occur during the x-ray beam interaction with tissue?
   1. Absorption
   2. Photon transmission
   3. Scattering
      - **A.** 1 and 2 only
      - **B.** 1 and 3 only
      - **C.** 2 and 3 only
      - **D.** 1, 2, and 3

3. The ability of an x-ray photon to remove an atom's electron is a characteristic known as _____.
   - **A.** attenuation
   - **B.** scattering

    C. ionization

    D. absorption

4. The x-ray interaction responsible for absorption is _____.

    A. differential

    B. photoelectric

    C. attenuation

    D. Compton

5. The x-ray interaction responsible for scattering is _____.

    A. differential

    B. photoelectric

    C. attenuation

    D. Compton

6. Remnant radiation is composed of which of the following?

    1. Transmitted radiation

    2. Absorbed radiation

    3. Scattered radiation

        A. 1 and 2 only

        B. 1 and 3 only

        C. 2 and 3 only

        D. 1, 2, and 3

7. What interaction causes unwanted exposure to the image, known as fog?

    A. Compton

    B. Transmitted

    C. Photoelectric

    D. Absorption

8. Which of the following factors would affect beam attenuation?

    1. Tissue atomic number

    2. Beam quality

    3. Fog

        A. 1 and 2 only

        B. 1 and 3 only

        C. 2 and 3 only

        D. 1, 2, and 3

9. The high brightness areas on a radiographic image are created by _____.

    A. transmitted radiation

    B. scattered radiation

    C. absorbed radiation

    D. primary radiation

10. An anatomic part that transmits the incoming x-ray photon would create an area of _____ on the radiographic image.

    A. fog

    B. high brightness

    C. low brightness

    D. noise

11. The process of creating a radiographic image by differential absorption varies for film-screen and digital imaging.

    A. True

    B. False

12. Which attribute(s) of a radiographic image affect(s) the visibility of sharpness?
    A. Distortion
    B. Contrast
    C. Brightness
    D. B and C

13. A radiographic image with many shades of gray but few differences among them is said to have _____.
    A. high contrast
    B. low contrast
    C. saturation
    D. excessive noise

14. Which of the following is defined as the range of exposure intensities that an image receptor can accurately detect?
    A. Saturation
    B. Spatial resolution
    C. Quantum noise
    D. Dynamic range

15. Fluoroscopy uses a continuous beam of x-rays to create images of moving internal anatomic structures.
    A. True
    B. False

Digital Image Characteristics, Receptors, and Image Acquisition

CHAPTER OUTLINE

Digital Image Characteristics
  Spatial Frequency and Spatial
    Resolution
  Dynamic Range
  Dose Monitoring

Modulation Transfer
    Function
Detective Quantum Efficiency
Signal-to-Noise Ratio
Contrast-to-Noise Ratio

**Digital Image Receptors and
  Image Acquisition**
  Computed Radiography
  Direct Radiography
Quality Control

OBJECTIVES

*After completing this chapter, the reader will be able
to perform the following:*

1. Define all the key terms in this chapter.
2. State all the important relationships in this
   chapter.
3. Compare and contrast the attributes of a digital
   image.
4. Explain the digital characteristics of matrix and
   pixels.
5. Recognize the relationship among pixel size,
   display field of view, and matrix size.
6. State the relationship between spatial frequency
   and spatial resolution.
7. Explain the importance of dynamic range and
   exposure latitude in exposure technique selection, image quality, and patient exposure.
8. Define *modulation transfer function* and

   detective quantum efficiency and explain their
   relationship to digital image quality.
9. Define *signal-to-noise ratio* and explain its
   importance to digital image quality.
10. Define *contrast-to-noise ratio* and explain its
    importance to digital image quality.
11. Differentiate between computed radiography
    (CR) and direct radiography image receptors
    (IRs) in acquiring the digital image.
12. Explain the importance of sampling frequency
    in reproducing a quality digital image.
13. Describe how the size of a CR imaging plate
    can affect spatial resolution.
14. Recognize the differences between indirect and
    direct conversion digital IRs.
15. List quality control checks the radiographer can
    do to evaluate digital equipment performance.

KEY TERMS

air kerma
bit
bit depth
byte
cassette
charge-coupled device
  (CCD)

complementary metal oxide
  semiconductor (CMOS)
contrast resolution
contrast-to-noise ratio (CNR)
CR fading
detective quantum efficiency
  (DQE)

dose area product (DAP)
dynamic range
exposure latitude
field of view (FOV)
fill factor
flat-panel detectors (FPDs)
grayscale

KEY TERMS—cont'd

imaging plate (IP)
kerma-area product (KAP)
luminescence
matrix
modulation transfer function
   (MTF)
Nyquist frequency

photostimulable luminescence
photostimulable phosphor
   (PSP)
pixel density
pixel pitch
pixels
quantum noise

sampling frequency
sampling pitch
scintillator
signal-to-noise ratio (SNR)
spatial frequency

During radiographic imaging, the radiation exiting a patient is composed of a range of intensities that reflect the absorption and transmission characteristics of the anatomic tissues. The image receptor (IR) receives the exit radiation and creates the latent or invisible image. The latent image is differently acquired depending on the type of IR. This chapter describes the digital image characteristics, common types of digital IRs used in radiography, and how the image is acquired.

DIGITAL IMAGE CHARACTERISTICS

In digital imaging, the latent image is stored as digital data, referred to as an electronic data set, and must be processed by a computer for viewing on a display monitor. Digital imaging can be accomplished using a specialized IR that can produce a computerized radiographic image. Two types of digital radiographic systems are in common use today: computed radiography (CR) and direct radiography (DR). Regardless of whether the imaging system is CR or DR, the computer can manipulate the radiographic image in various ways after the image has been digitally created.

Digital images are composed of numerical data that can be easily manipulated by a computer. When displayed on a computer monitor, there is tremendous flexibility in terms of altering the brightness and contrast of a digital image. The practical advantage of such capability is that regardless of the original exposure technique factors (within reason), any anatomic structure can be independently and well visualized. Computers can also perform various pre- and postprocessing image manipulations to further improve the visibility of the anatomic region.

A digital image is recorded as a **matrix** or combination of rows and columns (array) of small, usually square, "picture elements" called **pixels**. The size of a pixel is measured in microns (100 microns = 0.1 mm). Each pixel is recorded as a single numerical value, which is represented as a single brightness level on a display monitor. The location of the pixel within the image matrix corresponds to an area within the patient or volume of tissue (Fig. 4-1).

Given the dimensions of an anatomic area of interest, or **field of view (FOV)**, a matrix size of 1024 × 1024 has 1,048,576 individual pixels; a matrix size of 2048 × 2048 has 4,194,304 pixels. Digital image quality is improved with a larger matrix size that includes a greater number of smaller pixels (Fig. 4-2 and Box 4-1). Although image quality is improved for a larger matrix size and smaller pixels, computer processing time, network transmission time, and digital storage space increase as the matrix size increases.

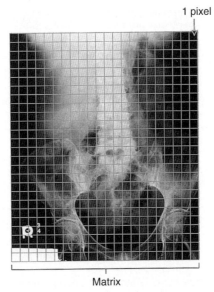

1 pixel

Matrix

FIG. 4-1 Location of the pixel within the image matrix corresponds to an area within the patient or volume of tissue. Note: Pixel size is not to scale and is used for illustration only.

FIG. 4-2 For a given field of view (FOV), the larger the matrix size, the greater the number of smaller individual pixels. Increasing the number of pixels improves the quality of the image. **A,** Matrix size is 64 × 64. **B,** Matrix size is 215 × 215. **C,** Matrix size is 2048 × 2048.

There is a relationship among pixel size, displayed FOV (the dimensions of an anatomic area displayed on the computer monitor), and matrix size, as demonstrated in the following formula:

$$\text{Pixel size} = \frac{\text{FOV}}{\text{Matrix size}}$$

This relationship demonstrates that if the FOV displayed on the monitor is increased for a fixed matrix size, then the pixel size is also increased (direct relationship). However, if the matrix size is increased for a fixed FOV, then the pixel size is decreased (inverse relationship).

BOX 4-1   Digital Imaging Terminology

Matrix—image displayed as a combination of rows and columns (array); a larger matrix size improves spatial resolution

Pixel—smallest component of the matrix; a greater number of smaller pixels improves spatial resolution

Pixel bit depth—number of bits that determines the precision with which the exit radiation is recorded and controls the exact pixel brightness that can be displayed

---

≫ MATHEMATICAL APPLICATION

Pixel Size and FOV

FOV = 17 inches (431.8 mm) and matrix size = 1024:

$$\frac{431.8}{1024} = 0.42 \text{ mm pixel size}$$

If the FOV was decreased to 12 inches (304.8 mm) for the same matrix size of 1024:

$$\frac{304.8}{1024} = 0.30 \text{ mm pixel size}$$

Decreasing the displayed FOV for a given matrix size will decrease the size of the pixels and increase spatial resolution.

≫ MATHEMATICAL APPLICATION

Pixel Size and Matrix Size

FOV = 17 inches (431.8 mm) and matrix size = 1024:

$$\frac{431.8}{1024} = 0.42 \text{ mm pixel size}$$

If the matrix size was increased to 2048 for the same FOV:

$$\frac{431.8}{2048} = 0.21 \text{ mm pixel size}$$

Increasing the matrix size for a given FOV displayed will decrease the size of the pixels and increase spatial resolution.

IMPORTANT RELATIONSHIP

Pixel Size, FOV, and Matrix Size

The pixel size is directly related to the FOV displayed and inversely related to the matrix size. Increasing the FOV for the same matrix size will increase the size of the pixel and decrease spatial resolution, whereas increasing the matrix size for the same FOV will decrease the pixel size and increase spatial resolution.

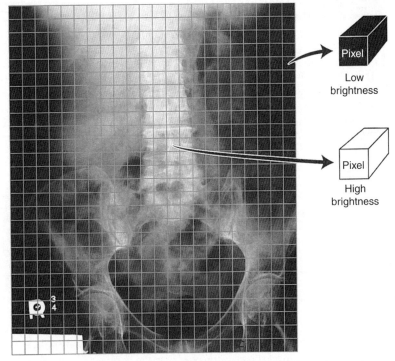

FIG. 4-3 Each pixel value represents a volume of tissue imaged.

The numerical value assigned to each pixel is determined by the relative attenuation of x-rays passing through the corresponding volume of tissue. Pixels representing highly attenuating tissues (increased absorption) such as bone are assigned a different numerical value for higher brightness than pixels representing tissues of low x-ray attenuation (decreased absorption) (Fig. 4-3). Each pixel also has a **bit depth**, or number of bits (Box 4-2), that determines the amount of precision in digitizing the analog signal and therefore the number of shades of gray that can be displayed in the image. Bit depth is determined by an analog-to-digital converter (ADC), which is an integral component of every digital imaging system. Because the binary system is used, bit depth is expressed as 2 to the power of n, or the number of bits (2^n). A larger bit depth allows a greater number of shades of gray to be displayed on a computer monitor. For example, a 12-bit depth (2^{12}) can display 4096 shades of gray, a 14-bit depth can display 16,384 shades of gray, and a 16-bit depth can display 65,536 shades of gray. A system that can digitize and display a greater number of shades of gray has better **contrast resolution**. An image with increased contrast resolution increases the visibility of anatomic details and the ability to distinguish among small anatomic areas of interest (Fig. 4-4).

IMPORTANT RELATIONSHIP

Pixel Bit Depth and Contrast Resolution

The greater the pixel bit depth (i.e., 16-bit), the more precise the digitization of the analog signal and the greater the number of shades of gray available for image display. Increasing the number of shades of gray available to display in a digital image improves its contrast resolution.

BOX 4-2 **Binary Digits**

Computers operate and communicate through the binary number system, which uses combinations of zeros and ones to process and store information. A digital transistor can be operated in two states: off (0) or on (1). Each 0 and 1 is called a **bit** and refers to the computer's basic unit of information. When 8 bits are combined, they form a **byte**, and 2 bytes form a word.

Binary digits are used to display the brightness level (grayscale) of a digital image. The greater the number of bits, the greater the number of shades of gray that can be displayed, and the quality of the image is improved.

FIG. 4-4 Pixel bit depth determines the shades of gray displayed on the monitor. The greater the pixel bit a digital system can display, the greater is the contrast resolution displayed in the image. (From Sprawls P: *The Physical Principles of Medical Imaging Online*, ed 2, http://www.sprawls.org/ppmi2.)

A digital image is composed of discrete information in the form of pixels that display various shades of gray. As previously mentioned, the greater the number of pixels in an image matrix, the smaller is their size. An image consisting of a greater number of pixels per unit area, or **pixel density**, provides improved spatial resolution. In addition to its size, the pixel spacing, or distance measured from the center of a pixel to an adjacent pixel, determines the **pixel pitch** (Fig. 4-5). Smaller-sized pixels have decreased pixel pitch and improved spatial resolution.

 IMPORTANT RELATIONSHIP

Pixel Density and Pitch and Spatial Resolution

Increasing pixel density and decreasing pixel pitch increases spatial resolution. Decreasing pixel density and increasing pixel pitch decreases spatial resolution.

Spatial Frequency and Spatial Resolution

Spatial resolution in digital imaging is primarily limited to the size of the pixel; however, when measuring an imaging system's ability to resolve small objects, it is important to understand the concept of spatial frequency and its relationship with spatial resolution. **Spatial frequency** can be defined by the unit of line pairs per millimeter (lp/mm). A resolution test pattern is a device used to record and measure line pairs (Fig. 4-6). Anatomic details are composed of large and small objects, and radiographic images display these details as variations from white to black brightness levels. Small objects have higher spatial frequency, and large objects have lower spatial frequency.

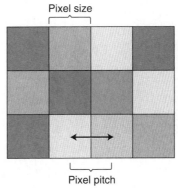

FIG. 4-5 The distance measured from the center of a pixel to an adjacent pixel determines the pixel pitch or spacing. (From Johnston JN, Fauber TL: *Essentials of Radiographic Physics and Imaging*, ed 3, St. Louis, 2020, Elsevier.)

FIG. 4-6 A resolution test pattern will record and measure line pairs per millimeter. (Courtesy of Fluke Biomedical.)

FIG. 4-7 A line pair is a high-contrast line separated by an interspace of equal width. The spatial frequency is shown for each of the line pairs. (From Bushong SC: *Radiologic Science for Technologists,* ed 10, St. Louis, 2013, Mosby.)

FIG. 4-8 Images showing how pixel size affects spatial resolution. **A,** Image with 20 pixels/cm; therefore, the pixel size is larger, and the spatial resolution is poor. **B,** Image with 40 pixels/cm. **C,** Image with 100 pixels/cm; therefore the pixel size is smaller than that in images *A* and *B*, and the spatial resolution is improved. (Courtesy of Andrew Woodward.)

It is more difficult to accurately image small anatomic objects (high spatial frequency) than to image large ones (low spatial frequency). An imaging system that can resolve a greater number of lp/mm (higher spatial frequency) has increased spatial resolution (Fig. 4-7). In digital imaging systems, the ability to resolve or demonstrate a specific spatial frequency is directly impacted by the size of the pixel. The images of the wrist (Fig. 4-8) demonstrate the impact that pixel size has on the spatial resolution visualized in an image.

IMPORTANT RELATIONSHIP

Spatial Frequency and Spatial Resolution

The unit of measure for spatial frequency is lp/mm. Increasing the number of lp/mm resolved in the imaging system (higher spatial frequency) results in improved spatial resolution.

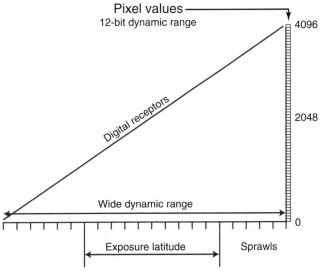

FIG. 4-9 The dynamic range of an imaging system refers to the ability of an image receptor to accurately capture the range of photon intensities exiting the patient. Exposure latitude is the range of exposures to produce a diagnostic image without under- or overexposure. (Modified from Sprawls P: *Physical Principles of Medical Imaging Online,* http://www.sprawls.org/resources.)

Dynamic Range

The **dynamic range** of an imaging system refers to the ability of an IR to accurately capture the range of photon intensities that exit the patient. Digital IRs have a wide dynamic range (Fig. 4-9). In practical terms, this wide dynamic range means that a small degree of underexposure or overexposure would still result in diagnostic image quality. This characteristic of digital receptors is advantageous in situations where automatic exposure control (AEC) may not be available, such as in mobile radiography. However, radiographers must make considerable effort to select exposure techniques that produce diagnostic images without insufficient or excessive exposure to the IR. Although digital detectors have a wide dynamic range, **exposure latitude** refers to the range of exposures that should be used to produce a diagnostic image (see Fig. 4-9) and is likely established by the preferences or needs of the imaging department.

During digitization of the image, a numerical value (bit depth) is assigned to the pixel that represents an x-ray intensity based on the attenuation characteristics of that volume of tissue. A larger pixel bit depth means the image displayed has a wide **grayscale**, and this illustrates the wide dynamic range of the digital detector. As noted in Fig. 4-9, the digital IR can accurately capture more than 4000 x-ray intensities exiting the patient. To display that range of brightness levels (grayscale), the pixel bit depth is 12. If the digital IR is able to capture over 16,000 x-ray intensities exiting the patient, the bit depth would be 14, and contrast resolution is improved compared with the 12-bit digital system.

Processing the digital data yields a radiographic image that can be viewed on a display monitor and altered in various ways. Even if optimal exposure techniques are not used, the image rescaling that occurs during the processing stage can produce images with the appropriate brightness levels. Digital image processing and display are discussed in detail in Chapter 5.

The ability of the IR to capture a wide range of exit photon intensities does not mean a quality image is always created. Although lower-than-necessary x-ray exposures can be detected and processed, image quality suffers because there is insufficient exposure to the IR, and quantum noise results. The computer can process the data resulting from an IR exposed to higher-than-necessary radiation and produce a quality image but at the expense of patient overexposure. It is the responsibility of the radiographer to select the amount of exposure necessary to produce a diagnostic digital image (exposure latitude).

IMPORTANT RELATIONSHIP

Digital Detectors, Dynamic Range, and Exposure Latitude

Digital IRs have a wide dynamic range; that is, they can accurately capture a wide range of x-ray intensities exiting the patient. The computer then processes the raw pixel data to compensate for an exposure error and create a diagnostic radiographic image. However, lower- or higher-than-necessary exposure techniques do not guarantee a quality digital image. Exposure latitude is the range of exposures that should be used to produce a diagnostic image.

! RADIATION PROTECTION ALERT

Digital Detectors and Dynamic Range

Because digital IRs have a wide dynamic range, a quality image can be produced when using more radiation exposure than necessary. Radiographers must take extra precautions to not unnecessarily overexpose patients and select exposure techniques within the exposure latitude established by the department.

Dose Monitoring

Air kerma (**k**inetic **e**nergy **r**eleased in **m**atter) specifies the intensity of x-rays at a given point in air at a known distance from the focal spot or source of x-rays. DR systems use **dose-area product (DAP)** as an indicator of exposure. DAP is a measure of exposure in air, followed by computation to estimate absorbed dose to the patient. It is measured by a DAP meter embedded in the collimator. The DAP value depends on the exposure factors and field size and reflects both the dose to the patient and the total volume of tissue being irradiated. **Kerma-area product (KAP)** is the same as DAP and is the product of the total air kerma and the area of the x-ray beam at the entrance of the patient. Units of DAP or KAP are expressed in micro, milli, or centigray per area squared but can vary by manufacturer. DAP and KAP provide indicators of patient radiation risk and may be documented in the patient's record.

Modulation Transfer Function

As previously stated, a radiographic image displays a range of brightness levels (grayscale) based on the variation in radiation intensities exiting the tissue. Anatomic detail is best visualized when the brightness level of the object is different than its surrounding tissue (high contrast). Larger sized objects (low spatial frequency) are more easily visualized. As the size of the object decreases, it attains higher spatial frequency and becomes more difficult to visualize in a radiographic image. **Modulation transfer function (MTF)** is a measure of the imaging system's ability to display the contrast of anatomic objects varying in size, and the value will be between 0 (no difference in brightness levels) and 1.0 (maximum difference in brightness levels). The formula for MTF is as follows:

$$MTF = \frac{(Maximum\ intensity - Minimum\ intensity)}{(Maximum\ intensity + Minimum\ intensity)}$$

An MTF of 1 (100% difference) would signify the difference between maximum and minimum brightness. An MTF of 1 is easier to achieve with large objects having low spatial frequency. It is more difficult to visualize smaller objects having high spatial frequency, and therefore most digital imaging systems' MTFs measure much lower than 1.0.

 IMPORTANT RELATIONSHIP

Modulation Transfer Function and Anatomic Detail

MTF is a measure of the imaging system's ability to accurately display small anatomic objects having high spatial frequency. An imaging system that has a high MTF can display anatomic detail with improved visibility.

Detective Quantum Efficiency

Detective quantum efficiency (DQE) is a measurement of the efficiency of an IR in converting the x-ray exposure it receives to a quality radiographic image. If an IR system can convert x-ray exposure into a quality image with 100% efficiency (meaning no information loss), the DQE would measure 100% or 1.0. However, no imaging system has 100% conversion efficiency. Nevertheless, the higher the DQE of a system, the lower the radiation exposure required to produce a quality image, thereby decreasing patient exposure. The system's DQE value is impacted by the type of material used in the IR to capture the exit radiation (e.g., DQE is higher for DR compared with CR IRs) and the energy of the x-ray beam (e.g., DQE is higher for amorphous selenium coated [a-Se] at higher kilovoltage peak levels compared with cesium iodide [CsI]). The DQE is also impacted by spatial frequency and MTF. Some conversion efficiency is lost when imaging at higher spatial frequencies; therefore, DQE is directly proportional to the MTF of the detector.

 IMPORTANT RELATIONSHIP

Detective Quantum Efficiency and X-ray Exposure

An IR with a higher DQE requires less x-ray exposure to produce a quality radiographic image when compared to an IR with a lower DQE value.

Signal-to-Noise Ratio

Signal-to-noise ratio (SNR) is a method of describing the strength of the radiation exposure compared with the amount of noise apparent in a digital image. Noise is a concern with any electronic data set, in this case digital image noise. Because the photon intensities are converted to an electronic signal that is digitized by the ADC, the term *signal* refers to the strength or amount of radiation exposure captured by the IR to create the image. The varying x-ray intensities exiting the patient are converted to varying signal strengths. Increasing the SNR improves the quality of the digital image; this means that the strength of the signal is high in comparison with the amount of noise, and therefore, image quality is improved. Decreasing the SNR means that there is increased noise compared with the strength of the signal, and therefore, the quality of the radiographic image is degraded. **Quantum noise** results when there are too few x-ray photons captured by the IR to create a latent image. In addition to quantum noise, sources of noise include the electronics that capture, process, and display the digital image.

The ability to visualize anatomic tissues is affected by the SNR. Noise interferes with the signal strength just as background static would interfere with the clarity of music heard. When the digital image displays increased noise, regardless of the source, anatomic details have decreased visibility.

 IMPORTANT RELATIONSHIP

Signal-to-Noise Ratio and Image Quality

Increasing the SNR increases the visibility of anatomic details, whereas decreasing the SNR decreases the visibility.

Contrast-to-Noise Ratio

Contrast-to-noise ratio (CNR) is a method of describing the contrast resolution compared with the amount of noise apparent in a digital image. Just as increased noise affects the SNR and visibility of the anatomic details, it also impacts the contrast displayed within the digital image. Brightness or signal differences in the digital image are a result of varying exit-radiation intensities from the attenuation of the x-ray beam in anatomic tissue (differential absorption). As previously stated, digital imaging systems have high contrast resolution. A system with higher contrast resolution means that anatomic tissues that attenuate the x-ray beam similarly (low subject contrast) can be better visualized. However, if the image has increased noise, the low subject contrast tissues will not be as well visualized. Digital images with a higher CNR increase the visibility of anatomic tissues (Fig. 4-10).

FIG. 4-10 Contrast-to-noise ratio (CNR). **A,** Image of a contrast detail phantom showing an increased CNR. Phantom objects are more visible. **B,** Image of contrast detail phantom showing a decreased CNR. Phantom objects are less visible. (Courtesy of Andrew Woodward.)

Contrast-to-Noise Ratio and Image Quality

Increasing the CNR increases the visibility of anatomic details, whereas decreasing the CNR decreases the visibility.

Different types of digital IRs use various methods of transforming the continuous exit radiation intensities into the array of discrete pixel values for image display. Some digital IRs use a sampling technique, whereas others have fixed detector elements (DELs) that are used to capture the exit radiation intensities. Regardless of the type used, a major determinant of the spatial resolution of digital images is the pixel size and spacing.

DIGITAL IMAGE RECEPTORS AND IMAGE ACQUISITION

Two types of digital IRs are typically used in radiography: CR and DR. These IRs differ in their construction and how they acquire latent images. After the latent image is acquired and the raw data are digitized, image processing and display are essentially the same, regardless of the type of IR.

Computed Radiography

CR IRs come in many sizes and can be portable and used in a table or upright x-ray unit or fixed in a dedicated chest unit. The CR IR includes a **cassette** that houses the **imaging plate (IP)** (Fig. 4-11). The radiation exiting the patient interacts with the IP, where the photon intensities are absorbed by the phosphor layer of the IP. Although some of the absorbed energy is released as visible light (luminescence), a sufficient amount of energy is stored in the phosphor to produce a latent image. **Luminescence** is the emission of light when stimulated by radiation.

The IP primarily consists of support, phosphor, and protective layers (Fig. 4-12). The phosphor layer is composed of barium fluorohalide crystals doped with europium, referred to as the **photostimulable phosphor (PSP)**. This type of phosphor emits visible light when stimulated by a high-intensity laser beam, a phenomenon termed **photostimulable luminescence**.

The phosphor (active layer) may be either a turbid or structured phosphor layer. A turbid phosphor has a random distribution of phosphor crystals within the active layer and can be used

FIG. 4-11 Typical computed radiography (CR) cassette showing the imaging plate (IP) housed within.

Cross-section of PSP plate

FIG. 4-12 Cross-section of a CR photostimulable phosphor (PSP) plate. (From Johnston JN, Fauber TL: *Essentials of Radiographic Physics and Imaging*, ed 3, St. Louis, 2020, Elsevier.)

FIG. 4-13 A turbid type phosphor layer. (From Leblans P, Vandenbroucke D, Willems P: Storage Phosphors for Medical Imaging. *Materials.* 2011; 4(6):1034-1086. https://doi.org/10.3390/ma4061034.)

with both CR and DR IRs (Fig. 4-13). A structured phosphor layer has columnar phosphor crystals within the active layer resembling needles standing on end and packed together (Fig. 4-14). The reflective layer reflects light released during the reading phase toward the photodetector. The conductive layer reduces and conducts away static electricity. The support layer is a sturdy material to give some rigidity to the plate. Finally, the soft backing layer protects the back of the plate and assists in preventing backscatter (x-rays scattered back from the plate) from *fogging* the phosphor layer during exposure.

CR imaging requires a two-step process for image acquisition: image capture in the IP and image readout. The latent image is formed in the PSP when the exit x-ray intensities are absorbed by the phosphor and the europium atoms become ionized by the photoelectric effect. The absorbed energy excites the electrons, elevating them to a higher energy state, where they become stored or trapped in the conduction band (Fig. 4-15). The conduction band is an energy level just beyond the valence band (outermost energy band of an atom). The number and distribution of these trapped electrons (which form the latent image) are proportional to the exit exposure intensity as a result of the tissue's differential x-ray absorption. Some of these excited electrons immediately return to their normal state, and the excess energy is released as visible light. A percentage

FIG. 4-14 A structured phosphor layer with columnar phosphor crystals. (From Leblans P, Vandenbroucke D, Willems P: Storage Phosphors for Medical Imaging. *Materials.* 2011; 4(6):1034-1086. https://doi.org/10.3390/ma4061034.)

**Phosphor layer of a PSP
plate during exposure**

FIG. 4-15 During exposure of the PSP phosphor layer, the higher-energy electrons will become trapped in the conduction band. A percentage of the higher-energy electrons will return to their normal state and release the excess energy as visible light. (From Johnston JN, Fauber TL: *Essentials of Radiographic Physics and Imaging*, ed 2, St. Louis, 2016, Mosby.)

of electrons remain in this higher-energy state until released during laser beam scanning of the readout stage. The acquired image data (released energy) are extracted from the digital receptor, converted to digital data, and computer processed for image display. Exposed IPs should be processed within a relatively short amount of time (within 1 h) because the latent image dissipates over time (**CR fading**). CR fading occurs because some of the signal (released energy) captured in the IP is lost.

FIG. 4-16 The exposed CR IP is placed in a reader unit to release the stored image, convert the analog image to digital, and send the data to a computer monitor, laser printer for a hard copy, or both. The reader unit also erases the exposed IP in preparation for the next exposure. (Courtesy of Fujifilm Medical Systems, Stamford, CT.)

IMPORTANT RELATIONSHIP

Computed Radiography Digital Image Receptors

The CR latent image is acquired in the PSP layer of the IP. Most energy from the exit radiation intensities is stored in the PSP for extraction in the reader unit.

The exposed IP is placed in or sent to a reader unit that converts the analog data into digital data for computer processing (Fig. 4-16). Reader units are available in single- or multiplate configurations. The major components of a typical reader unit are a drive mechanism to move the IP through the scanning process; an optical system, which includes the laser, beam-shaping optics, collecting optics, and optical filters; a photodetector, such as a photomultiplier tube (PMT); and an ADC. Manufacturers differ in the CR reader mechanics. Some devices move the IP, and some move the optical components. There are three important stages in digitizing the CR latent image: scanning, sampling, and quantization.

The purpose of scanning is to convert the latent image (released energy) into an electrical signal (voltage) that can be subsequently digitized and displayed as a manifest digital image. Once in the reader unit, the IP is removed from the cassette and scanned with a helium–neon laser beam or a solid-state laser diode to release the stored energy as visible light (Fig. 4-17). Absorption of the laser beam energy releases the trapped electrons, and they return to a lower energy state. During this process, the excess energy is emitted as visible light (photostimulable luminescence). The scanning of the plate results in a continuous pattern of light intensities being sent to the PMT or photodetector, whose output is directed to the ADC for sampling and quantization.

A photodetector collects, amplifies, and converts the visible light to an electrical signal proportional to the range of energies stored in the IP. The collected electronic signal values are of low voltage and therefore need to be amplified by the photodetector in order to travel to the ADC.

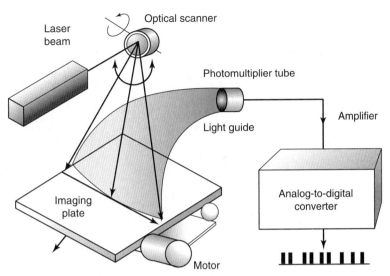

FIG. 4-17 A neon–helium laser beam scans the exposed CR IP to release the stored energy as visible light. The photomultiplier tube collects, amplifies, and converts the light to an electrical signal. The analog-to-digital converter converts the analog data to digital data. (Courtesy of Fujifilm Medical Systems, Stamford, CT.)

FIG. 4-18 Sampling and pixel pitch. The sampling frequency determines the distance between the midpoint of one pixel and the midpoint of an adjacent pixel.

The signal output from the photodetector is digitized by an ADC in order to produce a digital image. To digitize the analog signal from the photodetector, it must first be sampled. An important performance characteristic of an ADC is the **sampling frequency**, which determines how often the analog signal is reproduced in its discrete digitized form (Fig. 4-18).

As mentioned previously, small anatomic details have higher spatial frequency and would therefore need a higher sampling frequency than low spatial frequency anatomic details. The **Nyquist frequency** is a standard formula for converting analog data into to discreet digital units to accurately represent the analog signal or imaging data in digital radiography. To accurately reproduce an image from the continuous analog signal, the sampling rate must be at least two times the highest spatial frequency in the exit x-ray intensities (signal). If the sampling frequency is too low, an improper waveform (aliasing) may result, which is considered an image artifact and reduces the visibility of small anatomic detail (Fig. 4-19).

Increasing the sampling frequency of the analog signal increases the pixel density of the digital data and improves the spatial resolution of the digital image. The closer the samples are to each other

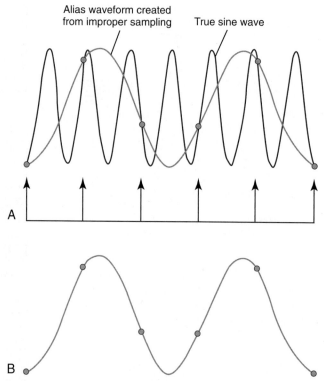

FIG. 4-19 CR sampling and its effect on the digital data. **A,** The sampling points of the analog waveform. **B,** The improper digital waveform (alias) that results from low sampling frequency.

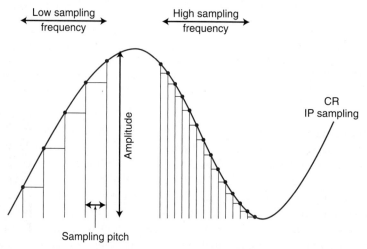

FIG. 4-20 CR sampling frequency and sampling pitch. (Courtesy of Richard Sanders.)

(increased sampling frequency), the smaller the **sampling pitch**, or distance between the sampling points (Fig. 4-20). Increasing the sampling frequency decreases the sampling pitch and results in smaller-sized pixels. The distance between the midpoint of one pixel to the midpoint of an adjacent pixel describes the pixel pitch. Spatial resolution is improved with an increased number of smaller pixels, resulting in a more faithful digital representation of the acquired analog image.

FIXED SAMPLING FREQUENCY

Large matrix

Small matrix

Pixel size

FIG. 4-21 Fixed sampling frequency. A fixed sampling frequency will maintain a fixed spatial resolution. A larger IP size will have a larger matrix to maintain the same pixel size. Note: Pixel size is not to scale and is used for illustration only.

IMPORTANT RELATIONSHIP
Sampling Frequency and Spatial Resolution

Increasing the sampling frequency results in more sampling points and decreased pixel pitch, which improves the spatial resolution of the digital image. Decreasing the sampling frequency results in fewer sampling points and increased pixel pitch and decreased spatial resolution.

Manufacturers of CR equipment vary in the method of sampling IPs of different sizes. Some manufacturers fix the sampling frequency to maintain a fixed spatial resolution, whereas others vary the sampling frequency to maintain a fixed matrix size. If the spatial resolution is fixed, the image matrix size is simply proportional to the IP size. A larger IP has a larger matrix to maintain spatial resolution (Fig. 4-21). If the matrix size is fixed, changing the size of the IP would affect the spatial resolution of the digital image. For example, under a fixed matrix size system, changing from a 14 × 17 inch (35 × 43 cm) IR size to a 10 × 12 inch (25 × 30 cm) IR would result in improved spatial resolution for the same FOV (Fig. 4-22). Spatial resolution is improved because in order to maintain the same matrix size and number of pixels, the pixels must be smaller in size. It is recommended to use the smallest IR size reasonable for the anatomic area of interest.

IMPORTANT RELATIONSHIP
Image Receptor Size and Matrix Size

For a fixed matrix size CR system, using a smaller IR for a given FOV results in improved spatial resolution of the digital image. Increasing the size of the IR for a given FOV results in decreased spatial resolution.

FIXED MATRIX SIZE

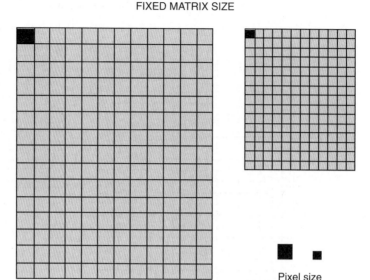

Pixel size

FIG. 4-22 Fixed matrix size. A fixed matrix size will vary the sampling frequency for a different IP size. A larger IP size results in a larger pixel size and decreased spatial resolution. Note: Pixel size is not to scale and is used for illustration only.

Another important ADC performance characteristic is degree of quantization or pixel bit depth, which controls the number of gray shades or contrast resolution of the image. During the process of quantization, each pixel, representing a brightness value, is assigned a numerical value. Quantization reflects the precision with which each sampled point is recorded. As previously discussed, the pixel size and pitch determine the spatial resolution, and the pixel bit depth determines the system's ability to display a range of shades of gray to represent anatomic tissues. Pixel bit depth is fixed by the choice of ADC, and CR systems manufactured with a greater pixel bit depth (i.e., 16-bit [in which 2^{16} bits can display 65,536 shades of gray]) improve the contrast resolution of the digital image.

Before the IP is returned to service, the plate is exposed to an intense white light to release any residual energy that could affect future exposures. PSPs can be reused and are estimated to have a life of 10,000 readings before requiring replacement. Advancements in PSP material, laser beam technology, and dual-sided IP scanning will continue to improve the process of CR image acquisition.

Direct Radiography

DR IRs have a self-scanning readout mechanism that uses an array of x-ray detectors that receive the exit radiation and convert the varying x-ray intensities into proportional electronic signals for digitization (Fig. 4-23). In contrast to CR, which requires a two-step image acquisition process and results in a longer delay between image capture and image readout, DR imaging combines the two processes. As a result, DR images are available almost instantly after exposure. However, DR receptors are more fragile and much more expensive than CR IRs. Several types of electronic detectors are available for DR.

Flat-Panel Detectors

Flat-panel detectors (FPDs) are solid-state IRs that use a large-area active matrix array of electronic components ranging in size from 43 × 35 cm to 43 × 43 cm (17 × 14 inch to 17 × 17 inch).

FIG. 4-23 A direct radiography digital detector assembly. (From Johnston JN, Fauber TL: *Essentials of Radiographic Physics and Imaging*, ed 3, St. Louis, 2020, Elsevier.)

FIG. 4-24 Flat-panel-detector (FPD) array. *A/D,* analog-to-digital; *a-SI,* amorphous silicon. (From Johnston JN, Fauber TL: *Essentials of Radiographic Physics and Imaging*, ed 2, St. Louis, 2016, Mosby.)

FPDs are constructed with layers to receive x-ray photons and convert them to electrical charges for storage and readout (Fig. 4-24). Signal storage, signal readout, and digitizing electronics are integrated into the flat-panel device. The top layer is composed of an x-ray converter, the second layer houses the thin-film transistor (TFT) array, and the third layer is a glass substrate. The TFT array is divided into square DELs, each having a capacitor to store electrical charges and a switching transistor for readout. Electrical charges are separately read out from each DEL. The electronic signal is then sent to the ADC for digitization.

Advancements in DEL technology have incorporated the ADC within the DEL. Digitizing the electrical signal within the DEL creates a more accurate signal. Having the analog electrical signal digitized before it leaves the DEL reduces its susceptibility to external disturbances. That is, the digital signal is not impacted by extraneous energy such as magnetic or radiofrequency disturbances in the surroundings. These energy disturbances can distort the original electrical signal.

The DEL has an x-ray-sensitive area representing each pixel in the image matrix. The pixel is therefore smaller than the DEL and can only capture a percentage of the x-rays reaching the

X-ray
tube

Computer
workstation

Laser printer

Flat-panel
direct capture
detector

Modified
radiographic
table

FIG. 4-25 FPD detector fixed in a modified x-ray table.

detector. This percentage of x-ray capture (~80%–95%) is known as the **fill factor**. Although FPDs with smaller DELs have smaller pixel sizes represented on the visible image and therefore improved spatial resolution, the fill factor is decreased and becomes a limitation. Efforts to further decrease size of the DEL for improved spatial resolution would require more radiation exposure to reach the IR to create the digital image. However, advancements in FPD technology, such as increasing the fill factor to 95% and improved detector materials, generally require less radiation exposure for optimum image quality. The detector system is usually dedicated to a single room and can be permanently mounted within the table or an upright Bucky system. Flat-panel digital detectors are also available as mobile IRs and can be removed from the Bucky and used on the tabletop or a stretcher. After exposure, the digital image is available within milliseconds on a viewing monitor, and no separate reader unit is involved for image processing (Fig. 4-25). Flat-panel systems are highly dose efficient and provide quicker access to images compared with CR. The spatial resolution of flat-panel receptors is generally superior to that of CR. Because a pixel detector is built into the DR flat-panel IR, the size and pitch of the pixel are determined by the DEL and are fixed. Therefore, spatial resolution for flat-panel-detector IRs is limited to the DEL. A system that uses a smaller DEL size has improved spatial resolution. FPDs are manufactured in two different ways to create electrical charges proportional to the x-ray exposure: indirect and direct conversion methods.

Indirect Conversion Detectors

Indirect conversion detectors use a **scintillator** such as CsI or gadolinium oxysulfide (Gd_2O_2S) to convert the exit radiation into visible light. This phosphor-type material used in a scintillator produces light following the absorption of the x-rays. The visible light, in proportion to the x-ray

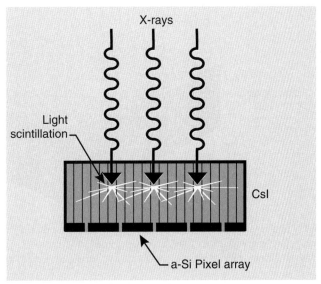

FIG. 4-26 FPD–indirect conversion. (Modified from Bushong SC: *Radiologic Science for Technologists*, ed 10, St. Louis, 2013, Mosby.)

exposure, is then converted to electrical charges by photodetectors (layer of amorphous silicon in the TFT array). The electrical charges are temporarily stored by capacitors in the TFT array before being digitized by the ADC and processed in the computer (Fig. 4-26).

The design of the scintillator used to convert the x-ray intensities into visible light can be structured or unstructured. Structured scintillator phosphors (in the form of needles or columns), usually crystalline CsI, reduce the spread of visible light, thus yielding images with higher spatial resolution than that of images obtained from unstructured scintillators and requiring less radiation to produce a quality image.

Other types of DR indirect conversion detectors include a **charge-coupled device (CCD)** and the **complementary metal oxide semiconductor (CMOS)**. The CCD is very light sensitive and can respond to very low light intensities. It also has a wide dynamic range and can respond to a wide range of light intensities. The scintillator for this form of indirect capture is a CsI phosphor plate. A scintillator is a material that absorbs x-ray energy and emits visible light in response. CsI is a hygroscopic material (it readily absorbs moisture) that must be hermetically sealed to avoid water absorption and prevent rapid degradation but is otherwise a high-efficiency scintillation material. The CsI phosphor plate may be coupled to the CCD using either a fiberoptic bundle or an optical lens system (Fig. 4-27). With this form of indirect capture, x-rays are absorbed by the scintillator and converted to light. This light energy is then transmitted to the CCD, where it is converted to an electronic signal and sent to the computer workstation for processing and display. Because there are currently technical limits to how large a single CCD device can be, an x-ray receptor may consist of an array of closely spaced CCDs. One challenge of this design is the seams at which the CCDs are joined (called *tiling* or *tiled*). Tiling is a process in which several CCD detectors adjoin to create one larger detector. This process results in seams with unequal response. This is addressed with computer preprocessing correction software that interpolates (averages) the pixel values along the seams (flat-field correction), in effect making the seams disappear.

FIG. 4-27 The basic components of a charge-coupled-device (CCD) array. The cesium iodide phosphor plate is coupled to the CCD using fiberoptic bundles. (From Johnston JN, Fauber TL: *Essentials of Radiographic Physics and Imaging*, ed 3, St. Louis, 2020, Elsevier.)

FIG. 4-28 A, Complementary metal oxide semiconductor (CMOS) detector array layers. **B,** CMOS device. (Part A courtesy of RIKEN and JASRI. Part B courtesy of Teledyne DALSA.)

Serving a similar purpose as the CCD is the CMOS. CMOS devices are scintillators made up of a crystalline silicon matrix. Each DEL has its own amplifier, photodiode, and storage capacitor and is surrounded by transistors (Fig. 4-28). They do not have quite the light sensitivity or resolution of CCDs, but they use a fraction of the power to run, are very inexpensive to manufacture, and are improving. The newest versions have very fast image acquisition times because of their random pixel access capabilities. This feature also makes for AEC functions that are not as easy to achieve with CCDs. Creation of CMOS detectors of large enough size for general radiography have been its limitation, but this is changing. Recent advances in CMOS technology, particularly the creation of crystal light tubes that prevent light spread and methods for increasing their size, make them applicable for radiographic imaging.

Indirect conversion detectors are so named because they involve a two-stage process of converting x-ray intensities first to visible light and then to electrical charges during image acquisition. The electrical signals are then directed to amplifiers and the ADC to produce a raw digital image.

FIG. 4-29 FPD–direct conversion. *a-Se,* Amorphous selenium coated; *TFT,* thin-film transistor. (Modified from Bushong SC: *Radiologic Science for Technologists*, ed 10, St. Louis, 2013, Mosby.)

IMPORTANT RELATIONSHIP

Indirect Conversion Detectors in Direct Radiography

Indirect conversion detectors involve a two-stage process of converting x-ray intensities first to visible light and then to electrical charges. A scintillator type material is used to absorb the x-ray energy, emits light in response, and then the light is converted to electrical signals. The electrical signals are then directed to amplifiers and the ADC to produce a raw digital image. Flat-panel TFT detectors are common in DR, but CCD and CMOS indirect conversion detectors are also used in digital radiography.

Direct Conversion Detectors

Direct conversion detectors use an a-Se detector to directly convert the exit radiation to electrical charges (Fig. 4-29). To compensate for the moderately low atomic number of selenium (Z = 34), the thickness of the amorphous selenium is relatively high (1 mm). An electrical field is applied across the selenium layer to limit the lateral diffusion of electrons as they migrate toward the TFT array. By this means, excellent spatial resolution is maintained. Similar to indirect conversion detectors, the electronic charge is stored in a TFT array before it is amplified, digitized, and processed in the computer.

IMPORTANT RELATIONSHIP

Direct Conversion Detectors in Direct Radiography

Direct conversion uses a-Se detectors to directly convert the exit radiation to electrical charges. Similar to indirect conversion detectors, the electronic charge is stored in a TFT array before it is amplified, digitized, and processed in the computer.

Regardless of the type of digital imaging system, the varying electrical signals are sent to the ADC for conversion into digital data. The digitized pixel intensities are patterned in the computer to form the image matrix. The image matrix is a digital composite of the varying x-ray intensities exiting the patient. Each pixel has a brightness level representing the attenuation characteristic of the volume of tissue imaged. After the varying x-ray intensities are converted to numeric data, the digital image can be electronically processed, manipulated, transported, or stored.

QUALITY CONTROL

Ensuring the digital equipment is performing as expected is an important goal of a quality control (QC) program. Equipment acceptance testing and routine equipment maintenance are accomplished by qualified medical physicists or vendor service personnel. However, many daily, weekly, and monthly QC activities should be performed by the radiographer. In addition to the routine QC checks on the x-ray equipment discussed in other chapters, visual inspection of IRs for potential image artifacts caused by IP scratches, blood, contrast media, dirt, and damage as a result of daily use are necessary regardless of the type of digital imaging system. Routine cleaning (according to the manufacturer) and inspection of the digital IR by the radiographer can identify potential problems that may impact radiographic quality. Box 4-3 lists common QC activities for digital IRs that can be performed by the radiographer. Most of these QC checks evaluate the performance of the digital imaging system and the display monitor. QC checks specific to the performance of the display monitor will be discussed in Chapter 5.

BOX 4-3 Quality Control Check: Digital Imaging Systems

Manufacturers of digital imaging equipment have developed quality control procedures specific to their equipment; however, there are basic universal procedures for CR and DR IRs that the radiographer can perform.

Several QC Phantom devices are available to assess the performance of the PSP and FPD imaging systems.

- IRs need to be visually inspected for any dirt, blood, contrast media, or scratches that could result in image artifacts. In addition, they should be regularly cleaned according to the manufacturer's specifications.
- The sensitivity of each PSP and FPD should be routinely checked to ensure the consistency of the exposure indicator value calibration.
- Shading or uniformity evaluates brightness consistency throughout the image.
- Linearity of the system can be evaluated by proportionally increasing and decreasing the radiation exposure to the IR and validating that the exposure indicator responds accordingly.
- Contrast resolution can be measured by imaging a contrast detail phantom to assess the visibility of low-contrast objects.
- Spatial resolution can be monitored by imaging a line-pair resolution test tool.
- For CR systems, the laser beam performance can be evaluated by imaging an opaque straight-edged object and visually checking for any jitter along the edges of the object.
- The measurement tool available at the workstation should be checked for accuracy.
- The thoroughness of the IP erasure function can be evaluated by performing a secondary erasure on the IP and checking for any residual exposure (ghosting).
- The FPD can be evaluated to confirm that no charges remain from the previous exposure.

CHAPTER SUMMARY

- A digital image with a larger matrix and smaller-sized pixels has improved quality.
- The pixel size is directly related to the FOV displayed and inversely related to matrix size.
- A pixel's bit depth determines the available shades of gray to display the digital image or its contrast resolution.
- Spatial resolution is improved by increasing the pixel density and decreasing the pixel pitch.
- lp/mm is the unit of measurement for spatial frequency. Increasing the number of resolved lp/mm (higher spatial frequency) increases spatial resolution.
- Digital IRs have a wide dynamic range, which means that they can accurately capture the wide range of photon energies that exit a patient. However, lower- or higher-than-necessary exposure techniques do not guarantee a quality digital image with reasonable radiation exposure to the patient.
- Digital imaging systems with a wider dynamic range have higher pixel bit depths to display the range of grayscale. A 12-bit pixel depth system can display 4096 shades of gray, whereas a 14-bit pixel depth system can display 16,384 shades of gray, therefore improving the quality of the displayed image.
- Radiographers should select exposure techniques within the exposure latitude of the digital imaging system and departmental standards.
- The MTF is a measure of an imaging system's ability to display contrast of anatomic objects varying in size, and the value ranges between 0 (no difference in brightness levels) and 1.0 (maximum difference in brightness levels).
- DQE is a measurement of the efficiency of an IR in converting the x-ray exposure it receives to a quality radiographic image. The higher the DQE of a system, the lower the radiation exposure required to produce a quality image, and therefore, patient exposure is decreased.
- SNR is a method of describing the strength of the radiation exposure compared with the amount of noise apparent in a digital image. When the digital image displays increased noise, regardless of the source, anatomic details will have decreased visibility.
- CNR is a method of describing the contrast resolution compared with the amount of noise apparent in a digital image. Digital images having a higher CNR will increase the visibility of anatomic tissues.
- CR and DR IRs differ in their construction and how they acquire latent images. After the latent image is acquired and the raw data are digitized, image processing and display are essentially the same for CR and DR.
- In CR, the IP has a photostimulable phosphor layer that absorbs the exit radiation and excites electrons, which become elevated to a higher energy state and get trapped.
- The exposed IP is placed in a reader unit where the trapped electrons are released during the laser beam scanning, and the excess energy is emitted as visible light. A photodetector collects, amplifies, and converts the visible light to an electrical signal proportional to the range of energies stored in the IP.
- The signal output from the photodetector is digitized by an ADC converter to produce a digital image.
- The sampling frequency in CR determines how often the analog signal is reproduced in its discrete digitized form. Increasing the sampling frequency increases the pixel density of the digital data and improves the spatial resolution of the digital image.
- After data extraction, CR IPs must be erased by exposure to an intense white light to release any residual energy before reuse.
- In contrast to CR, DR IRs combine image capture and readout.

- Signal storage, signal readout, and digitizing electronics are integrated into a solid-state FPD.
- FPDs use both indirect and direct conversion methods to create proportional electrical charges that are sent to the ADC for conversion to digital data.
- Indirect conversion detectors use a scintillator to convert the exit radiation to visible light, and then the visible light is converted to electrical charges for storage in the TFTs.
- Other indirect conversion detectors include CCDs and CMOS.
- Direct conversion detectors directly convert the exit radiation into electrical charges for storage in the TFTs.
- After the varying x-ray energies are converted to numerical data, the digital image can be electronically processed, manipulated, transported, or stored.
- Routine quality control checks on the digital imaging system should be performed by the radiographer.

REVIEW QUESTIONS

1. Which of the following would improve spatial resolution?
   A. Small matrix and large pixel size
   B. Decreased pixel density and increased pixel pitch
   C. Large matrix and large pixel size
   D. Large matrix and increased pixel density

2. The type of image receptor (IR) that uses a photostimulable phosphor to acquire the latent image is _____.
   A. an intensifying screen
   B. a flat-panel detector
   C. computed radiography
   D. direct radiography

3. Which of the following is used to extract the latent image from an imaging plate (IP)?
   A. Laser beam
   B. Photomultiplier tube
   C. Analog-to-digital converter
   D. Thin-film transistor

4. Which of the following will improve the spatial resolution of the digital image?
   A. Decreased sampling frequency and increased sampling pitch
   B. Decreased sampling frequency and decreased sampling pitch
   C. Increased sampling frequency and increased sampling pitch
   D. Increased sampling frequency and decreased sampling pitch

5. Which of the following would improve the spatial resolution of the digital image for a given field of view (FOV)?
   A. A fixed matrix size and larger IP
   B. A decreased sampling frequency and larger IP
   C. A small matrix size and larger pixel size
   D. A fixed matrix size and small IP

6. What is the process of assigning a numerical value to represent a brightness value?
   A. Dynamic range
   B. Signal-to-noise ratio
   C. Quantization
   D. Spectral sensitivity

7. Which of the following pixel bit depths would display a greater range of shades of gray to represent anatomic tissues?
   A. 8 bit
   B. 10 bit
   C. 14 bit
   D. 16 bit

8. Small anatomic detail has _____.
   A. decreased pixel density
   B. increased spatial resolution
   C. high spatial frequency
   D. low signal to noise ratio

9. Digital imaging systems have a wide dynamic range.
   A. True
   B. False

10. _____ refers to the range of exposures that should be used to produce a diagnostic image.
    A. Modulation transfer function
    B. Bit depth
    C. Exposure latitude
    D. Dynamic range

11. A lower signal-to-noise ratio (SNR) improves the quality of a digital image.
    A. True
    B. False

12. Decreasing the displayed FOV for a given matrix size will decrease the size of the pixels and increase spatial resolution.
    A. True
    B. False

13. Which of the following is a measurement of the efficiency of an IR in converting the x-ray exposure it receives to a quality radiographic image?
    A. DAP
    B. MTF
    C. DQE
    D. SNR

14. A higher sampling frequency during CR latent image digitization will
    A. increase spatial resolution.
    B. decrease pixel density.
    C. increase pixel pitch.
    D. increase CNR.

15. A 16-bit digital system would have a narrow dynamic range compared to a 12-bit system.
    A. True
    B. False

16. Which of the following provide an indication of patient radiation risk during a radiographic procedure?
    A. DQE
    B. DAP
    C. KAP
    D. B and C only

17. Digital detectors that require a two-stage process to acquire and digitize the latent image include
    A. flat-panel detectors indirect conversion.
    B. CCD.
    C. CMOS.
    D. all the above.

18. Image artifacts can be caused by
    1. dirty CR IPs.
    2. low sampling frequency.
    3. increased pixel density.
        A. 1 and 2 only
        B. 1 and 3 only
        C. 2 and 3 only
        D. 1, 2, and 3

Digital Image Processing, Display, and Data Management

OBJECTIVES

*After completing this chapter, the reader will be able
to perform the following:*

1. Define all the key terms in this chapter.
2. State all the important relationships in this chapter.
3. State the purpose of digital image processing.
4. Identify preprocessing corrections performed on the raw image data.
5. Describe the construction of a histogram.
6. Explain histogram analysis, automatic rescaling, and lookup tables and their role during image preprocessing to create a quality digital image.
7. Differentiate among the vendor-specific and the universal standard types of exposure indicators and recognize their importance to digital image quality.
8. Recognize default and postprocessing operations and their impact on image display.
9. Comprehend how over- and reprocessing image data could reduce the diagnostic and archival quality of the data.
10. Identify the important features of monitors that may affect the quality of the displayed image.
11. Explain the difference between luminance and luminance ratio.
12. Define data management and its role in providing radiology services.
13. Recognize the HIPAA standard in protecting health information.
14. Define *picture archival and communication system (PACS)* and state the major components.
15. Explain the role of Digital Imaging and Communications in Medicine (DICOM) in PACS.
16. Recognize the challenges of teleradiology, data transmission, storage, archives, and security.

KEY TERMS

alternative algorithms
aspect ratio
automatic rescaling
contrast enhancement
contrast resolution
data management

deviation index (DI)
digital image processing
Digital Imaging and Communications in Medicine (DICOM)
disaster recovery
display workstation

dual-energy subtraction
edge enhancement
electronic health record (EHR)
electronic masking
equalization
exposure indicator

Acquisition of the latent image can be accomplished with different types of image receptors (IRs), most commonly computed radiography (CR) and direct radiography (DR), as discussed in Chapter 4. After the raw image data (released energy) are extracted from the digital receptor and converted to digital data (digitization), the image must be computer processed before its display and diagnostic interpretation. This chapter describes how digital data are processed to reproduce a quality image for display on a computer monitor. When displayed on a computer monitor, there is tremendous flexibility in altering the appearance of the digital image. In digital form, images can be transmitted, stored, and archived. Managing imaging data is an enormous responsibility, and important issues regarding data management are briefly discussed in this chapter.

DIGITAL IMAGE PROCESSING

The term **digital image processing** refers to various computer algorithms (mathematical computations) applied to digital data for the purpose of optimizing the image for display. Although many digital image processing operations are proprietary (manufacturer specific) and outside the scope of this textbook, several commonly used processing methods are described. Generally, digital image processing can be described in stages, preprocessing to prepare the data for processing and display, and default (preset) or postprocessing, which includes computer operations available before and after the image is displayed.

When the released energy from the IR is digitized, several operations occur to the raw data to account for flaws or imperfections in the electronic IR and to prepare the image data for processing and display. Bad or dead pixel and flat fielding corrections are just two examples of computer operations applied to the raw image data. Because of the electronic components of a DR IR, imperfections can lead to artifacts and malfunctioning pixels (bad or dead pixels). Software corrections can be applied to account for these imperfections, which only occur with DR-type IRs. Flat fielding correction is discussed in Chapter 4 regarding charge-coupled device–type IRs and is a process of correcting the nonuniformity of pixel values throughout the entire image. The anode heel effect discussed in Chapter 2 is an example of how pixel values can become nonuniform across the digital IR.

To process the latent digital image, the computer creates a **histogram** (or graphic representation of a data set) of the image. This graph (data set) includes all the pixel values that represent the latent image (released energy) after the software corrections were applied and sometimes referred to as the *exposure* histogram. The *x*-axis represents the range of pixel values assigned, and the *y*-axis represents the number (frequency) of pixels for each value (Fig. 5-1). The location of the graph along the *x*-axis represents image brightness levels, and the shape of the graph represents image contrast (grayscale).

Because the entire CR imaging plate (IP) is scanned to extract the image from the photostimulable phosphor, the computer identifies the exposure field brightness levels and the edges of the collimated image so all the exposure data outside the collimated image can be excluded (exposure field recognition and segmentation). Ideally, all four edges of a collimated field should be recognized. If at least three edges are not identified, all data, including raw exposure or scatter outside the x-ray field, may be included in the histogram, resulting in a processing error. See Fig. 5-2 for an example of a processing error.

FIG. 5-1 Exposure histogram. Illustration of the raw exposure data histogram before preprocessing. The exposure data outside the collimated image needs to be excluded from the histogram to prevent a processing error. (Modified from Seibert JA. [1999]. Physics of Computed Radiography, AAPM 1999 Annual Meeting, Nashville [PowerPoint slides]. Retrieved from https://www.aapm.org/meetings/99AM/pdf/2795-64903.pdf, accessed June 17, 2019.)

FIG. 5-2 Histogram-analysis error. **A,** Poor quality computed radiography (CR) image resulting from a histogram error caused by incorrect collimation. **B,** Image showing correctly collimated borders resulting in a quality CR image. (Courtesy of Andrew Woodward.)

In newer CR imaging systems, the collimated borders may not have the same impact on data processing as in older CR systems. Processing errors are less likely to occur with DR IRs than with CR IRs because the image data are extracted only from the exposed detector elements (DELs); however, the collimated edges of the image still need to be recognized.

> ### IMPORTANT RELATIONSHIP
> #### Preprocessing: Corrections and Histogram
>
> Several operations occur on the raw image data to prepare for further processing in order to display a quality image. Software corrections can be applied to account for imperfections (bad or dead pixels) that only occur with DR type IRs, and flat fielding is a process of correcting the non-uniformity of pixel values throughout the entire image. A histogram is created that represents the range of digital pixel values versus the relative prevalence of the pixel values in the latent image. Scanning the entire IR to identify the exposure field brightness levels and the edges of the collimated image (exposure field recognition and segmentation) is necessary to identify only the image data representing the anatomic area.

Histogram Analysis

Histogram analysis is an important processing technique to identify the edges of an image and assess the exposure data (pixel values) before image processing and display. The location and shape of the exposure histogram are impacted by the anatomic area imaged, the exposure technique, positioning, and collimation. The computer analyzes the histogram using processing algorithms and compares it with a preestablished (reference) histogram specific to the anatomic part being imaged. This process is called **histogram analysis**. The computer software has stored histogram models, each having a shape characteristic of the selected anatomic region and projection. These stored histogram models have **values of interest (VOIs)**, which determine the range of the histogram data set that should be included in the displayed image (Fig. 5-3).

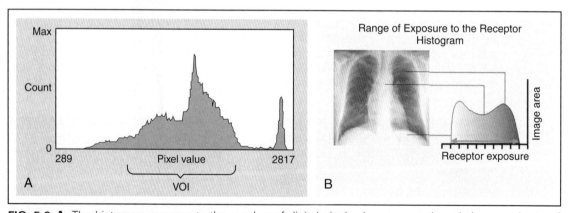

FIG. 5-3 A, The histogram represents the number of digital pixel values versus the relative prevalence of those values in the latent image. The *x*-axis represents the amount of exposure and the *y*-axis the incidence of pixels for each exposure level. **B,** Range of exposure to the receptor histogram. Each image has its own histogram. *VOI,* Value of interest. (Part A from Cesar LJ: Computed radiography: its impact on radiographers, *Radiol Technol* 68(3):225-232, 1997. Part B modified Sprawls P: *Physical Principles of Medical Imaging Online,* ed 2, http://www.sprawls.org/ppmi2.)

> ### IMPORTANT RELATIONSHIP
> #### Histogram Analysis
>
> During histogram analysis, the exposure histogram is compared with a stored (reference) histogram for that anatomic part; VOIs are identified in preparation for image processing and display.

Exposure Indicator

An important feature of digital image processing is its ability to create an image with the appropriate amount of brightness, regardless of the exposure to the IR. As a result of the histogram analysis, the average value of the VOI is determined and used to provide important information to the radiographer regarding the exposure to the digital IR. The **exposure indicator** provides a numeric value indicating the level of radiation exposure to the digital IR. See Table 5-1 for a list of CR vendor-specific exposure indicators.

In CR, the exposure indicator value represents the exposure level to the IP, and the values are vendor specific. Fuji and Konica use sensitivity (S) numbers, and the value is inversely related to the exposure to the IR. An S number of 200 is equal to 10 µGy (1 mR) of exposure to the IR. If the S number increases from 200 to 400, this would indicate a decrease in exposure to the IR by half. Conversely, a decrease in the S number from 200 to 100 would indicate an increase in exposure to the IR by a factor of 2 or doubling of the exposure. Carestream (Kodak) uses exposure index (EI) numbers; their value is directly related to the exposure to the plate and the changes are logarithmic expressions. For example, a change in EI from 2000 to 2300, a difference of 300, is equal to a factor of 2 and represents twice as much exposure to the plate. Agfa uses log median (lgM) numbers; their value is directly related to exposure to the plate and the changes are logarithmic expressions. For example, a change in lgM from 2.5 to 2.8, a change of 0.3, is equal to a factor of 2 and represents twice as much exposure to the IR. Optimal ranges of the exposure indicator values are vendor specific and vary among the types of procedures, such as abdomen and chest imaging versus extremity imaging. DR imaging systems also display an exposure indicator and use differing methods to calculate the exposure indicator and are manufacturer specific.

This variability among the manufacturer-specific exposure indicator values and relationship to the IR exposure has been challenging to radiographers. As a result, the industry has recommended a universal standard exposure indicator. Although there are some variations between the standard exposure indicators, there is common terminology. The **deviation index (DI)** is a value that reflects the difference between the desired or target exposure to the IR and the actual exposure to the IR. A DI of 0 would indicate there is no difference between the desired (target) EI and the actual EI. A DI between −0.5 and +0.5 is within the target range. DIs greater than +1.0 are

TABLE 5-1	Computed Radiography Vendor-Specific Exposure Indicators				
Vendor	Exposure Indicator	Scale	EI Value, 10 µGy (1mR) exposure	2× Exposure	½ Exposure
Fuji and Konica	Sensitivity (S)	Inverse	200	100	400
Carestream (Kodak)	Exposure index (EI)	Logarithmic	2000	2300	1700
Agfa	Log median value (lgM)	Logarithmic	2.5	2.8	2.2

BOX 5-1　Deviation Index

The deviation index (DI) is a value that reflects the difference between the desired or target exposure to the image receptor (IR) and the actual exposure to the IR.

DI Value	Actual Exposure to IR
>+3.0	Excessive exposure
>+1.0	Overexposed
<+0.5	Exposure within target range
0	No difference between target (desired) and actual exposure to IR
>−0.5	Exposure within target range
<−1.0	Underexposed
<−3.0	Insufficient exposure

considered overexposed (a DI of greater than +3.0 has excessive exposure), and DIs less than −1.0 are considered underexposed (a DI less than −3.0 has insufficient exposure). See Box 5-1.

It is important to note that all EIs, even the recommended standard DI, have limitations. Variables such as collimation, kilovoltage peak (kVp), and centering may influence the EI, and therefore the level of noise and image quality should be evaluated along with the EI or DI value. The radiographer needs to be knowledgeable about the EI value on the equipment she or he uses in digital imaging and how exposure techniques can be altered to correct for exposure errors. In addition, the department standards should be followed for how over- and underexposures are to be handled before repeating the image.

The radiographer should monitor the exposure indicator values as a guide for proper exposure techniques. If the exposure indicator value is within the acceptable range, adjustments can be made for contrast and brightness with postprocessing functions, and this will not degrade the image. However, if the exposure is outside of the acceptable range, attempting to adjust the image data with postprocessing functions would not correct for improper IR exposure and may result in noisy or suboptimal images that should not be submitted for interpretation.

The radiographer has a role in the selection of the appropriate anatomic part and projection before computer processing. This step prepares the computer for the type of data being supplied for histogram analysis. If the radiographer selects a part other than the imaged one, a histogram-analysis error may occur. In addition, any errors that occur, such as during data extraction from the IR or rescaling during computer processing, could affect the exposure indicator and provide a false value. It is important for radiographers not only to consider the exposure indicator value carefully but also to recognize its limitations.

 IMPORTANT RELATIONSHIP

Exposure Indicator

The exposure indicator provides a numeric value indicating the level of radiation exposure to the digital IR. These values may be vendor specific and have a direct, logarithmic, or inverse relationship to the IR exposure. A universal standard exposure indicator (DI) has been developed and provides the radiographer with important information about the IR exposure. The radiographer should assess the exposure indicator along with image quality before considering a repeat image.

! RADIATION PROTECTION ALERT

Exposure Indicators

The radiographer should strive to select techniques that result in exposure indicator values falling within the indicated optimum range for the corresponding digital imaging system. However, the radiographer also needs to recognize the limitations of exposure indicators for providing accurate information.

Lookup Tables

During histogram analysis, **lookup tables (LUTs)** provide a method of processing the image data, based on the reference histogram, to transform the image data into a quality image for display. Because digital IRs have a linear exposure response and a wide dynamic range, raw data images exhibit low contrast and must be altered to improve the visibility of anatomic structures. LUTs provide the means to alter the brightness and grayscale of the digital image using computer algorithms.

Histogram analysis is used to maintain consistent image brightness despite over- or underexposure of the IR. This procedure is known as **automatic rescaling**. The computer rescales the image (Fig. 5-4) based on the comparison of the histograms. Although automatic rescaling is a convenient feature, radiographers should be aware that rescaling errors can occur because of positioning and collimation errors and with image artifacts, such as a hip prosthesis, and can result in poor-quality digital images.

LUTs also provide a means to adjust the contrast or grayscale necessary to adequately view the anatomic region. Fig. 5-5 visually compares pixel values of the original image with those of a

FIG. 5-4 Effect of exposure on image quality. Automatic rescaling is used during histogram analysis to maintain a consistent image brightness despite over- or underexposure of the image receptor (IR). (Modified Sprawls P: *Physical Principles of Medical Imaging Online*, ed 2, http://www.sprawls.org/ppmi2.)

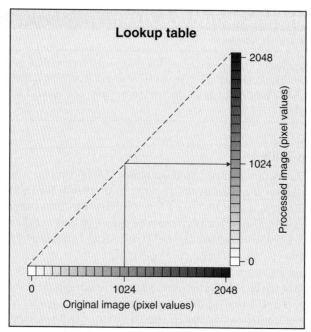

FIG. 5-5 Straight line graph demonstrating no change in the pixel values from the original to the processed image. (Modified Sprawls P: *Physical Principles of Medical Imaging Online*, ed 2, http://www.sprawls.org/ppmi2.)

processed image. If the image is not altered, the graph would be a straight line. If the original image is altered, the original pixel values would be different in the processed image, and the graph would no longer be a straight line but resemble an S-shaped curve (Fig. 5-6). For example, each pixel value could be altered to display the digital image with a change in contrast (grayscale). New pixel values would be calculated that result in the image being displayed with higher contrast (Fig. 5-7). Fig. 5-8 shows the original image, the graph after changes in the pixel values, and the processed higher-contrast image. LUTs provide a method of processing digital images to change the displayed brightness and contrast required for each anatomic area (Fig. 5-9). Fig. 5-10 is an example of how the brightness and contrast of the exposure histogram can be realigned to match the reference histogram to display a quality radiographic image.

IMPORTANT RELATIONSHIP

Lookup Tables

LUTs provide the means to alter the original pixel values to improve the brightness and contrast of the displayed image.

Some of the newer digital imaging systems provide a mechanism for the radiographer to re-process the image data to improve its presentation at the display monitor, known as **alternative algorithms**. Selecting an alternative anatomical region or projection will apply a different algorithm to the original image data, and the reprocessed image will be displayed with a change in brightness and/or contrast at the radiographer's workstation. This could prevent the need for a repeat image causing additional exposure to the patient. However, the reprocessed image is

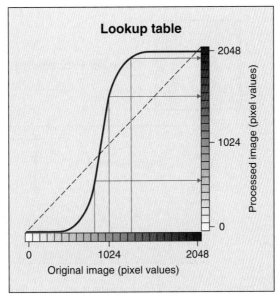

FIG. 5-6 Graph demonstrating a change in pixel values from the original image to the processed image. The shape of the graph resembles an S-shaped curve. (Modified Sprawls P: *Physical Principles of Medical Imaging Online*, ed 2, http://www.sprawls.org/ppmi2.)

FIG. 5-7 Lookup table (LUT) altering the pixel values of a low-contrast image to display an image with higher contrast. (Modified Sprawls P: *Physical Principles of Medical Imaging Online*, ed 2, http://www.sprawls.org/ppmi2.)

not assured to have improved quality and if sent to PACS (discussed later) for display on the radiologist's workstation, it would limit her or his ability to further postprocess and manipulate the image because some of the original image data are lost. Additionally, information about the reprocessing of the original image data would be identified on the displayed image and could cause problems with storage and retrieval of the imaging procedure. Use of alternative algorithms is not a standard practice for radiographers and should only be performed within the established policies of the department.

FIG. 5-8 The original low-contrast chest image is altered to have higher contrast. The graph shows a change in the pixel values from the original image. (Modified Sprawls P: *Physical Principles of Medical Imaging Online*, ed 2, http://www.sprawls.org/ppmi2.)

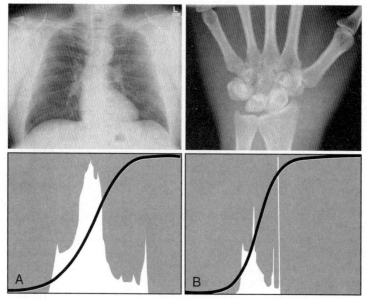

FIG. 5-9 A, Chest image with its histogram and LUT graph, which differs from **B,** image of the wrist with its histogram and LUT graph. (Courtesy of Andrew Woodward.)

Depending on the software available, a digital image can be additionally manipulated in a variety of ways. The following are common default (preset) or postprocessing techniques:

1. **Dual-energy subtraction** (Fig. 5-11) is a technique that can remove superimposed structures so that the anatomic area of interest becomes more visible. Because the image is in a digital format, the computer can subtract selected brightness values to create an image without superimposed structures.

FIG. 5-10 Histogram realignment. **A**, Illustration showing underexposure to the IR. Notice the location of the histogram and LUT graph along the *x*-axis and the shape of the LUT graph. **B**, Illustration showing how the histogram and LUT graph has been realigned to display an improved quality image. **C**, Illustration showing overexposure to the IR. Notice the location of the histogram and LUT curve along the *x*-axis and the shape of the LUT curve before its realignment in *B*. The LUT graph is created in *A* and *C* for illustration only.

FIG. 5-11 Subtraction postprocessing techniques. **A**, Skeletal areas are removed. **B**, Lungs and soft tissue are removed.

2. **Contrast enhancement** (Fig. 5-12) is a postprocessing technique that alters the pixel values to increase image contrast.
3. **Edge enhancement** (also known as high-pass filtering) (Fig. 5-13) is a postprocessing technique that improves the visibility of small, high-contrast structures. However, image noise may be slightly increased.
4. **Inversion** (also known as black/white reversal) (Fig. 5-14) is a postprocessing technique that reverses the grayscale from the original image.

FIG. 5-12 Postprocessing adjustment in radiographic contrast. **A,** Longer-scale contrast typical of chest radiography. **B,** Contrast has been adjusted to present a higher scale.

FIG. 5-13 A radiographic image demonstrates an edge-enhancement postprocessing technique.

FIG. 5-14 Radiographic image demonstrates a black/white reversal postprocessing technique.

FIG. 5-15 Smoothing (also known as low-pass filtering). **A,** Image without applying smoothing processing. **B,** Image after smoothing processing. (Courtesy of Andrew Woodward.)

5. **Smoothing** (also known as low-pass filtering) (Fig. 5-15) is a postprocessing technique that suppresses image noise (quantum noise). However, spatial resolution is degraded.
6. **Equalization** (Fig. 5-16) is a postprocessing function whereby underexposed areas (light areas) are made darker and overexposed areas (dark areas) are made lighter. The effect is an image that appears to have lower contrast so that dense and lucent structures can be better seen within the same image.

Other postprocessing functions include **region of interest (ROI)**, which provides calculation of selected pixel values within the area of interest to provide quantitative information about the tissue. Additional software can provide **stitching** of multiple images into one image for viewing anatomic areas such as for a scoliosis series.

A word of caution is warranted regarding postprocessing: overuse of these functions can drastically and negatively alter the data set, which is the digital image. Overwriting the original image with a postprocessed replica may reduce the diagnostic and archival quality of the data. One should also keep in mind that in many facilities, the radiographers' workstations use monitors of significantly lower quality and viewing conditions that are very different compared with the radiologists' workstations. How an image looks on the radiographer's workstation in a brightly lit work area may be very different from the way it looks on the radiologist's high-resolution monitor in a darkened reading room. Therefore, care should be taken in the postprocessing of an image before forwarding it for interpretation.

Advancement in digital image processing continues to improve image quality and diagnostic interpretation. Grid subtraction and virtual grids are just two examples of these software advancements. Grids are discussed in Chapter 7 and improve image quality by removing scatter (fog) that

FIG. 5-16 Equalization. **A,** Image without equalization. **B,** Image with equalization. (Courtesy of Andrew Woodward.)

serves no useful purpose and only degrades image quality. However, the use of grids provides challenges in terms of grid artifacts, grid positioning errors, and increased radiation exposure to the patient. Computer software is being developed that can remove unwanted artifacts caused by the grid pattern (grid subtraction), such as the moiré effect, or remove the scatter radiation (fog) visualized in a digital image produced without a grid (virtual grid). There are many radiographic procedures that could prevent the use of a grid especially during mobile or operating room procedures caused by grid alignment challenges. Advancements in computer software algorithms can remove the scatter radiation (virtual grid) and display the digital image with improved grayscale (contrast).

DIGITAL IMAGING ARTIFACTS

Digital imaging artifacts occur for various reasons and generally have a bright or dark appearance. The complexity of the electronics involved in creating the digital image often makes it difficult to isolate the cause of the problem because the level of brightness of digital artifacts does not necessarily provide an indication of the source. Digital artifacts may be classified as detectors (CR plate, thin-film transistor array), occurring during image data extraction before the analog-to-digital converter (ADC) or during the ADC process and subsequent signal processing performed by the computer up to the point of image display. Examples of CR detector–related artifacts include IP stains, particulates, scratches, cracks, and fogging. Artifacts occurring during data extraction on CR systems are related to issues with the laser optics, transport mechanisms, light guide, and laser sampling and stationary grid frequencies. See Fig. 5-17 for examples of CR artifacts.

DR detector artifacts may be related to calibration of an individual DEL, row, or column of the detector matrix. Artifacts occurring during data extraction are related to electronic readout mechanisms associated with the rows and columns of the DELs comprising the detector matrix.

FIG. 5-17 CR image artifacts. **A,** Bright lines in the shoulder region as a result of scratches on the imaging plate. **B,** Bright specs between the fourth and fifth metacarpals as a result of dirt on the image plate. (Courtesy of Andrew Woodward.)

FIG. 5-18 Direct radiography image artifacts. **A,** Erasure error. **B,** Improper alignment of central-ray and IR in a Bucky table.

DR detector artifacts can also occur from an erasure error or if the technologist improperly centers the CR to table grid. See Fig. 5-18 for examples of DR artifacts. If the source of the artifact is not related to the detector or extraction of image data up to the ADC, the remaining sources are likely to be the electronic components starting within the ADC and subsequent circuits that are involved with transmitting the digital signal to the computer for processing or processed image data sent to the display monitor. A discussion of artifacts related to the electronic readout mechanisms or occurring within the ADC and subsequent components of the imaging system is beyond the scope of this book.

IMAGE DISPLAY

After computer processing, the digital image is ready to be displayed for viewing. The quality of the digital image is also affected by important features of the display monitor, such as its luminance and resolution, and viewing conditions such as ambient lighting and monitor placement. Specialized post-processing software is used at the display workstation to aid the radiologist in image interpretation. In addition to soft-copy viewing, the digital image can be printed on specialized film by a laser printer.

Postprocessing

Postprocessing functions are computer software operations available to the radiographer and radiologist that allow manual manipulation of the displayed image. These functions allow the operator to manually adjust many presentation features of the image to enhance the diagnostic value.

Electronic Masking

After the image is processed, regions viewed on the image can be altered further by **electronic masking**, also known as *shuttering*. For example, when the area of interest is properly collimated, the image may display increased brightness surrounding the radiation-exposed field. This region of brightness provides no useful information and can be removed from the displayed image, which is automatic in newer digital equipment. In addition, electronic masking can remove regions surrounding the exposure field that provide no useful information or may negatively impact the histogram analysis. However, it is not within the standards of practice for radiographers to make decisions about removing information within the radiation-exposed field. Proper collimation before radiation exposure is important and should not be replaced with electronic masking. A properly collimated x-ray field preexposure and automatic electronic masking of the bright intensities outside the radiation-exposed field should show a thin white line around the edges of the image, which indicates the image was collimated smaller than the size of the IR. Electronic masking has no effect on the overall image quality (removing scatter) or on patient exposure.

Brightness

Because the image is composed of numerical data, the brightness level displayed on the computer monitor can be easily altered to visualize the range of the recorded anatomic structures. This adjustment is accomplished using a basic windowing function. The **window level** (or center) sets the midpoint of the range of brightness visible in the image. Changing the window level on the display monitor allows the image brightness to be increased or decreased throughout the entire range (Fig. 5-19). When the range of brightness displayed is less than the maximum, the processed image presents only a subset of the total information contained within the computer (Fig. 5-20).

IMPORTANT RELATIONSHIP
Window Level and Image Brightness

A relationship exists between window level and image brightness on the display monitor. Changing the window level on the display monitor allows the image brightness to be increased or decreased throughout the entire range.

Contrast

The number of different shades of gray that can be stored and displayed by a computer system is termed **grayscale**. **Contrast resolution** is another term associated with digital imaging and is

FIG. 5-19 Window level. **A,** Original image without additional postprocessing. **B,** Image with a change in the window level to make the image displayed with less brightness (darker).

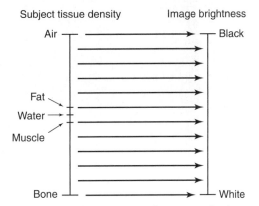

FIG. 5-20 Changing the window level increases or decreases the image brightness throughout the range of densities recorded in the image. (From Kuni C: *Introduction to Computers and Digital Processing in Medical Imaging*, Chicago, 1988, Year Book Medical Publishers.)

used to describe the ability of the imaging system to distinguish between objects that exhibit similar brightness levels because they attenuate the x-ray beam similarly. An important distinguishing characteristic of a digital image is its improved contrast resolution. As previously mentioned, the brightness level of a pixel is determined by the bit depth or number of bits (i.e., 12, 14, or 16), which affects the number of shades of gray available for image display. Increasing the number of shades of gray increases the contrast resolution within the image. An image with increased contrast resolution, when optimally windowed, increases the visibility of very subtle anatomic features.

After the digital image is processed, radiographic contrast can be adjusted to vary the visualization of the area of interest; this is necessary because the contrast resolution of the human eye is limited. **Window width** is a basic control that adjusts the radiographic contrast. Because the digital image can display shades of gray ranging from black to white, the display monitor can vary the range or number of shades of gray visible on the image to show the desired anatomy. Adjusting the range of visible shades of gray varies the image contrast (Fig. 5-21). When the entire number of shades of gray is displayed (wide window width), the image has lower contrast; when a smaller number of shades of gray is displayed (narrow window width), the image has higher contrast (Fig. 5-22).

In digital imaging, an inverse relationship exists between window width and image contrast. A wide window width displays an image with lower contrast than the same area of interest displayed with a narrow window width.

FIG. 5-21 Window width. **A**, Original image without additional postprocessing. **B**, Image with an increase in window width to make the image displayed with decreased (lower) contrast.

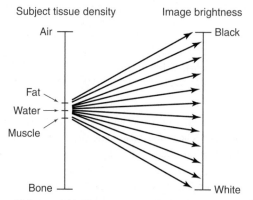

FIG. 5-22 Changing the window width increases or decreases the range of visible brightness levels. A narrow window width decreases the range of brightness levels and increases contrast. A wider window width increases the range of brightness levels and reduces contrast. (From Kuni C: *Introduction to Computers and Digital Processing in Medical Imaging*, Chicago, 1988, Year Book Medical Publishers.)

FIG. 5-23 The level or center of the window and the window width change the visual display of the digital image. (Modified Sprawls P: *Physical Principles of Medical Imaging Online*, ed 2, http://www.sprawls.org/ppmi2.)

FIG. 5-24 Changing the window level for a chest x-ray varies the visibility of the anatomic detail or contrast for both low- and high-brightness levels. (Modified Sprawls P: *Physical Principles of Medical Imaging Online*, ed 2, http://www.sprawls.org/ppmi2.)

The center or midpoint of the window level and the width of the window determine the brightness and contrast of the displayed image (Fig. 5-23). Fig. 5-24 demonstrates how the image is altered when the window level is changed for a given window width.

IMPORTANT RELATIONSHIP

Window Width and Image Contrast

A narrow (decreased) window width displays higher radiographic contrast, whereas a wider (increased) window width displays lower radiographic contrast.

The ability to optimize image display in real time using the window level and width controls is a major advantage of soft-copy (versus hard copy) viewing of digital images. It is important to note that windowing does not alter the original stored pixel values of an image but rather alters only how they are displayed. However, more complex image manipulations available on primary display monitors use preset LUTs for windowing (level and width) and other operations. It is advised to save the original image and one for display so complex operations on the display image will not affect the original image.

Display Characteristics

As previously discussed, the quality of the digital image is affected by its acquisition parameters and subsequent computer processing. In addition, the quality of the digital image is affected by the performance of the display monitor. The quality of display monitors may not be equal among all those used for viewing digital images. Monitors used by radiologists for diagnostic interpretation, referred to as *primary*, must be of higher quality than the monitors used only for routine image review (*secondary*). However, the radiographer's monitor should be of sufficiently high quality to accurately discern all the image quality characteristics before sending the image to the radiologist for diagnostic interpretation. Display monitors used for radiographic diagnostic interpretation are typically monochrome high-resolution monitors and can be set to portrait or landscape formats and configured with one, two, or four monitors (Fig. 5-25). The construction of common display monitors used in routine imaging is discussed in Chapter 10.

Several important features of display monitors (used in digital radiography) affect their performance. Digital images are captured and processed to display a specific matrix size. As previously discussed, an image created with a large matrix having many smaller-sized pixels improves the spatial resolution of the digital image (pixel image). If the monitor used for viewing the digital

FIG. 5-25 A set of portrait display monitors used for soft-copy viewing. (©Barco.)

image cannot display a matrix of that size (because it has too few display pixels), image quality is decreased.

It is recommended that a high-resolution 5-megapixel (2048 × 2560 pixels) display monitor be used for diagnostic interpretation. However, the display size (dimensions) along with the pixel pitch is another method to assess the capabilities of the display monitor. A display monitor having diagonal dimensions of 54 cm (21 inches) is adequate for viewing images sized 35 × 43 cm (14 × 17 inch) with a recommended pixel pitch of 0.200 mm at a standard viewing distance of about 60 cm (24 inches). According to the ACR-AAPM-SIIM *Technical Standards for Electronic Practice of Medical Imaging* (2017), suitable visualization of the entire digital image will occur when the diagonal display distance is 80% of the viewing distance. At 67-cm (26-inch) viewing distance, 80% would yield a 54-cm (21-inch) diagonal sized display monitor. However, depending on the type of device used to display the digital image (workstation, tablet, laptop), the display dimensions and viewing distances could change.

IMPORTANT RELATIONSHIP

Display Monitor

A high-resolution 5-megapixel (2048 × 2560 pixels) display monitor is recommended for diagnostic interpretation. In addition, a display monitor having diagonal dimensions of 54 cm (21 inches) is adequate for viewing images sized 35 × 43 cm (14 × 17 inch) with a recommended pixel pitch of 0.200 mm at a standard viewing distance of about 60 cm (24 inches).

Another important display feature is the **aspect ratio** (width to height dimension). Display monitors with 3:4 or 4:5 aspect ratios are appropriate for viewing radiographic digital images. Newer display monitors may have a wider format such as 16:9 or 16:10, which would provide for presentation of multiple images, similar to dual monitors.

Because anatomic tissue is visualized using various brightness levels, the amount of light emitted from the monitor (luminance) affects the quality of the displayed image. **Luminance** is a measurement of the light intensity (brightness) emitted from the surface of the monitor and is expressed in units of candela per square meter (cd/m^2). There are different measurements of luminance: ambient, minimum, maximum, and ratio. Ambient luminance is the light that reflects off the display surface from the room (ambient) lighting after the monitor has been turned off and is added into the other measurements. Primary display monitors should exhibit a minimum luminance of 1.0 cd/m^2 and a maximum luminance of 350 cd/m^2. A ratio of the maximum to minimum luminance, luminance ratio (LR), is recommended to be greater than 250, and a display monitor with an LR of 350 has improved image contrast.

The contrast resolution of a digital image is determined by the pixel bit depth. A digital imaging system capable of displaying 16,384 shades of gray (14 bit) requires a monitor capable of displaying a large grayscale range. Monitors that have a higher LR are capable of displaying a greater grayscale range. It is recommended that display monitors used for image interpretation have a graphic bit depth of 8, yielding 256 shades of gray. The DICOM **grayscale standard display function (GSDF)** as recommended by the American Association of Physicists in Medicine (AAPM) Task Group 18 should not vary by more than 10%.

Additional concerns of display monitors include geometrical distortions, such as concavity and convexity; veiling glare, which adversely affects image contrast; and display noise, which is typically a result of statistical fluctuations or luminance differences in the image. Routine quality control (QC) of the display monitor is just as important as monitoring the digital

---

BOX 5-2   Quality Control Check: Display Monitor

Quality control (QC) test devices for evaluating the performance of the display monitor include the American Association of Physicists in Medicine (AAPM) TG18-QC test pattern and the Society of Motion Picture and Television Engineers test pattern (SMPTE). Several aspects of a display monitor can be evaluated with these test patterns, including geometric distortion, luminance, resolution, contrast resolution, noise, and veiling glare.

---

imaging acquisition and processing devices. Box 5-2 describes QC methods for evaluating display monitors.

 IMPORTANT RELATIONSHIP

Display Monitor Luminance

Luminance is a measurement of the light intensity (brightness) emitted from the surface of the monitor and is expressed in cd/m². Primary display monitors should exhibit a minimum luminance of 1.0 cd/m² and a maximum luminance of 350 cd/m². A ratio of the maximum to minimum luminance, LR, is recommended to be greater than 250, and a display monitor with an LR of 350 has improved image contrast.

Laser Printers

Although not commonly needed for interpretation, hard-copy records of digital images may still occasionally be desired. Digital images can be windowed while being viewed on a display monitor and then printed onto film by a laser printer. Multiple images can be printed on a single sheet, and multiple copies of images processed differently can be printed. Laser printers that use either wet or dry printing methods are available. Wet laser printers use liquid chemicals (developer and fixer) to process the image. In dry processing, the chemicals are part of the film. The image is created by use of heat instead of liquid chemicals.

DATA MANAGEMENT

Because of the advancement and use of electronic information in health care, **data management** is a complex system-wide effort to ensure that people, equipment, and processes are in place to expand health care communication and improve patient outcomes. Modern radiology practice requires efficient and effective methods for acquisition, storage, retrieval, transmission, and display of digital image data from multiple imaging modalities and throughout health care systems. Digital communication needs in radiology also include the processing and delivery of patient data and subsequent interpretation of radiologic procedures. The ability to simultaneously integrate digital images, speech, and patient medical information involves a very complex system.

Imaging Informatics

Imaging informatics, also known as radiology informatics, involves data management for radiology services both within and outside the health care system. Managing electronic health information along with digital images (acquisition, storage, retrieval, and transmission) and their interpretation and consultation is essential to providing effective and efficient health care to improve patient outcomes. In addition, the safety and security of **protected health information (PHI)**

must be ensured and adhere to local, state, and federal guidelines. PHI is any health-related information collected, stored, and shared that can be linked to an individual. One of the purposes of the US **Health Insurance Portability and Accountability Act (HIPAA)** (passed in 1996), is "the establishment of national standards for electronic health care transactions and national identifiers for providers, health insurance plans, and employers." These standards are an effort to protect the privacy and confidentiality of patients' health information while making PHI available to individuals who need access to this information for patient care, insurance, or billing.

IMPORTANT RELATIONSHIP
Data Management

Data management is a complex system-wide effort to ensure that people, equipment, and processes are in place to expand health care communication and improve patient outcomes. Imaging informatics requires efficient and effective methods for acquisition, storage, retrieval, transmission, and display of digital image data from multiple imaging modalities and throughout health care systems. HIPAA established national standards to protect the privacy and confidentiality of patients' PHI.

When a patient comes to a facility for health care, personal information is gathered that will assist in his or her care. Information gathered from the patient (demographic data, relevant history, physician orders, and so on) at the facility will be collected and stored in the **hospital information system (HIS)**. If the patient is scheduled for a radiology procedure, some of this patient information becomes a part of the radiology workflow and stored in the **radiology information system (RIS)**. The RIS is similar to the HIS but specific to the radiology department. All this electronic information (demographics, relevant history, digital images and interpretations) is included in the HIS and available to authorized personnel at the facility. **The electronic health record (EHR)** is the system for patient PHI that can be shared outside the facility and among many health care systems.

IMPORTANT RELATIONSHIP
Patient Health Information

Patient health information is collected and stored in the HIS and shared with the RIS. The EHR is the system for patient PHI that can be shared outside the facility and among many health care systems.

Picture Archival and Communication System

A **picture archival and communication system (PACS)** is a computer system designed for digital imaging that can receive, store, archive, distribute, and display digital images. The major components of PACS include the imaging modalities, digital communication networks, display workstations, and archival capabilities for storage and retrieval. Integration of HIS and RIS can be accomplished by networks. A network system links all these computer systems so that images, patient data, and interpretations can be viewed simultaneously by people at different workstations (Fig. 5-26). An important goal of a radiology network system is to provide the referring physician with the radiology report, patient data, and radiographic images at a convenient location and in a timely manner.

FIG. 5-26 Communication among the computer system for medical information (RIS), the computer systems for imaging (input modalities), radiology workstations, and archive storage. Referring physicians can receive radiology reports, patient data, and radiographic images through the Internet (web server). (Carter C, Veale B: *Digital Radiography and PACS*, ed 3, St. Louis, 2019, Elsevier, Inc.)

IMPORTANT RELATIONSHIP

Picture Archival and Communication System

A PACS is a computer system designed for digital imaging that can receive, store, archive, distribute, and display digital images. The major components of PACS include the imaging modalities, digital communication networks, display workstations, and archival capabilities for storage and retrieval.

Digital Imaging and Communications in Medicine (DICOM) is an international communication standard for information sharing between PACS and imaging modalities to transmit, store, retrieve, print, process, and display medical imaging information. All digital image data management equipment should conform to the DICOM standard so that the features and performance of the devices are consistent throughout health care systems.

The **Health Level Seven standard (HL7)** is a communication standard for medical information. Connectivity and communication among these systems are necessary for radiology to realize the full potential of imaging informatics. Network systems are currently being marketed to meet the demands in radiology. A well-integrated system would improve patient care through cost-effective, reliable, secure, and timely delivery of patient and digital imaging information. **Integrating the Healthcare Enterprise (IHE)** "is an initiative by healthcare professionals and industry to improve the way computer systems in healthcare share information. IHE promotes the coordinated use of established standards such as DICOM and HL7 to address specific clinical needs in support of optimal patient care."

As the complexity of medical images and patient data have grown, new approaches to PACS have developed. One challenge has been expansion and maintenance of PACS systems, access to and storage of data over decades, and changes in vendors. One latest solution is the trend toward

vendor neutral archives (VNAs). VNAs allow for images and data from different systems and in different formats to be stored using a singular system on a common infrastructure. VNAs may be used as replacements to existing PACS to avoid very expensive transition costs. They may also be used to consolidate several systems that exist within a single facility or across a system of facilities. Another growing trend is the creation of health information exchanges (HIEs) for the purpose of sharing patient information across systems and creating networks of service providers.

 IMPORTANT RELATIONSHIP

Digital Communication Networks

> DICOM is an international communication standard for information sharing between PACS and imaging modalities to transmit, store, retrieve, print, process, and display medical imaging information. HL7 is a communication standard for medical information. Connectivity and communication among these systems are necessary for radiology to realize the full potential of imaging informatics. IHE promotes the coordinated use of established standards such as DICOM and HL7 to address specific clinical needs in support of optimal patient care.

A **display workstation** is simply a desktop computer that allows for the retrieval and viewing of medical images from one of the modalities or storage components of the PACS (Fig. 5-27). The quality and function of one of these stations depends on the user. The software loaded to each display station also depends on the user. For general viewing by non-interpreting physicians and other health care workers, a very basic package allowing minimal adjustment may be all that is available. QC display stations and interpreting stations have greater function and capability, such as more advanced image manipulation (windowing: level and width), annotation, patient demographic information, cropping, panning, and magnification (zoom). Even among radiographers, each may have access to different functions protected by login and password to limit which aspects of a medical image may be changed, and by whom, so as to prevent accidentally damaging or negatively altering the record.

In addition to other standards of communication, DICOM specifies information included as a header on digital images (DICOM header), such as accession number, patient name and identification number, date and time of examination, radiographic procedure, and total number of images in the study. It is also recommended that exposure-related information be included in the DICOM header such as kVp, milliamperage-seconds, exposure indicator, and any post- or reprocessing of the digital data. A modality worklist can assist the radiographer in maintaining the accuracy of the information.

It is important that the display of digital images be consistent among the monitors used within and outside the health care system. The **Grayscale Standard Display Function (GSDF)** is the DICOM recommended standard for consistent display characteristics such as grayscale appearance and image quality.

 IMPORTANT RELATIONSHIP

Display Workstation

> A display workstation is simply a desktop computer that allows for the retrieval and viewing of medical images from one of the modalities or storage components of the PACS. QC display stations and interpreting stations have greater function and capability, such as more advanced image manipulation (windowing: level and width), annotation, patient demographic information, cropping, panning, and magnification (zoom). In addition to other standards of communication, DICOM specifies information included as a header on digital images (DICOM header), and the GSDF is the DICOM recommended standard for consistent display characteristics, such as grayscale appearance and image quality.

FIG. 5-27 Primary workstation. A four-bank monitor workstation and a two-bank monitor workstation. (Carter C, Veale B: *Digital Radiography and PACS*, ed 3, St. Louis, 2019, Elsevier, Inc.)

Transmission, Storage, and Archives

To improve transmission of the data to the various end users of the imaging data, compression may be used. Image compression can be reversible or irreversible. **Reversible compression** means that there is no loss of image data (lossless) at the end user. **Irreversible compression** means that there is some loss of image data (lossy) at the end user and may be used to decrease transmission time and or storage space. However, irreversible compression is only used in circumstances in which the loss of image data does not impact the job of the end user. If irreversible compression is used, the image displayed must be labeled as such, and irreversible compression cannot be used for diagnostic interpretation of images. Transmission devices need to have the capacity to handle the volume of images, delivered within a reasonable time frame and, can check for errors.

One of the biggest challenges of a PACS is storage. With increasingly complex modalities feeding large image files (data sets) into the system, the demand for storage is ever increasing and must comply with local, state, and federal guidelines. This is further complicated by the HIPAA requirement to store images and data for years. Policies and procedures are also needed to effectively and appropriately archive (current and previous exams) and store digital image data.

There is also the requirement to address **disaster recovery** processes. This is basically a requirement to duplicate all files in a remote location so that recovery is possible in the event of a disaster and the primary files are lost.

To support this ever-increasing demand for data storage, PACS has taken on new directions. Traditionally, PACS systems were created and maintained in house (within the facility). This required the purchase and maintenance of very large computer servers and storage systems. One recent trend to address storage space and expense is cloud-based storage. This process consists of offsite storage and servers supported by a secure network and third-party vendor. This also shifts the disaster recovery requirement to the vendor along with the maintenance and storage equipment purchase. The user basically pays for the service and storage space as needed.

There are also hybrid versions of this configuration whereby the facility maintains current image and patient data in house and longer-term storage externally or in the cloud. The advantages and disadvantages of these systems are facility dependent and change according to the imaging volume, facility size, and need for access. The speed of access, for example, depends on connectivity speed and file size.

 IMPORTANT RELATIONSHIP

Transmission, Storage, and Archive

Transmission devices need to have the capacity to handle the volume of images, delivered within a reasonable time frame, and can check for errors. To improve transmission of the data to the various end users of the imaging data, compression (reversible or irreversible) may be used. Policies and procedures are also needed to effectively and appropriately archive (current and previous exams) and store digital image data for years.

Teleradiology

Teleradiology is the practice of diagnostic image interpretation outside the facility (offsite) from where the imaging data are acquired. It can be used for preliminary diagnosis for referring and emergency department physicians, after-hours interpretations and consultations, and subspecialty expertise (e.g., cardiovascular or neuroradiology), and it can solve manpower issues such as vacations and rural facilities having limited access to radiologists. There is a growing number of large companies using radiologists for teleradiology both within and outside the United States.

Although teleradiology can address many of the challenges facing imaging departments as described previously, there are issues that need to be considered. The ACR *White Paper on Teleradiology Practice* outlines many of these issues and reports important best-practice guidelines, a few of which will be discussed.

The main goal of any radiology health care system is to focus on patient care and improve patient outcomes. In most radiology departments, the radiologist is an integral part of the workflow and can communicate with radiographers, patients, and other staff involved in the care of patients. Because of the nature of teleradiology, radiologists' interpreting imaging studies outside the radiology department (teleradiologists) are not physically present, and communication among the imaging professionals could be problematic. Communication needs between teleradiologists and the imaging professionals include providing timely and relevant patient information, the ability to answer questions regarding the procedure, and maintaining standard QC practices. Poor communication can have negative results and impact the patient's care and outcomes.

Having onsite radiologists is preferred; however, there is a need for teleradiology, and it can serve a valuable supplemental purpose in radiology. The practice of teleradiology should maintain the same high standards, safety, and quality as onsite radiology services.

 IMPORTANT RELATIONSHIP

Teleradiology

Teleradiology is the practice of diagnostic image interpretation outside the facility (offsite) from where the imaging data are acquired. Communication needs between teleradiologists and the imaging professionals include providing timely and relevant patient information, the ability to answer questions regarding the procedure, and maintaining standard QC practices. The practice of teleradiology should maintain the same high standards, safety, and quality as onsite radiology services.

QUALITY CONTROL AND SECURITY

QC is an important activity to ensure that radiographic equipment is functioning properly and should occur routinely and consistently. QC activities are equally important for digital image data management. According to the ACR-AAPM-SIIM *Technical Standard for Electronic Practice of Medical Imaging* (revised in 2017), "Any facility using a digital image data management system must have documented policies and procedures for monitoring and evaluating the effective management, safety, and proper performance of acquisition, digitization, processing, compression, transmission, display, archiving, and retrieval functions of the system. The QC program should be designed to maximize the quality and accessibility of diagnostic information." Basic and universal QC procedures for both CR and DR equipment have been discussed previously in this chapter. QC test devices for evaluating the performance of the display monitor include the AAPM TG18-QC (Fig. 5-28) test

FIG. 5-28 The American Association of Physicists in Medicine (AAPM) TG18-QC test pattern. (Johnston J, Fauber T: *Essentials of Radiographic Physics and Imaging*, St. Louis, 2012, Mosby, Inc., an affiliate of Elsevier Inc.)

FIG. 5-29 The Society of Motion Picture and Television Engineers test pattern (SMPTE). (Bushong SC: *Radiologic Science for Technologists*, ed 9, St. Louis, MO, 2008, Mosby, Inc., an affiliate of Elsevier Inc.)

pattern and the Society of Motion Picture and Television Engineers test pattern (SMPTE) (Fig. 5-29). Several aspects of a display monitor can be evaluated with these test patterns, including geometric distortion, luminance, resolution, contrast resolution, noise, and veiling glare.

QC activities for digital image data management, including, compression, transmission, archiving, and retrieval functions of the system, are beyond the scope of this textbook and would most likely be performed by an imaging informatics professional.

IMPORTANT RELATIONSHIP

Quality Control

QC is an important activity to ensure that radiographic equipment is functioning properly and should occur routinely and consistently. QC activities are equally important for digital image data management and are most likely performed by an imaging informatics professional.

Security of PHI is an ever-growing concern in health care and radiology. Policies and procedures must be in place and adhered to by all health care workers who have access to PHI. Some of the recommended procedures that will ensure privacy and security include *anonymization* (patient identifiable information is removed from the PHI) if performing clinical research, *authentication* to verify the identity of the user of PHI, *authorization* (which limits access to PHI for approved users only, maintaining records of interactions with PHI [auditing]), and *confidentiality* to prevent unauthorized users from access to PHI.

Radiographers have routine access to PHI in performance of their duties and must take responsibility for adhering to the department's policies and procedures. Patients must be confident that radiographers have the skills to perform their imaging procedures and believe that their PHI will be secure.

IMPORTANT RELATIONSHIP

Security of Patient Health Information

Radiographers have routine access to PHI in performance of their duties and must take responsibility for adhering to the department's policies and procedures. Patients must be confident that radiographers have the skills to perform their imaging procedures and believe that their PHI will be secure.

CHAPTER SUMMARY

- Digital image processing refers to various computer algorithms applied to digital data for the purpose of optimizing the image for display.
- Preprocessing operations such as bad or dead pixel and flat fielding corrections occur to the raw data to prepare the image data for processing and display.
- A histogram is a graphic representation of the image data set. This graph includes all the pixel values that represent the latent image after the software corrections were applied. The location of the graph along the x-axis represents image brightness levels, and the shape represents image contrast or grayscale.
- Histogram analysis is an important processing technique used to identify the edges of the image and assess the exposure data (pixel values) prior to image processing and display.
- The computer analyzes the histogram using processing algorithms and compares it with a preestablished (reference) histogram specific to the anatomic part being imaged.
- Automatic rescaling is a process employed to maintain a consistent image brightness despite over- or underexposure.
- During histogram analysis, the exposure indicator provides a numerical value that indicates the level of radiation exposure to the digital IR.
- After histogram analysis, LUTs provide the means to alter the original pixel values to improve the brightness and contrast of the image.
- Default and postprocessing functions, such as electronic masking, window level and width, subtraction, contrast enhancement, edge enhancement, smoothing, and equalization, allow manipulation of the displayed image.
- Display monitors provide soft-copy viewing of digital radiographs. Primary monitors are high-quality monitors used for diagnostic interpretation.
- Important features regarding display monitors used for interpretation include viewing conditions, matrix size, pixel pitch, luminance, LR, and contrast resolution.
- Laser printers that use either wet or dry methods to print hard-copy images are available.
- Imaging informatics involves data management for radiology services both within and outside the health care system.
- HIPAA establishes standards for PHI.
- PACS is the communication system for digital imaging modalities and can receive, store, distribute, and display digital images.
- DICOM is a communication standard for information sharing among PACS, imaging modalities, and display, and HL7 is a communication standard for medical information.
- Image compression may be used to transmit image date but should be reversible so no data are lost.
- Digital data storage has challenges, and policies and procedures are needed to effectively and appropriately archive and store digital image data.

- Teleradiology is the practice of diagnostic image interpretation outside the facility from where the imaging data are acquired.
- QC activities are important to ensure that digital radiographic equipment and systems are functioning properly.
- Security of PHI must be in place and adhered to by all health care workers.

REVIEW QUESTIONS

1. Which of the following is defined as a graphic representation of the pixel values?
   A. Automatic rescaling
   B. Values of interest
   C. Histogram
   D. Exposure indicator

2. What process is employed to maintain consistent digital image brightness for over- or underexposure?
   A. Automatic rescaling
   B. Histogram
   C. Exposure indicator
   D. Lookup tables (LUTs)

3. Which of the following is not a numerical value indicating the level of radiation exposure to a digital image receptor (IR)?
   A. Sensitivity number
   B. Exposure indicator
   C. Window level
   D. Exposure index

4. Which of the following may impact the location and shape of the histogram?
   1. Exposure technique
   2. Positioning
   3. Collimation
      A. 1 and 2 only
      B. 1 and 3 only
      C. 2 and 3 only
      D. 1, 2, and 3

5. What digital process alters image brightness and grayscale to improve the visibility of anatomic structures?
   A. Automatic rescaling
   B. Histogram analysis
   C. Exposure indicator
   D. LUTs

6. Maintaining a low level of ambient lighting can improve soft-copy viewing of digital images.
   A. True
   B. False

7. Display monitors used for soft-copy viewing of digital images should have _____.
   A. increased ambient lighting
   B. decreased matrix size
   C. high pixel pitch
   D. high luminance

8. Which of the following is not a function during postprocessing of a displayed digital image?
   A. Histogram analysis
   B. Electronic masking
   C. Windowing
   D. Edge enhancement

9. Wider window width _____.
   A. increases brightness
   B. decreases brightness
   C. increases contrast
   D. decreases contrast

10. What postprocessing technique suppresses image noise?
    A. Edge enhancement
    B. Equalization
    C. Inversion
    D. Smoothing

11. What is the communication standard for information sharing between PACS and imaging modalities?
    A. DQE
    B. DICOM
    C. SMPTE
    D. HL7

12. The deviation index (DI) is a value that reflects the difference between the desired or target exposure to the IR and the actual exposure to the IR.
    A. True
    B. False

13. A DI of −0.75 reflects insufficient exposure to the IR.
    A. True
    B. False

14. Which of the following may occur as a result of the DI value greater than +3.0?
    1. Excessive noise visible
    2. Saturation
    3. Patient overexposure
       A. 1 and 2 only
       B. 1 and 3 only
       C. 2 and 3 only
       D. 1, 2, and 3

15. What standard was enacted to protect privacy and confidentiality of patient's health information?
    A. Electronic health record
    B. Health Insurance Portability and Accountability Act
    C. Protected health information
    D. Integrating the Healthcare Enterprise

16. To transmit and store large amounts of imaging data, what may occur?
    A. Compression
    B. Disaster recovery
    C. Teleradiology
    D. Vendor neutral archives

Exposure Technique Factors

CHAPTER OUTLINE

Primary Factors
  Milliamperage and Exposure
    Time
  Kilovoltage Peak
Secondary Factors
  Focal Spot Size
  Source-to-Image-Receptor
    Distance

Object-to-Image-Receptor
  Distance
Calculating Magnification
Central Ray Alignment
Grids
Beam Restriction
Generator Output
Tube Filtration

Compensating Filters
Patient Factors
  Body Habitus
  Part Thickness

OBJECTIVES

*After completing this chapter, the reader will be able
to perform the following:*

1. Define all the key terms in this chapter.
2. State all the important relationships in this chapter.
3. Explain the relationship between milliamperage (mA) and exposure time with radiation production and image receptor (IR) exposure.
4. Calculate changes in milliamperage and exposure time to change or maintain exposure to the IR.
5. Describe the effect of changes in mA and exposure time on digital images.
6. Recognize how to correct factors for an exposure error.
7. Explain how kilovoltage peak (kVp) affects radiation production and IR exposure.
8. Calculate changes in kVp to change or maintain exposure to the IR.
9. Describe the effects of changes in kVp on digital images.
10. Recognize the factors that affect spatial resolution and distortion.
11. Calculate changes in mAs for changes in source-to-image-receptor distance.
12. Calculate the magnification factor and determine image and object size.
13. Describe the use of grids and beam restriction and their effect on IR exposure and image quality.
14. Calculate changes in mAs when adding or removing a grid.
15. Recognize patient factors that may affect IR exposure.
16. Identify exposure factors that can affect patient radiation exposure.
17. State exposure technique modifications for the following considerations: body habitus and patient thickness.

KEY TERMS

15% rule
body habitus
direct square law
exposure indicator
exposure maintenance formula

inverse-square law
magnification factor (MF)
object-to-image-receptor
    distance (OID)

source-to-image-receptor
    distance (SID)
source-to-object distance
    (SOD)

In Chapter 2, variables that affect both the quantity and the quality of the x-ray beam are presented. Milliamperage (mA) and exposure time affect the quantity of radiation produced, and kilovoltage affects both the quantity and the quality. Chapter 3 emphasizes that a good-quality radiographic image accurately represents the anatomic area of interest. The characteristics evaluated for image quality are brightness, contrast, spatial resolution, distortion, and noise. This chapter focuses on exposure techniques and the use of accessory devices and their effects on the radiation reaching the patient, image receptor (IR), and the image produced. Radiographers have the responsibility of selecting the combination of exposure factors to produce a good-quality image. Knowledge of how these factors affect the exposure to the IR individually and in combination assists radiographers in producing a radiographic image with the amount of information desired for a diagnosis. In addition, the patient should be exposed to the least amount of radiation reasonable to produce a diagnostic-quality image. This chapter discusses all the primary and secondary factors and their effects on the radiation reaching the patient, IR, and image quality.

PRIMARY FACTORS

The primary exposure technique factors selected by the radiographer on the control panel are mA, exposure time (s), and kilovoltage peak (kVp). Depending on the type of control panel, mA and exposure time may be selected separately or combined as one factor, milliamperage-seconds (mAs). Regardless, it is important to understand how changing each factor separately or in combination affects the radiation reaching the patient, IR, and the radiographic image.

Milliamperage and Exposure Time

The quantity of radiation exiting the x-ray tube and reaching the patient affects the amount of remnant radiation reaching the IR. The product of mA and exposure time is directly proportional to the quantity of x-rays produced (Fig. 6-1). When an anatomic part is adequately penetrated, the exposure to the IR will increase in proportion to increases in the quantity of x-rays (Fig. 6-2). Conversely, when the quantity of x-rays is decreased, the exposure to the IR decreases. Therefore, exposure to the IR can be increased or decreased by adjusting the amount of radiation (mAs).

 IMPORTANT RELATIONSHIP
mAs and Quantity of Radiation

As mAs increases, the quantity of radiation reaching the IR increases. As mAs decreases, the amount of radiation reaching the IR decreases.

FIG. 6-1 Milliamperage (mA) and radiation quantity. Changing the mA results in a proportional change in the quantity (amplitude) of x-rays produced. (From Johnston JN, Fauber TL: *Essentials of Radiographic Physics and Imaging*, ed 2, St. Louis, 2016, Mosby.)

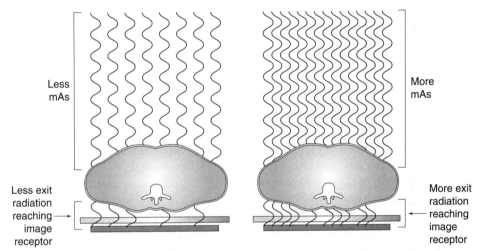

FIG. 6-2 Milliamperage-seconds (mAs) and radiation exposure. As the quantity of x-rays is increased mAs, the exposure to the image receptor (IR) proportionally increases.

Because the mAs is the product of mA and exposure time, increasing either mA or time will increase the amount of radiation exposure to the IR.

⟩⟩ **MATHEMATICAL APPLICATION**

Adjusting mA or Exposure Time

$$200 \, mA \times 0.100 \, s = 20 \, mAs$$

To increase the mAs to 40, one could use the following formulas:

$$400 \, mA \times 0.100 \, s = 40 \, mAs$$

$$200 \, mA \times 0.200 \, s = 40 \, mAs$$

As demonstrated in the previous Mathematical Application, mAs can be doubled by doubling either the mA or the exposure time. A change in either milliamperage (mA) or exposure time (s) proportionally changes the mAs. To maintain the same mAs, the radiographer must increase the mA and proportionally decrease the exposure time or decrease the mA and proportionally increase the exposure time.

IMPORTANT RELATIONSHIP
mA and Exposure Time

mA and exposure time have an inverse proportional relationship when maintaining the same mAs.

MATHEMATICAL APPLICATION
Adjusting mA and Exposure Time to Maintain mAs

$$200 \, mA \times 100 \, ms \, (0.100 \, s) = 20 \, mAs$$

To maintain mAs, use the following formulas:

$$400 \, mA \times 50 \, ms \, (0.050 \, s) = 20 \, mAs$$

$$100 \, mA \times 200 \, ms \, (0.200 \, s) = 20 \, mAs$$

It is important for the radiographer to determine the appropriate mAs level needed to produce a diagnostic image. This is not an easy task because there are so many variables that can affect the required mAs. For example, single-phase generators produce less radiation with the same mAs compared with high-frequency generators. A patient's age, the general condition of the patient, and the thickness of the anatomic part also affect the mAs required for a procedure. In addition, IRs respond differently for a given mAs level. For example, mAs does not control the amount of brightness displayed within a digital image. Digital IRs can detect a wider range of radiation intensities (wider dynamic range) exiting the patient and therefore are not dependent on the mAs. However, exposure errors can adversely affect the quality of a digital image. If the mAs is too low (low exposure to the digital IR), image brightness is adjusted during computer processing to achieve the desired level. Even after adjusting the level of brightness, there may be increased quantum noise visible within an image (Fig. 6-3). If the selected mAs is too high (high exposure to the digital IR), the brightness can also be adjusted; however, the patient will receive more radiation than necessary.

IMPORTANT RELATIONSHIP
mAs and Digital Image Brightness

The level of mAs does not control image brightness when using digital IRs. During computer processing, image brightness is maintained when the mAs is too low or too high. A lower-than-needed mAs produces an image with increased quantum noise, and a higher-than-needed mAs exposes a patient to unnecessary radiation.

The brightness of a digital image can be altered during image processing; hence, information about the exposure to the IR is important. Manufacturers of each type of digital system

FIG. 6-3 A, Radiographic image obtained with high mAs showing decreased quantum noise. **B,** Radiographic image obtained with low mAs showing increased quantum noise. (From Johnston JN, Fauber TL: *Essentials of Radiographic Physics and Imaging,* ed 3, St. Louis, 2020, Elsevier.)

specify the expected range of x-ray exposure sufficient to produce a quality image. A numerical value (**exposure indicator**) is displayed on the processed image to indicate the level of x-ray exposure received (incident exposure) on the digital IR. It is important for the radiographer to consider the indicated value because exposure errors, as previously stated, affect the quality of the digital image and the radiation dose to the patient. Exposure errors are not obvious by simply looking at the digital image because the digital data are normalized to provide images with diagnostic brightness levels (Fig. 6-4). Most manufacturers of digital IRs suggest a range for the exposure indicator on the basis of the radiographic procedure. If the exposure indicator value falls outside this range, exposure to the digital IR, image quality, and patient exposure could be affected.

IMPORTANT RELATIONSHIP
Exposure Indicator Value

A numerical value or exposure indicator is displayed on the processed digital image to indicate the level of x-ray exposure received (incident exposure) on the IR. If the exposure indicator value falls outside the manufacturer's suggested range, exposure to the digital IR, image quality, and patient exposure could be affected.

Generally, for repeat images necessitated by exposure errors, the mAs is adjusted by a factor of 2; therefore, a minimum change involves doubling or halving the mAs. If a radiographic image must be repeated because of another error, such as positioning, the radiographer may use the

FIG. 6-4 Exposure errors can be computer adjusted to maintain image brightness. **A**, Image created with sufficient mAs. **B**, Image created with insufficient mAs, resulting in increased quantum noise visible. **C**, Image created with excessive mAs, resulting in decreased quantum noise visible. The exposure indicator value reflected the exposure errors to the IR for images *B* and *C*. (From Johnston JN, Fauber TL: *Essentials of Radiographic Physics and Imaging*, ed 3, St. Louis, 2020, Mosby.)

opportunity to make an adjustment in the exposure to the IR to produce an image of diagnostic quality. A radiographic image repeated because of insufficient or excessive exposure requires a change in mAs by a factor of at least 2.

To best visualize the anatomic area of interest, the selected mAs must produce a sufficient amount of radiation that reaches the IR. An excessive or insufficient amount of mAs adversely affects image quality and patient radiation exposure. The radiographer should be diligent in monitoring exposure indicator values to ensure that quality images are obtained with the lowest reasonable radiation dose to the patient.

Kilovoltage Peak

The kVp affects the exposure to the IR because it alters the amount and penetrating ability of the x-ray beam (Fig. 6-5). The area of interest must be adequately penetrated before the mAs can be adjusted to produce a quality radiographic image. When adequate penetration is achieved, increasing the kVp further results in more radiation reaching the IR (Fig. 6-6). In addition to affecting the amount of radiation exposure to the IR, the kVp affects subject contrast.

> **IMPORTANT RELATIONSHIP**
>
> ### *kVp and the Radiographic Image*
>
> Increasing or decreasing the kVp changes the amount of radiation exposure to the IR and the subject contrast produced within the image.

FIG. 6-5 Kilovoltage peak (kVp) and radiation quality and quantity. Increasing the kVp from 72 to 82 shows an increase in the quantity of x-rays (amplitude), and the x-ray emission shifts toward the right, indicating an increase in the energy or quality of the beam. (From Johnston JN, Fauber TL: *Essentials of Radiographic Physics and Imaging,* ed 2, St. Louis, 2016, Mosby.)

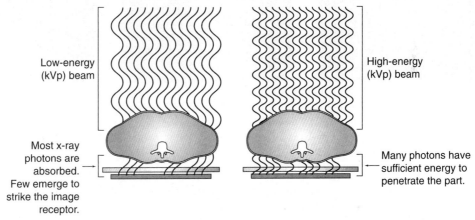

FIG. 6-6 The kVp and radiation exposure. Increasing the kVp increases the penetrating power of the radiation and increases the exposure to the IR.

Kilovoltage Peak and Exposure to the Image Receptor

Because kVp affects the amount of radiation reaching the IR, its effect on the digital image is similar to the effect of mAs. Assuming that the anatomic part has been adequately penetrated, too much radiation reaching the IR (within reason) will still produce a digital image with the appropriate level of brightness as a result of computer adjustment during image processing; however, the patient will be overexposed. Similarly, too little radiation reaching the IR (within reason) will produce a digital image with the appropriate level of brightness, but the increased quantum noise will decrease the image quality.

A diagnostic-quality image (Fig. 6-7A) was produced using 70 kVp at 2 mAs. Fig. 6-7B was produced using 50 kVp at 2 mAs, and Fig. 6-7C was produced using 93 kVp at 2 mAs. Although the brightness was adjusted by the computer, the exposure indicator for each of the images varied greatly and reflected the exposure to the IR. When a kVp that is too low is selected, the brightness is adjusted, but quantum noise may be visible. Additionally, when a kVp that is too high is selected without an appropriate decrease in mAs, the image brightness is adjusted, but patient exposure may be increased because of increased x-ray quantity and scatter within the tissues. Although brightness can be computer adjusted when using a kVp that is too high, increased scatter radiation can also reach the IR and may adversely affect image quality.

FIG. 6-7 A, Image produced using 70 kVp at 2 mAs. **B**, Image produced using 50 kVp t 2 mAs, resulting in higher subject contrast and computer adjusted to maintain brightness but increased quantum noise visible. **C**, Image produced using 93 kVp at 2 mAs, resulting in lower subject contrast and computer adjusted to maintain brightness, but patient exposure is increased. (From Johnston JN, Fauber TL: *Essentials of Radiographic Physics and Imaging*, ed 3, St. Louis, 2020, Mosby.)

Excessive or insufficient radiation exposure to the digital IR, as a result of the mAs or kVp, should be reflected in the exposure indicator value.

IMPORTANT RELATIONSHIP
Exposure Errors in Digital Imaging

kVp and mAs exposure errors should be reflected in the exposure indicator value; however, image brightness can be maintained during computer processing.

RADIATION PROTECTION ALERT
Excessive Radiation Exposure and Digital Imaging

Although the computer can adjust image brightness for technique exposure errors, routinely using more radiation than required for the procedure in digital radiography unnecessarily increases patient exposure. Even though the digital system can adjust overexposure, it is an unethical practice to knowingly overexpose a patient.

Kilovoltage is not a factor that is typically manipulated to vary the amount of IR exposure because the kVp also affects subject contrast. However, it is sometimes necessary to manipulate the kVp to maintain the required exposure to the IR. For example, using portable or mobile x-ray equipment may limit the choice of mAs settings, and the radiographer must adjust the kVp to maintain sufficient exposure to the IR.

Maintaining or adjusting exposure to the IR can be accomplished with kVp using the **15% rule**. The 15% rule states that increasing or decreasing the kVp by 15% has the same effect as doubling or halving the mAs; for example, increasing the kVp from 82 to 94 (15%) produces a similar exposure to the IR as increasing the mAs from 10 to 20.

 IMPORTANT RELATIONSHIP

kVp and the 15% Rule

A 15% increase in kVp has the same effect on exposure to the IR as doubling the mAs. A 15% decrease in kVp has the same effect on exposure to the IR as halving the mAs.

Increasing the kVp by 15% increases the exposure to the IR unless the mAs is decreased. In addition, decreasing the kVp by 15% decreases the exposure to the IR unless the mAs is increased.

 MATHEMATICAL APPLICATION

Using the 15% Rule

To increase exposure to the IR, multiply the kVp by 1.15 (original kVp + 15%):
$$75\,kVp \times 1.15 = 86\,kVp$$

To decrease exposure to the IR, multiply the kVp by 0.85 (original kVp − 15%):
$$75\,kVp \times 0.85 = 64\,kVp$$

To maintain exposure to the IR, when increasing the kVp by 15% (kVp × 1.15), divide the original mAs by 2:
$$75\,kVp \times 1.15 = 86\,kVp \text{ and mAs}/2$$

When decreasing the kVp by 15% (kVp × 0.85), multiply the mAs by 2:
$$75\,kVp \times 0.85 = 64 \text{ and mAs} \times 2$$

! RADIATION PROTECTION ALERT

kVp/mAs

Whenever possible, a higher kilovoltage and lower mAs should be used to reduce patient exposure. Increasing kilovoltage requires a lower mAs to maintain the desired exposure to the IR and decreases the radiation dose to the patient. For example, changing kVp from 75 to 86 when imaging a pelvis is a 15% increase and would require half the mAs needed for the original 75 kVp. Higher kVp increases the beam penetration; therefore, less radiation is needed to achieve a desired exposure to the IR.

Kilovoltage Peak and Subject Contrast

Altering the penetrating power of the x-ray beam affects its absorption and transmission through the anatomic tissue being radiographed. Higher kVp increases the penetrating power of the x-ray beam and results in less absorption and more transmission in the anatomic tissues, which results in less variation in the x-ray intensities exiting the patient (lower subject contrast). As a result, images with lower subject contrast (more shades of gray) are produced (Fig. 6-8). When a low kVp is used, the x-ray beam penetration is decreased, resulting in more absorption and less transmission, which results in greater variation in the x-ray intensities exiting the patient. This produces an image with higher subject contrast (Fig. 6-9).

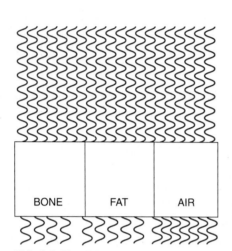

FIG. 6-8 The kVp and exit-beam intensities. Higher kVp increases the penetrating power of the x-ray beam and results in less absorption and more transmission in the anatomic tissues, resulting in less variation in the x-ray intensities exiting the patient. As a result, images with lower subject contrast are produced.

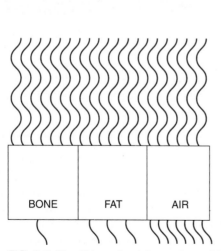

FIG. 6-9 The kVp and exit-beam intensities. Lower kVp decreases the x-ray beam penetration, resulting in more absorption and less transmission, which results in greater variation in the x-ray intensities exiting the patient. As a result, images with higher subject contrast are produced.

IMPORTANT RELATIONSHIP

kVp and Subject Contrast

A high kVp results in less absorption and more transmission in anatomic tissues, which results in less variation in the x-ray intensities exiting (remnant) the patient, producing lower subject contrast. A low kVp results in more absorption and less x-ray transmission in the anatomic tissues but with more variation in the x-ray intensities exiting the patient, resulting in higher subject contrast.

Changing the kVp affects the beam's absorption and transmission as it interacts with anatomic tissue; however, using a higher kVp reduces the total number of interactions and increases the amount of x-rays transmitted. In these interactions, Compton scattering increases, photoelectric absorption decreases, and more scatter exits the patient. It is important to understand that in addition to kVp affecting subject contrast, increasing kVp increases the amount of scatter (fog) reaching the IR and consequently, the radiographic contrast.

 IMPORTANT RELATIONSHIP

Kilovoltage, Scatter Radiation, and Radiographic Contrast

At higher kVp, more x-rays are transmitted with fewer overall interactions; however, a greater proportion of the interactions are from Compton scattering (fog) than photoelectric absorption, which decreases the radiographic contrast. Decreasing the kVp will increase photoelectric absorption and increase the number of interactions, but the proportion of Compton scattering (fog) will decrease compared with photoelectric absorption, increasing radiographic contrast.

The level of radiographic contrast desired and the kVp selected depend on the type and composition of the anatomic tissue, the structures that must be visualized, and (to some extent) the diagnostician's preference. For most anatomic regions, an accepted range of kVp provides an appropriate level of subject contrast. As long as the selected kVp is sufficient to penetrate the anatomic part, radiographic contrast can be further adjusted by the computer to display the desired contrast for the anatomic region.

Radiographic images are generally not repeated because of contrast errors. If a repeat radiograph is necessary and kVp is to be adjusted either to increase or decrease the level of subject contrast, the 15% rule provides an acceptable method of adjustment. In addition, whenever a change of 15% is made in the kVp to maintain the exposure to the IR, the radiographer must adjust the mAs by a factor of 2. The selection of kVp alters its absorption and transmission through the anatomic part, regardless of the type of IR used; therefore, kVp must be wisely selected. Exposure techniques using higher kVp with lower mAs settings are recommended in digital imaging because contrast is primarily controlled during computer processing.

SECONDARY FACTORS

Many secondary or influencing factors affect the x-ray beam, amount of radiation reaching the IR, and image quality. It is important for the radiographer to understand their effects individually and in combination.

Focal Spot Size

On the control panel, the radiographer can select whether to use a small or large focal spot size. The physical dimensions of the focal spot on the anode target in x-ray tubes used in standard radiographic applications usually range from 0.5 to 1.2 mm. Small focal spot sizes are usually 0.5

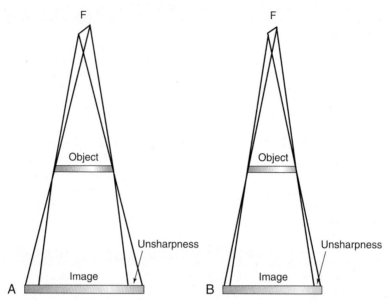

FIG. 6-10 Focal spot size and spatial resolution. Focal spot size influences the amount of unsharpness recorded in the image. As focal spot size changes, so does the amount of unsharpness. **A,** Larger focal spot. **B,** Smaller focal spot.

or 0.6 mm, and large focal spot sizes are usually 1 or 1.2 mm. Focal spot size is determined by the filament size. When the radiographer selects a particular focal spot size, he or she is actually selecting a filament size that is energized during x-ray production. Lower mA settings are associated with the small filament, whereas higher mA settings energize the large filament. Focal spot size is an important consideration for the radiographer because it affects spatial resolution (Fig. 6-10).

IMPORTANT RELATIONSHIP

Focal Spot Size and Spatial Resolution

As focal spot size increases, unsharpness increases and spatial resolution decreases; as focal spot size decreases, unsharpness decreases and spatial resolution increases.

Generally, the smallest available focal spot size should be used for every exposure. However, exposure is limited for a small focal spot size. When a small focal spot is used, the heat created during the x-ray exposure is concentrated into a smaller area and could cause tube damage. The radiographer must weigh the importance of improved spatial resolution for a particular examination or anatomic part against the amount of radiation exposure used. Modern radiographic x-ray generators are equipped with safety circuits that prevent an exposure from being made if the exposure exceeds the tube loading capacity for the selected focal spot size. Repeated exposures made just under the limit over a long period can still jeopardize the life of the x-ray tube.

Source-to-Image-Receptor Distance

The distance between the radiation source and the IR, known as **source-to-image-receptor distance (SID)**, affects the amount of radiation reaching the patient and subsequently the IR. Because of the divergence of the x-ray beam, the intensity of the radiation varies at different distances.

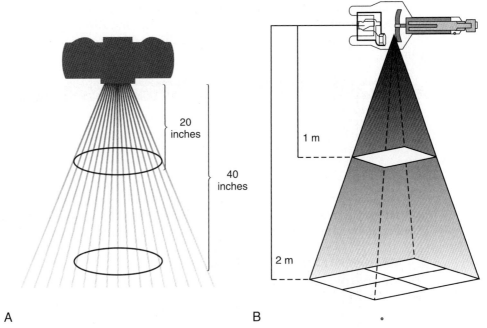

A   B

FIG. 6-11 Source-to-image-receptor distance (SID) and radiation intensity. **A** and **B,** Changing SID and its effect on the intensity of the x-ray beam reaching the IR (**A**) and on the divergence of the beam (**B**).

This relationship between distance and x-ray beam intensity is best described by the **inverse-square law**. This law states that the intensity of an x-ray beam is inversely proportional to the square of the distance from the source. Because beam intensity varies as a function of the square of the distance, SID affects the quantity of radiation reaching the IR. As SID increases, the x-ray intensity becomes spread over a larger area, decreasing the overall intensity of the x-ray beam reaching the IR (Fig. 6-11).

>> **IMPORTANT RELATIONSHIP**

SID and X-ray Beam Intensity

As SID increases, the x-ray beam intensity becomes spread over a larger area. This decreases the overall intensity of the x-ray beam reaching the IR.

>> **MATHEMATICAL APPLICATION**

Inverse-Square Law Formula

$$\frac{I_1}{I_2} = \frac{(D_2)^2}{(D_1)^2}$$

If the intensity of radiation at an SID of 40 inches is equal to 400 mR, what is the intensity of radiation when the distance is increased to 72 inches?

$$\frac{400\,\text{mR}}{X} = \frac{(72)^2}{(40)^2}; \ 400\,\text{mR} \times 1600 = 640{,}000 = 5184X; \ \frac{640{,}000}{5184} = X; \ 123.5\,\text{mR} = X$$

Because increasing the SID decreases x-ray beam intensity, the mAs must be accordingly increased to maintain proper exposure to the IR. When the SID is decreased, the beam intensity increases; therefore, the mAs must be accordingly decreased to maintain proper exposure to the IR.

 IMPORTANT RELATIONSHIP

SID and mAs

Increasing the SID requires the mAs to be increased to maintain exposure to the IR, and decreasing the SID requires a decrease in the mAs to maintain exposure to the IR.

Maintaining consistent radiation exposure to the IR when the SID is altered requires the mAs to be adjusted to compensate. The **direct square law** or **exposure maintenance formula** provides a mathematical calculation for adjusting the mAs when changing the SID.

 MATHEMATICAL APPLICATION

Direct Square Law or Exposure Maintenance Formula

$$\frac{mAs_1}{mAs_2} = \frac{(SID_1)^2}{(SID_2)^2}$$

Optimal exposure to the IR is achieved at an SID of 40 inches using 25 mAs. The SID must be increased to 72 inches. What adjustment of mAs is needed to maintain exposure to the IR?

$$\frac{25}{X} = \frac{(40)^2}{(72)^2}; 1600X = 129,600; \frac{129,600}{1600}; X = 81mAs_2$$

Standard distances are used in radiography to provide more consistency in radiographic quality. Most diagnostic radiography is performed at an SID of 40, 48, or 72 inches. Certain circumstances, such as trauma or mobile radiography, do not permit the use of standard distances. In these circumstances, the radiographer must determine the change needed in the mAs to obtain a quality radiograph. When a 72-inch (180-cm) SID cannot be used, adjusting the SID to 56 inches (140 cm) requires half the mAs. When a 40-inch (100-cm) SID cannot be used, adjusting the SID to 56 inches (140 cm) requires twice the mAs. This quick method of calculating mAs changes should produce sufficient exposure to the IR.

In addition to altering the intensity of radiation, SID affects size distortion and spatial resolution. As the distance between the source and the IR increases, the diverging x-rays become more perpendicular to the object being radiographed and thus reduce the size distortion (magnification) produced on the image (Fig. 6-12).

 IMPORTANT RELATIONSHIP

SID, Size Distortion, and Spatial Resolution

As SID increases, size distortion (magnification) decreases, and spatial resolution increases; as SID decreases, size distortion (magnification) increases, and spatial resolution decreases.

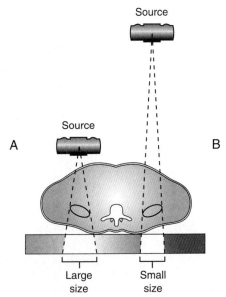

FIG. 6-12 SID and size distortion. **A** and **B,** A long SID creates less magnification than a short SID. The image in *A* is larger than that in *B* because the object is closer to the source.

Standard distances for SID are used in radiography to accommodate equipment limitations. Except for chest and cervical spine radiography, a 40-inch (100-cm) or 48-inch (120-cm) SID is standard. A greater 72-inch (180-cm) SID, such as that used for chest imaging, decreases the magnification of the heart and records its size more accurately. Increasing the SID from the standard distances may be recommended for positions that result in increased OID. For example, increase the SID when imaging the cervical spine between 60 inches (150 cm) and 72 inches (180 cm) for positions that have an increased OID, such as the lateral and oblique positions. Increasing the SID improves spatial resolution.

Object-to-Image-Receptor Distance

When distance is created between the object being radiographed and the IR, known as **object-to-image-receptor distance (OID)**, a decrease in beam intensity may result. As the exit radiation continues to diverge, less overall intensity of the x-ray beam reaches the IR. Decreasing the exposure to the IR may require an increase in the mAs to compensate.

When sufficient distance between the object and IR exists, an air gap is created, also reducing the amount of scatter radiation from striking the IR (Fig. 6-13). Whenever the amount of scatter radiation reaching the IR is reduced, the radiographic contrast is increased. The amount of OID required to increase image contrast depends in part on the percentage of scatter radiation exiting the patient. For anatomic areas that produce a high percentage of scatter radiation, more OID is needed to increase image contrast than for anatomic areas that produce less scatter.

In addition to affecting the intensity of radiation reaching the IR, the OID affects the amount of size distortion (magnification) and spatial resolution. Optimal spatial resolution is achieved when the OID is zero. However, this OID cannot realistically be achieved in radiographic imaging because there is always some distance created between the area of interest and the IR. As the exit beam leaves the patient, it continues to diverge. When distance is created between the area

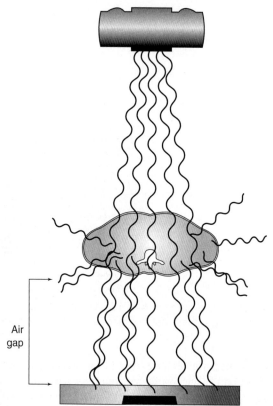

Air gap

FIG. 6-13 Object-to-image-receptor distance (OID) and air gap. The distance created between the object and the IR reduces the amount of scattered radiation reaching the IR.

of interest (within the body) and the IR, the diverging exit beam records the anatomic part with increased size distortion or magnification (Fig. 6-14).

IMPORTANT RELATIONSHIP

OID, Size Distortion, and Spatial Resolution

Increasing the OID increases magnification and decreases the spatial resolution, whereas decreasing the OID decreases magnification and increases the spatial resolution.

OID is a factor that affects the intensity of radiation reaching the IR, image contrast, magnification, and spatial resolution. The distance between the area of interest and the IR has the greatest effect on the amount of size distortion. The radiographer must position the area of interest as close to the IR as possible to minimize the distortion. Although the OID necessary to adversely affect image quality has not been standardized, the radiographer should minimize the OID whenever possible. In certain situations, it is difficult to minimize OID because of factors or conditions beyond the radiographer's control. In these situations, size distortion can still be reduced by increasing the SID.

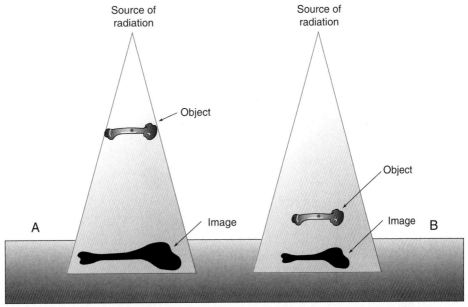

FIG. 6-14 OID and size distortion. **A** and **B,** A long OID creates more magnification than a short OID. The image in *A* is larger than that in *B* because the object is farther from the IR.

Calculating Magnification

To observe the effect of distance (SID and OID) on size distortion, it is necessary to consider the **magnification factor (MF)**. This factor indicates how much size distortion or magnification is demonstrated on a radiographic image. The MF can be mathematically expressed by the following formula:

$$MF = SID \div SOD$$

Source-to-object distance (SOD) refers to the distance from the x-ray source (focal spot) to the object being imaged. SOD can be mathematically expressed as follows:

$$SOD = SID - OID$$

SOD is demonstrated in Fig. 6-15.

An MF of 1 indicates no magnification, meaning that the image size matches the true object size. True object size on an image is impossible to achieve because some magnification exists on every image. MF values greater than 1 can be expressed as percentages of magnification. For example, an MF of 1.15 indicates that the image size is 15% larger than the object size.

▶▶ MATHEMATICAL APPLICATION

Magnification Factor

An anteroposterior projection (AP) of the knee is produced with an SID of 40 inches and an OID of 3 inches (SOD is equal to 37 inches). What is the MF?

$$SOD = SID - OID, \quad MF = \frac{40}{37}; \quad MF = 1.081,$$

$$37 = 40 - 3$$

$$MF = \frac{SID}{SOD}$$

FIG. 6-15 Source-to-object distance (SOD). The SOD is the distance between the source of the x-ray and the object being radiographed.

In the case of the Mathematical Application for MF, an MF of 1.081 means that the image size is 8.1% larger than the true object size. It should be noted that the MF computed here is a minimum. A 3-inch OID implies that the posterior surface of a patient's knee was 3 inches away from the IR for an AP projection. Anatomy that is anterior to the posterior surface of the knee, such as the patella, is farther away from the IR and is magnified even more.

It may be helpful to know the measurement of the true object size in comparison with its size on a radiographic image. After the MF is known, the object size can be determined. This requires the use of another formula:

$$\text{Object size} = \frac{\text{Image size}}{MF}$$

▶ MATHEMATICAL APPLICATION
Determining Object Size

On an AP image of a knee taken with an SID of 40 inches and an OID of 3 inches (SOD = 37 inches), the size of a lesion measures 0.5 inches in diameter on the radiographic image. The MF has been determined to be 1.081. What is the object size of this lesion?

$$\frac{40}{37} = 1.081\,MF \qquad \text{Object size} = \frac{0.5\,\text{inch}}{1.081}$$

The object size is 0.463 inches.

If the sizes of both the object and the image are known, then the percentage of magnification of the object can be calculated by the following formula:

$$\text{Object \% of magnification} = \frac{\text{Image size} - \text{Object size}}{\text{Object size}} \times 100$$

MATHEMATICAL APPLICATION

Determining Object % of Magnification

A lesion on the radiographic image measures 1.16 cm and the lesion's (object's) true size measures 1.06 cm. What is the object % of magnification?

$$\text{Object \% of magnification} = \frac{1.16 - 1.06}{1.06 \text{ cm}} = 100$$

$$\frac{0.10}{1.06} = 0.09434 \times 100 = 9.43 \text{ \% Object magnification}$$

Perhaps the most practical use of these formulas is to observe how changing the SID and OID affects the image size. Size distortion or magnification can be increased by decreasing the SID or increasing the OID. This increase in magnification can be mathematically demonstrated using the MF and then calculating the change in the size of the object on the radiographic image. Any time magnification is increased, spatial resolution decreases.

Central Ray Alignment

Shape distortion of the anatomic area of interest can occur from inaccurate central ray (CR) alignment of the x-ray tube, the part being radiographed, or the IR. Any misalignment of the CR among these three factors alters the shape of the part recorded on the image.

For example, Fig. 6-16 demonstrates shape distortion when the anatomic part and the IR are misaligned. In addition, shape distortion can occur if the CR of the primary beam is not directed to enter or exit the anatomy as required for the particular projection or position (off centering). This shape distortion occurs because the path of individual photons in the primary beam becomes more divergent as the distance increases from the CR. The radiographer must properly control alignment of the x-ray tube, part, and IR, and he or she must properly direct the CR to minimize shape distortion. In addition to creating shape distortion, CR angulation and misalignment of the tube, part, and IR could affect the exposure to the IR. For example, when the CR is angled, the distance between the source of the radiation and the IR is increased. Generally, when the CR is angled, the SID is accordingly decreased to maintain exposure to the IR. If misalignment occurs among the tube, part, or IR, the distance between the source of radiation and the IR or the part, and the IR could be increased or decreased. This change could affect the amount of exposure to the IR, and the mAs may need adjustment.

Grids

A radiographic grid is a device that is placed between the part of interest and the IR to absorb scatter radiation exiting the patient. Limiting the amount of scatter radiation that reaches the IR improves the quality of the image. Much of the scatter radiation exiting the patient does not reach the IR when absorbed by a grid (Fig. 6-17). The effect of less scatter, or unwanted exposure, on the image is to increase the radiographic contrast. Grids are typically used only when the anatomic part is 10 cm (4 inches) or greater in thickness, and more than 60 kVp is needed for the exam.

IMPORTANT RELATIONSHIP

Grids, Scatter, and Contrast

Placing a grid between the anatomic part and the IR absorbs scatter radiation exiting the patient and increases radiographic contrast.

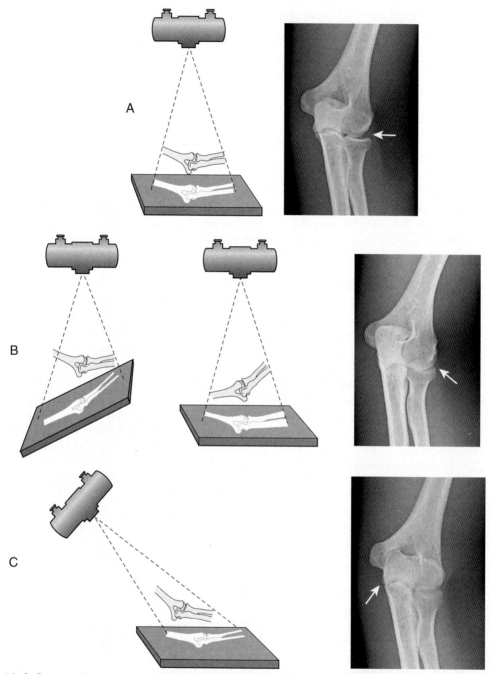

FIG. 6-16 A, Proper alignment among the x-ray tube, part, and IR. This is a quality image with minimal distortion. Note the proper alignment of the radial head with the capitulum in the image. **B,** Improper alignment among the x-ray tube, part, and IR. The illustration on the *left* shows the IR misaligned to the part, and the one on the *right* shows the part not parallel to the IR. This image has a distorted shape because of misalignment of the part and IR. Note the improper alignment of the radial head with the capitulum in the image. **C,** Improper alignment among the x-ray tube, part, and IR. This image has shape distortion because of the central ray not being perpendicular to the part. Note the elongation of the olecranon process. (From Johnston JN, Fauber TL: *Essentials of Radiographic Physics and Imaging,* ed 2, St. Louis, 2016, Mosby.)

Primary
x-ray beam

Scatter radiation
hits the lead strip
and is absorbed

Grid

Image receptor

FIG. 6-17 Grids and scatter absorption. When a grid is used, much of the scatter radiation toward the IR is absorbed. (From Johnston JN, Fauber TL: *Essentials of Radiographic Physics and Imaging*, ed 3, St. Louis, 2020, Mosby.)

The more efficient a grid is in absorbing scatter, the greater is its effect on radiographic contrast. Grids also absorb a certain amount of the transmitted radiation exiting the patient and therefore reduce the amount of radiation reaching the IR.

IMPORTANT RELATIONSHIP
Grids and IR Exposure

Adding, removing, or changing a grid requires an adjustment in mAs to maintain radiation exposure to the IR.

When grids are used, the mAs must be adjusted to maintain exposure to the IR. In addition, the more efficient a grid is in absorbing scatter, the greater is the increase in mAs. The grid conversion formula is a mathematical formula for adjusting the mAs for changes in the type of grid.

When a grid is added, the radiographer must multiply the mAs by the correct grid conversion factor (Table 6.1) to compensate for the decrease in exposure. When a grid is removed, the mAs must be divided by the correct conversion grid factor to compensate for the increase in exposure. When the grid ratio is changed, the following formula should be used to adjust the exposure:

$$\frac{mAs_1}{mAs_2} = \frac{\text{Grid conversion factor}_1}{\text{Grid conversion factor}_2}$$

TABLE 6-1 Grid Conversion Chart	
Grid Ratios	**Grid Conversion Factor (GCF)**
No grid	1
5:1	2
6:1	3
8:1	4
12:1	5
16:1	6

▶▶ MATHEMATICAL APPLICATION
Adjusting mAs for Changes in the Grid

A quality radiographic image is obtained using 5 mAs at 70 kVp without using a grid. What new mAs is needed when adding a 12:1 grid to maintain the same exposure to the IR?

$$\frac{5\,mAs}{X} = \frac{1}{5}; 1X = 25; X = 25\,mAs$$

The new mAs produces an exposure comparable to the IR without the grid.

❗ RADIATION PROTECTION ALERT
Grid Selection

Decisions regarding the use of a grid and grid ratio should be made by balancing image quality and patient protection. To keep patient exposure as low as reasonable, grids should be used only when appropriate, and the grid ratio should be the lowest that would provide sufficient contrast improvement.

It is important to note that brightness can be computer adjusted when the mAs is not properly adjusted for adding or changing a grid (Fig. 6-18). However, without proper mAs adjustment when adding or changing a grid, increased quantum noise or unnecessary patient radiation exposure could be the result.

Grid construction and efficiency are discussed in greater detail in Chapter 7.

Beam Restriction

Any change in the size of the x-ray field alters the amount of tissue irradiated. A larger field size (decreasing collimation) increases the amount of tissue irradiated, causing more scatter radiation to be produced, thus increasing the amount of radiation reaching the IR. The increased amount of scatter (fog) reaching the IR results in less radiographic contrast. Conversely, a smaller field size (increasing collimation) reduces the amount of tissue irradiated, the amount of scatter radiation produced, and the amount of radiation reaching the IR. The decreased amount of scatter radiation reaching the IR results in higher radiographic contrast but requires an increase in the mAs. The effect of collimation is greater when imaging large anatomic areas, performing examinations without a grid, and using a high kVp.

FIG. 6-18 A, A quality image created without a grid. **B,** An image created with a grid but no adjustment in mAs. This image has higher contrast but increased quantum noise visible. **C,** Image created with a grid and appropriate mAs adjustment. This image has higher contrast than image *A* and less quantum noise visible than image *B*. (From Johnston JN, Fauber TL: *Essentials of Radiographic Physics and Imaging*, ed 3, St. Louis, 2020, Elsevier.)

IMPORTANT RELATIONSHIP
Beam Restriction and IR Exposure

Changes in beam restriction alter the amount of tissue irradiated and therefore affect the amount of exposure to the IR. The effect of collimation is greater when imaging large anatomic areas, performing examinations without a grid, and using a high kVp.

! RADIATION PROTECTION ALERT
Beam Restriction

In performing a radiographic examination, the radiographer should be aware of the anatomic area of interest and limit the x-ray field size to just beyond this area. Collimating to the appropriate field size is a basic method for protecting patients from unnecessary exposure.

Generator Output

Exposure techniques and radiation output depend on the type of generator used. Generators with more efficient output, such as three-phase or high-frequency units, require lower exposure technique settings to produce an image comparable with single-phase units (Fig. 6-19). The radiographer must be aware of the generator output when using different types of equipment, especially when performing examinations in different departments. For example, imaging a knee using a

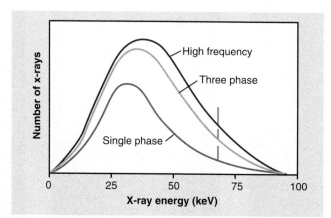

FIG. 6-19 Generators and radiation output. The quantity (amplitude) and the quality (shift to the right) of the x-ray beam are increased when using high-frequency and three-phase generators because they are more efficient in x-ray production. (From Johnston JN, Fauber TL: *Essentials of Radiographic Physics and Imaging*, ed 2, St. Louis, 2016, Mosby.)

FIG. 6-20 Tube filtration and radiation output. Increasing beam filtration decreases the quantity (amplitude) and increases the quality (shift to the right) of the x-ray beam. *Al*, Aluminum. (From Johnston JN, Fauber TL: *Essentials of Radiographic Physics and Imaging*, ed 2, St. Louis, 2016, Mosby.)

single-phase generator requires more mAs than imaging a knee using a three-phase generator. In addition, x-ray generators must be periodically calibrated to ensure that they are producing consistent radiation output.

Tube Filtration

Small variations in the amount of tube filtration should not have any effect on radiographic quality. Variability of the x-ray tube filtration should be checked as a part of routine quality control checks on the radiographic equipment. X-ray tubes with excessive or insufficient filtration may affect image quality. Increasing the amount of tube filtration increases the ratio of higher-penetrating x-rays to lower-penetrating x-rays. As a result, the average energy of the x-ray beam has been increased and can increase the amount of scatter radiation reaching the IR. The increased x-ray energy (kVp) and scatter production decrease radiographic contrast. In addition, increasing the tube filtration decreases the quantity of radiation reaching the patient (Fig. 6-20). Insufficient tube filtration increases the quantity of radiation and decreases the ratio of higher-penetrating x-rays to lower-penetrating x-rays. As a result, the average energy of the x-ray beam has been decreased, which can decrease the amount of scattered radiation reaching the IR. The decreased x-ray energy (kVp) and scatter production increase radiographic contrast. The amount of tube filtration should not vary greatly, and therefore, small changes would not have a visible effect on radiographic contrast.

 IMPORTANT RELATIONSHIP
Tube Filtration, Radiation Quantity, and Average Energy

Increasing tube filtration decreases radiation quantity and increases the average energy of the x-ray beam. Decreasing tube filtration increases radiation quantity and decreases the average energy of the x-ray beam.

Compensating Filters

When imaging an anatomic area that varies greatly in tissue thickness, a compensating filter (discussed in Chapter 2) can be placed in the primary beam to produce a more uniform exposure to the IR. The use of compensating filters requires an increase in the mAs to maintain the overall exposure to the IR. The amount of increase in the mAs depends on the thickness and type of compensating filter. In addition, the use of a compensating filter increases the exposure to the patient and is not typically used in routine radiography.

PATIENT FACTORS

Body Habitus

Body habitus refers to the general form or build of the body, including its size. It is important for the radiographer to consider body habitus when establishing exposure techniques. There are generally four types of body habitus: sthenic, hyposthenic, hypersthenic, and asthenic (Fig. 6-21).

The sthenic body habitus is commonly called a *normal* or *average* build. The hyposthenic type refers to a similar type of body habitus as sthenic but with a tendency toward a more slender and taller build. Together, the sthenic and hyposthenic types of body habitus are, in terms of establishing radiographic techniques, classified as *normal* or *average* for the adult population.

Hypersthenic and asthenic body habitus types are more extreme. The hypersthenic body habitus refers to a large, stocky build. These individuals have thicker part sizes compared with sthenic or hyposthenic individuals, so the exposure factors for their radiographic examinations are higher.

Asthenic refers to a very slender body habitus, and exposure factors for asthenic individuals are at the low end of technique charts because their respective part sizes are thinner than those of sthenic and hyposthenic individuals.

Part Thickness

The thickness of the anatomic part being imaged affects the amount of x-ray beam attenuation that occurs. A thick part absorbs more radiation, whereas a thin part transmits more radiation. Maintaining the exposure to the IR when imaging a thicker part requires the mAs to be accordingly increased (Fig. 6-22). In addition, when a thinner anatomic part is being radiographed, the mAs must be accordingly decreased.

Because x-rays are exponentially attenuated, a general guideline is that for every change in part thickness of 4 to 5 cm (1.6–2 inches), the radiographer should adjust the mAs by a factor

FIG. 6-21 Four types of body habitus. (From Johnston JN, Fauber TL: *Essentials of Radiographic Physics and Imaging*, ed 2, St. Louis, 2016, Mosby.)

FIG. 6-22 **A**, A quality image. **B**, Image created with added thickness and no mAs adjustment, which results in increased quantum noise visible. **C**, Image created with added patient thickness and appropriate mAs adjustment, which results in decreased quantum noise visible. (From Johnston JN, Fauber TL: *Essentials of Radiographic Physics and Imaging*, ed 3, St. Louis, 2020, Elsevier, Inc.)

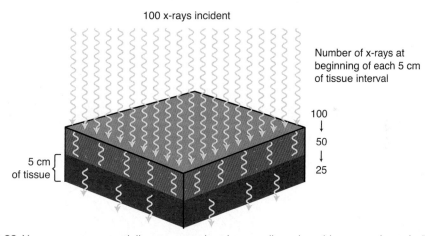

FIG. 6-23 X-rays are exponentially attenuated and generally reduced by approximately 50% for each 4 to 5 cm (1.6–2 inches) of tissue thickness. (From Johnston JN, Fauber TL: *Essentials of Radiographic Physics and Imaging*, ed 2, St. Louis, 2016, Mosby.)

of 2 (Fig. 6-23). For example, an optimal image is obtained using 20 mAs on an anatomic part measuring 18 cm (7 inches). The same anatomic part is radiographed in another similar patient and it measures 23 cm (9 inches). What new mAs is needed to expose the IR? Because the part thickness increased by 5 cm (2 inches), the original mAs is multiplied by 2, yielding 40 mAs. If the same part in another patient measures 28 cm (11 inches), what new mAs is needed? Because the part thickness increased by another 5 cm (2 inches), the mAs is multiplied by 2, yielding 80 mAs. This mAs is four times greater than that for the original patient's anatomic part, which measured 10 cm (4 inches) less.

As the thickness of a given type of anatomic tissue increases, the amount of scattered radiation increases, and radiographic contrast decreases. Using a higher kVp for a thicker part only adds to the increase in scatter radiation. Increased scatter radiation would continue degrading the quality of the image because it creates fog, which decreases the contrast.

The amount of radiographic contrast achieved is also influenced by the composition of the anatomic part to be radiographed. As mentioned in Chapter 3, subject contrast is a category of radiographic contrast. The thickness of the tissue, effective atomic number, and cell compactness (tissue density) affect its absorption characteristics. The absorption characteristics of the anatomic tissue create the brightness levels produced on a radiographic image. Tissues that have a higher effective atomic number absorb more radiation than tissues with a lower effective atomic number.

Anatomic structures having a wide range of tissue compositions, varying in parameters such as effective atomic number and tissue density, demonstrate high subject contrast (Fig. 6-24). Anatomic structures consisting of a similar type of tissue demonstrate low subject contrast (Fig. 6-25). The radiographer cannot control the composition of the anatomic part to be radiographed. Changing the kVp alters its absorption and transmission within anatomic tissues. Knowledge about the absorption characteristics of anatomic tissues and the effect of kVp helps the radiographer produce a desired level of radiographic contrast.

The quality of a radiographic image depends on a multitude of variables. Knowledge of these variables and their radiographic effect assists the radiographer in producing quality radiographs. Table 6.2 summarizes common exposure technique mathematical calculations. Table 6.3 is a chart demonstrating how the variables discussed in this chapter affect the primary beam and IR exposure, and Table 6.4 is a chart demonstrating how the variables discussed in this chapter affect image quality.

Higher contrast

FIG. 6-24 Higher subject contrast resulting from great differences in radiation absorption between tissues that vary greatly in composition.

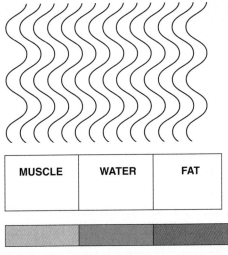

Lower contrast

FIG. 6-25 Lower subject contrast resulting from fewer differences in radiation absorption between tissues that are more similarly composed.

TABLE 6-2	**Exposure Technique Mathematical Calculations.**	
Exposure Technique Factor	**Relationship to Maintain Exposure to Image Receptor**	**Formula**
mAs	↑ mA and ↓ second	mA × second = mAs
kVp: 15% rule	↑ kVp and ↓ mAs	kVp × 1.15 and mAs/2 kVp × .85 and mAs × 2
Direct square law or exposure maintenance formula	↑ SID and ↑ mAs	$\dfrac{mAs_1}{mAs_2} = \dfrac{(SID_1)^2}{(SID_2)^2}$
Grid conversion factor (GCF): No grid = 1 5:1 = 2 6:1 = 3 8:1 = 4 12:1 = 5 16:1 = 6	↑ Grid ratio and ↑ mAs	$\dfrac{mAs_1}{mAs_2} = \dfrac{GCF_1}{GCF_2}$
Magnification factor (MF)	↑ OID and ↓ SID will ↑ magnification	$MF = \dfrac{SID}{SOD}$ $Object\ size = \dfrac{Image\ size}{MF}$ Image size = Object size × MF
Patient thickness	↑ Thickness and ↑ mAs	Every 4- to 5-cm change in thickness change mAs by a factor of 2

kVP, Kilovoltage peak; *mAs,* milliamperage-seconds; *OID,* object-to-image-receptor distance; *SID,* source-to-image-receptor distance; *SOD,* source-to-object distance.

TABLE 6-3 **Exposure Factors and Their Effects on the Primary and Remnant X-ray Beams**

	Primary Beam Reaching the Patient	Remnant Beam Reaching the Image Receptor
mAs		
Increasing mAs	↑ Quantity	↑ Quantity
Decreasing mAs	↓ Quantity	↓ Quantity
kVp		
Increasing kVp	↑ Quantity and quality	↑ Quantity and quality
Decreasing kVp	↓ Quantity and quality	↓ Quantity and quality
Focal Spot Size		
Smaller focal spot size	No effect	No effect
Larger focal spot size	No effect	No effect
SID		
Increasing SID	↓ Quantity	↓ Quantity
Decreasing SID	↑ Quantity	↑ Quantity
OID		
Increasing OID	No effect	↓ Quantity and scatter
Decreasing OID	No effect	↑ Quantity and scatter
CR Angle		
Increase CR Angle[a]	↓ Quantity	↓ Quantity
Grid		
Increasing grid ratio	No effect	↓ Quantity and scatter
Decreasing grid ratio	No effect	↑ Quantity and scatter
Beam Restriction		
Increasing collimation	↓ Quantity	↓ Quantity and scatter
Decreasing collimation	↑ Quantity	↑ Quantity and scatter
Generator Output		
Single-phase generator	↓ Quantity and quality	↓ Quantity and quality
High-frequency generator	↑ Quantity and quality	↑ Quantity and quality
Tube Filtration		
Adding Filtration	↓ Quantity and ↑ average energy	↓ Quantity and ↑ average energy
Removing Filtration	↑ Quantity and ↓ average energy	↑ Quantity and ↓ average energy
Compensating Filter		
Adding a compensating filter	↓ Quantity	↓ Quantity
Part Thickness		
Increasing part thickness	No effect	↓ Quantity
Decreasing part thickness	No effect	↑ Quantity

[a]Without a decrease in source-to-image-receptor distance (SID).
CR, Central ray; *kVP,* kilovoltage peak; mA, milliamperage; *mAs,* milliamperage-seconds; *OID,* object-to-image-receptor distance; *SID,* source-to-image-receptor distance.

TABLE 6-4 Exposure Technique Factors and Image Quality

INDIVIDUAL FACTOR CHANGE WITHOUT EXPOSURE TECHNIQUE COMPENSATION RESULTING IN A DIAGNOSTIC IMAGE

Exposure Factor	IR Exposure	Brightness[a]	Contrast[a,b]	Spatial Resolution	Distortion
mAs					
Increase	Increase	No effect	No effect	No effect	No effect
Decrease	Decrease	No effect	No effect	No effect	No effect
kVp[c]					
Increase	Increase	No effect	Decrease	No effect	No effect
Decrease	Decrease	No effect	Increase	No effect	No effect
Focal Spot Size					
Increase	No effect	No effect	No effect	Decrease	No effect
Decrease	No effect	No effect	No effect	Increase	No effect
SID					
Increase	Decrease	No effect	No effect	Increase	– Magnification
Decrease	Increase	No effect	No effect	Decrease	+ Magnification
OID					
Increase	Decrease	No effect	Increase[d]	Decrease	+ Magnification
Central Ray Angle					
Increase	Decrease	No effect	No effect	Decrease	+ Shape distortion
Grid Use					
Add grid	Decrease	No effect	Increase	No effect	No effect
Remove grid	Increase	No effect	Decrease	No effect	No effect
Collimation					
Increase	Decrease	No effect	Increase	No effect	No effect
Decrease	Increase	No effect	Decrease	No effect	No effect
Tube Filtration					
Excessive	Decrease	No effect	Decrease	No effect	No effect
Insufficient	Increase	No effect	Increase	No effect	No effect
Patient Thickness					
Increase	Decrease	No effect	Decrease	Decrease	+ Magnification
Decrease	Increase	No effect	Increase	Increase	– Magnification
Patient Motion	No effect	No effect	No effect	Decrease	No effect

[a] Brightness and contrast can be adjusted by the computer.
[b] Increase is higher contrast, and decrease is lower contrast.
[c] Kilovoltage peak (kVp) affects subject contrast.
[d] Increase (higher) contrast because of less scatter reaching image rector; effect dependent on anatomic region, thickness, and amount of object-to-image-receptor distance (OID).

IR, Image receptor; *mAs,* milliamperage-seconds; *SID,* source-to-image-receptor distance.

CHAPTER SUMMARY

- The product of mA and exposure time (mAs) is directly proportional to the quantity of x-rays produced and exposure to the IR.
- The mA and exposure time have an inverse relationship to maintain exposure to the IR.
- The kVp changes the penetrating power of the x-ray beam and has a direct effect on exposure to the IR.
- Changing the kVp by 15% has the same effect on exposure to the IR as changing the mAs by a factor of 2.
- A numerical value or exposure indicator is displayed on the processed digital image that indicates the level of x-ray exposure received (incident exposure) on the IR.
- The kVp has an inverse relationship with subject contrast: a high kVp creates an image with low subject contrast, and a low kVp creates an image with high subject contrast.
- Brightness and contrast are primarily controlled by computer processing in digital imaging.
- Focal spot size affects only spatial resolution. A smaller focal spot size increases spatial resolution.
- SID has an inverse squared relationship with the intensity of radiation reaching the patient and the IR.
- Increasing OID decreases exposure to the IR.
- Decreasing SID and increasing OID increases size distortion (magnification) and decreases spatial resolution.
- Grids absorb the scatter radiation exiting the patient and increase radiographic contrast.
- Beam restriction affects the amount of tissue irradiated, scatter produced, and exposure to the IR.
- Changes in SID, grids, and patient thickness require a change in mAs to maintain the exposure to the IR.
- Generators with more efficient output, such as three-phase or high-frequency generators, require lower exposure techniques to produce the same exposure to the IR as a single-phase generator.
- Excessive or insufficient tube filtration affects the exposure to the IR and contrast.
- Exposure factors may need to be modified for body habitus and part thickness.

REVIEW QUESTIONS

1. Which of the following is accurate regarding the relationship between milliamperage (mA) and exposure time to maintain the exposure to the image receptor (IR)?
   A. Direct proportional
   B. Direct
   C. Inverse
   D. Inverse proportional

2. The exposure indicator value reflects excessive exposure to the IR. Which of the following is the best for correcting the exposure error?
   A. Decrease kVp by 50%
   B. Increase mAs by 15%
   C. Decrease mAs by 50%
   D. Decrease mAs by 15%

3. What exposure factor affects both the quality and the quantity of the x-ray beam?
   A. kVp
   B. SID
   C. mA
   D. Focal spot size

4. Which of the following is not affected by kilovoltage?
   A. Compton interactions
   B. Spatial resolution
   C. Subject contrast
   D. Radiation quantity

5. Increasing the mAs has _____ effect on brightness displayed in digital imaging.
   A. a direct
   B. a proportional
   C. an inverse
   D. no

6. Which of the following would maintain radiation exposure to the IR when the kilovoltage is decreased by 15%?
   A. Increase mAs by 15%.
   B. Increase mAs by 50%.
   C. Double the mAs.
   D. Halve the mAs.

7. A quality image is produced using 70 kVp and 25 mAs at a 40-inch SID. What calculated change in the exposure technique is necessary to maintain radiation exposure to the IR when the SID is increased to 56 inches?
   A. 60 kVp at 25 mAs
   B. 70 kVp at 12.5 mAs
   C. 70 kVp at 50 mAs
   D. 60 kVp at 50 mAs

8. Without exposure technique compensation, increasing the OID by 4 for a knee film image would
   1. increase magnification.
   2. decrease exposure to IR.
   3. increase contrast.
      A. 1 and 2 only
      B. 1 and 3 only
      C. 2 and 3 only
      D. 1, 2, and 3

9. A quality image is produced using 80 kVp at 10 mAs with a 6:1 ratio grid. Calculate the change in exposure technique to maintain radiation exposure to the IR when changing to a 12:1 ratio grid.
   A. 80 kVp at 17 mAs
   B. 68 kVp at 20 mAs
   C. 80 kVp at 6 mAs
   D. 92 kVp at 5 mAs

10. Which of the following factors does not affect spatial resolution?
    A. Focal spot size
    B. SID
    C. OID
    D. Grid

11. Which of the following factors does not affect the radiation exposure to the IR?
    A. Collimation
    B. Focal spot size
    C. Compensating filters
    D. Body habitus

12. What exposure factor change is recommended to maintain radiation exposure to the IR when increasing the patient thickness by 5 cm?
    A. Double the kVp
    B. Double the mAs
    C. Decrease kVp by 15%
    D. Increase mAs by 15%

Scatter Control

CHAPTER OUTLINE

OBJECTIVES

After completing this chapter, the reader will be able to perform the following:

1. Define all the key terms in this chapter.
2. State all the important relationships in this chapter.
3. Explain how scatter radiation affects radiographic images.
4. State the purpose of beam-restricting devices.
5. Describe each type of beam-restricting device.
6. State the purpose of automatic collimators or positive beam-limiting devices.
7. Describe the purpose of a radiographic grid.
8. Describe the construction of grids, including the different types of grid patterns, dimensions, and grid focus.
9. Calculate grid ratio.
10. List the various types of stationary grids and describe the function and purpose of a moving grid.
11. Demonstrate the use of the grid conversion formula.
12. Describe the different types of grid alignment errors that can occur to cause grid cutoff.
13. Identify the factors to be considered in using a grid.
14. Recognize how beam restriction and the use of grids affect patient radiation exposure.
15. Explain the air gap technique and describe its use.

KEY TERMS

air gap technique
aperture diaphragm
automatic collimator
beam-restricting device
beam restriction
Bucky

Bucky factor
collimation
collimator
cone
convergent line
convergent point

crossed grid
crosshatched grid
cylinder
focal distance
focal range
focused grid

KEY TERMS—cont'd

grid	grid frequency	moiré effect
grid cap	grid pattern	nonfocused grid
grid cassette	grid ratio	parallel grid
grid conversion factor (GCF)	interspace material	positive beam-limiting device
grid cutoff	linear grid	short dimension
grid focus	long dimension	wafer grid

Controlling the amount of scatter radiation produced in a patient and ultimately reaching the image receptor (IR) is essential for creating a good-quality image. Scatter radiation is detrimental to radiographic quality because it adds unwanted exposure (fog) to the image without adding any patient information.

Digital IRs are sensitive to lower-energy levels of radiation such as scatter, which results in increased fog in the image and decreases radiographic contrast. However, image contrast can be computer manipulated by changing the window width. Increased scatter radiation, produced within the patient and the higher-energy scatter exiting the patient, affects the exposure to the patient and anyone within close proximity. The radiographer must act to minimize the amount of scatter radiation reaching the IR.

Beam-restricting devices and radiographic grids are tools that the radiographer can use to limit the amount of scatter radiation reaching the IR. Beam-restricting devices decrease the x-ray-beam field size and the amount of tissue irradiated, thereby reducing the amount of scatter radiation produced. Radiographic grids are used to improve radiographic image quality by absorbing scatter radiation exiting the patient, thereby reducing the amount of scatter reaching the IR. It should be noted that grids do nothing to prevent scatter *production*; they merely reduce the amount of scatter reaching the IR after scatter radiation is produced.

SCATTER RADIATION

Scatter radiation, as described in Chapter 3, is primarily the result of Compton interactions, in which an incoming x-ray photon loses energy and changes direction. Two major factors affect the amount and energy of scatter radiation exiting the patient: kilovoltage peak (kVp) and the volume of irradiated tissue. The volume of irradiated tissue depends on the thickness of the part and the x-ray-beam field size. Increasing the volume of irradiated tissue results in increased scatter production because there are more atoms available for Compton interactions. In addition, using a higher kVp increases x-ray transmission and reduces its overall absorption (photoelectric interactions); however, higher kVp increases the percentage of Compton interactions and the energy of scatter radiation exiting the patient. Using higher kVp or increasing the volume of irradiated tissue results in increased scatter radiation exiting the patient.

 IMPORTANT RELATIONSHIP

kVp and Scatter

The amount and energy of scatter radiation exiting the patient depends, in part, on the kVp selected. Examinations using higher kVp produce a greater proportion of higher-energy scattered x-rays than examinations using low kVp.

IMPORTANT RELATIONSHIP

X-ray-Beam Field Size, Thickness of the Part, and Scatter

The larger the x-ray-beam field size, the greater the amount of scatter radiation produced. The thicker the part being imaged, the greater the amount of scatter radiation produced.

IMPORTANT RELATIONSHIP

Volume of Tissue Irradiated and Scatter

The volume of tissue irradiated is affected by both the part thickness and the x-ray-beam field size. Therefore, the greater the volume of tissue irradiated, because of either or both factors, the greater the amount of scatter radiation produced.

BEAM RESTRICTION

It is the responsibility of the radiographer to limit the x-ray-beam field size to the anatomic area of interest. Beam restriction serves two purposes: limiting patient exposure and reducing the amount of scatter radiation produced within the patient.

The unrestricted primary beam is cone shaped and projects a round field onto the patient and IR (Fig. 7-1). If not restricted in some way, the primary beam goes beyond the boundaries of the

FIG. 7-1 The unrestricted primary beam is cone shaped, projecting a circular field. **A,** Side view. **B,** View from above.

FIG. 7-2 A, Full view of the abdomen with decreased collimation when compared with *B*. **B**, Increased collimation of the abdominal region to image the lumbar spine. (From Bontrager K, Lapignano J: *Textbook of Radiographic Positioning and Related Anatomy*, ed 7, St. Louis, 2010, Elsevier.)

IR, resulting in unnecessary patient exposure. Any time the x-ray field extends beyond the anatomic area of interest, the patient receives unnecessary exposure. Limiting the x-ray-beam field size is accomplished with a **beam-restricting device**. Located just below the x-ray tube housing, the beam-restricting device changes the shape and size of the primary beam.

The terms **beam restriction** and **collimation** are used interchangeably; they refer to a decrease in the size of the projected radiation field. The term *collimation* is used more often than the term *beam restriction* because collimators are the most popular type of beam-restricting device. Increasing collimation means decreasing the field size, and decreasing collimation means increasing the field size (Fig. 7-2).

IMPORTANT RELATIONSHIP
Beam Restriction and Patient Dose

As beam restriction or collimation increases, the field size and patient dose decrease. As beam restriction or collimation decreases, the field size and patient dose increase.

! RADIATION PROTECTION ALERT
Appropriate Beam Restriction

In performing a radiographic examination, the radiographer should be aware of the anatomic area of interest and limit the x-ray field size to just beyond this area. Collimating to the appropriate field size is a basic method for protecting patients from unnecessary exposure.

BEAM RESTRICTION AND SCATTER RADIATION

In addition to decreasing the patient dose, beam-restricting devices reduce the amount of scatter radiation produced within the patient and reduce the amount of scatter to which the IR is exposed, thereby increasing radiographic contrast. The relationship between collimation (field size) and the

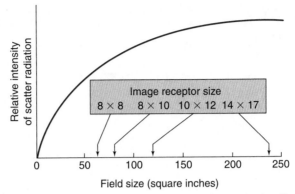

FIG. 7-3 As field size increases, the relative quantity of scattered radiation increases.

quantity of scatter radiation is illustrated in Fig. 7-3. As previously stated, collimation means decreasing the size of the projected x-ray field; hence, increasing collimation means decreasing x-ray field size, and decreasing collimation means increasing x-ray field size.

 IMPORTANT RELATIONSHIP

Collimation and Scatter Radiation

As collimation increases, the x-ray field size and quantity of scatter radiation decrease; as collimation decreases, the x-ray field size and quantity of scatter radiation increase.

Collimation and Contrast

Because collimation decreases the x-ray-beam field size, less scatter radiation is produced within the patient, and hence, less scatter radiation reaches the IR. As described in Chapter 3, this affects the radiographic contrast.

 IMPORTANT RELATIONSHIP

Collimation and Radiographic Contrast

As collimation increases, the quantity of scatter radiation decreases and radiographic contrast increases; as collimation decreases, the quantity of scatter radiation increases, and radiographic contrast decreases.

Compensating for Collimation

Increasing the collimation decreases the volume of tissue irradiated, the amount of scatter radiation produced, the number of photons that strike the patient, and the number of x-ray photons that reach the IR to produce the latent image. As a result, the exposure-technique factors (kVp, milliamperage-seconds [mAs], or both) may need to be increased when increasing collimation to maintain exposure to the IR.

 IMPORTANT RELATIONSHIP

Collimation and Exposure to the Image Receptor

As collimation increases, exposure to the IR decreases; as collimation decreases, exposure to the IR increases.

TABLE 7-1   Restricting the Primary Beam

Increased Factor	Result
Collimation	Patient dose *decreases*
	Scatter radiation *decreases*
	Radiographic contrast *increases*
	Exposure to the image receptor *decreases*
X-ray field size	Patient dose *increases*
	Scatter radiation *increases*
	Radiographic contrast *decreases*
	Exposure to the image receptor *increases*

It has been recommended that significant collimation requires the mAs to be increased by 30% to 50% to compensate for the decrease in IR exposure. Post-exposure electronic masking or cropping of the displayed digital image is a feature available at the radiographer's workstation. However, post-exposure electronic masking should never replace pre-exposure collimation because it does not reduce scatter production, improve image contrast, or reduce patient radiation exposure.

Important relationships regarding the restriction of the primary beam are summarized in Table 7-1.

> **⚠ RADIATION PROTECTION ALERT**
>
> ***Post-exposure Electronic Masking or Cropping***
>
> Post-exposure electronic masking or cropping the displayed image should never replace pre-exposure collimation because it does not reduce scatter production, reduce patient radiation exposure, or increase image contrast.

TYPES OF BEAM-RESTRICTING DEVICES

Several types of beam-restricting devices, which differ in sophistication and utility, are available. Most beam-restricting devices are made of metal or a combination of metals that readily absorb x-rays.

Aperture Diaphragms

The simplest type of beam-restricting device is the aperture diaphragm. An **aperture diaphragm** is a flat piece of lead (diaphragm) that contains a hole (aperture). Commercially made aperture diaphragms are available (Fig. 7-4), or hospitals can make their own for purposes specific to a radiographic unit. Aperture diaphragms are easy to use; they are placed directly below the x-ray tube window. An aperture diaphragm can be made by cutting rubberized lead into the size needed to create the diaphragm and cutting a hole of the appropriate shape and size into the center to create the aperture.

Although the size and shape of the aperture can be changed, the aperture cannot be adjusted from the designed size, and therefore, the projected x-ray field size is not adjustable. In addition, because of the aperture's proximity to the radiation source (focal spot), a large area of unsharpness surrounds the radiographic image (Fig. 7-5). Although aperture diaphragms are still used in some applications, their use is not as widespread as other types of beam-restricting devices.

FIG. 7-4 Commercially made aperture diaphragm.

FIG. 7-5 Radiographic image unsharpness using an aperture diaphragm.

Cones and Cylinders

Cones and cylinders are shaped differently (Fig. 7-6), but they have many similar attributes. A **cone** or **cylinder** is essentially an aperture diaphragm that has an extended flange attached to it. The flange can vary in length and can be shaped as either a cone or a cylinder. The flange can also be made to telescope, increasing its total length (Fig. 7-7). Like aperture diaphragms, cones and cylinders are easy to use but generally not in use today. They slide onto the tube, directly below the window. Cones and cylinders limit the unsharpness surrounding radiographic images more than aperture diaphragms do, with cylinders accomplishing this task slightly better

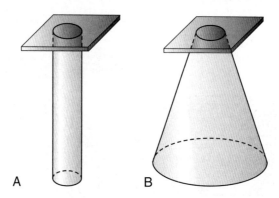

FIG. 7-6 A, Cylinder. **B,** Cone.

FIG. 7-7 Telescoping cylinder. (From *Mosby's Radiographic Instructional Series: Radiographic Imaging,* St. Louis, 1998, Mosby.)

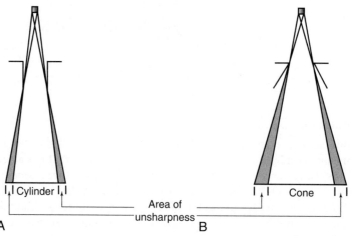

FIG. 7-8 A cylinder (**A**) is better at limiting unsharpness than a cone (**B**).

FIG. 7-9 Radiograph of the frontal and maxillary sinuses not using a cone (**A**) and using a cone (**B**). (From *Mosby's Radiographic Instructional Series: Radiographic Imaging*, St. Louis, 1998, Mosby.)

than cones (Fig. 7-8). However, they are limited in terms of available sizes, and they are not interchangeable among tube housings. Cones have a disadvantage compared with cylinders: if the angle of the flange of the cone is greater than the angle of divergence of the primary beam, the base plate or aperture diaphragm of the cone is the only metal restricting the primary beam. Therefore, cylinders generally were more useful than cones. Cones and cylinders are almost always made to produce a circular projected field and were advantageously used for some radiographic procedures (Fig. 7-9).

Collimators

The most sophisticated, useful, and accepted type of beam-restricting device for radiography today is the **collimator**. Beam restriction accomplished with the use of a collimator is referred to as *collimation*. The terms *collimation* and *beam restriction* are used interchangeably.

A collimator has two or three sets of lead shutters (Fig. 7-10). Located immediately below the tube window, the entrance shutters limit the x-ray beam much as the aperture diaphragm would. One or more sets of adjustable lead shutters are located 3 to 7 inches (8–18 cm) below the tube. These shutters consist of longitudinal and lateral leaves or blades, each with its own control. This design makes the collimator adjustable in terms of its ability to produce projected x-ray fields of varying sizes. The x-ray field shape produced by a collimator is always rectangular or square unless an aperture diaphragm, cone, or cylinder is slid in below the collimator. Collimators are equipped with a white light source and a mirror to project a light field onto the patient. This light is intended to accurately indicate where the primary x-ray beam will be projected during exposure. In case of failure of this light, an x-ray field measurement guide (Fig. 7-11) is present on the front of the collimator. This guide indicates the projected field size on the basis of the adjusted size of the collimator opening at source-to-image-receptor distances (SIDs). This guide helps to ensure that the radiographer does not open the collimator to produce an x-ray field that is larger than the IR. Another problem that may occur is the lack of accuracy of the light field. The mirror that reflects the light down toward the patient or the light bulb itself could be slightly out of position, projecting a light field that inaccurately indicates where the primary beam will be projected. There is a means of testing the accuracy of this light field and the location of the center of the projected beam (Box 7-1).

FIG. 7-10 Collimators have two sets of lead shutters that are used to change the size and shape of the primary beam.

FIG. 7-11 The x-ray field measurement guide on the front of a collimator.

BOX 7-1   Quality-Control Check: Collimator and Beam Alignment

- Lack of congruence of the x-ray field light and the exposure field and misalignment of the light and Bucky tray may affect the quality of the radiographic image. In addition, if the x-ray central ray is not perpendicular to the table and Bucky tray, radiographic quality may be compromised. A collimator and beam alignment test tool template and cylinder can be easily imaged and evaluated for proper alignment.
- Collimator misalignment should be less than ±2% of the SID used, and the perpendicularity of the x-ray central ray must be misaligned by no more than ±1% of the SID used.

A plastic template with crosshairs is affixed to the bottom of the collimator to indicate where the center of the primary beam (central ray) will be directed. This template is of great assistance to the radiographer in accurately centering the x-ray field to the patient.

Automatic Collimators

An **automatic collimator**, also called a **positive beam-limiting device**, automatically limits the size and shape of the primary beam to the size and shape of the IR. For a few years, automatic collimators were required by the US federal law on all new radiographic installations. This law has since been rescinded, and automatic collimators are no longer a requirement on any radiographic equipment. However, they are still widely used. Automatic collimators mechanically adjust the primary beam size and shape to the size and placement of the IR when the IR is placed in the Bucky tray, which is located just below the tabletop and behind the front of the upright unit. In newer direct radiography units with a single IR, automatic collimation may occur when the anatomic area to be imaged is selected. For example, if an anteroposterior (AP) shoulder is selected, the collimator may automatically adjust to an 8 × 12-inch (20 × 30-cm) x-ray field size, but if an AP lumbar spine is selected, the collimator will automatically adjust to a 10 × 14-inch (25 × 35-cm) x-ray field size.

Automatic collimation makes it difficult for the radiographer to increase the size of the primary beam to a field larger than that of the IR, which would result in increasing the patient's radiation exposure. Positive beam-limiting devices were seen as a way to protect patients from overexposure to radiation; however, it should be noted that automatic collimators have an override mechanism that allows the radiographer to disengage this feature.

> ## ❗ RADIATION PROTECTION ALERT
> ### *Limit X-ray Field Size to the Anatomic Area of Interest*
>
> The radiographer should always be sure that the size of the x-ray field is restricted to the anatomic area of interest. Digital IRs are typically of a similar size, and, in many instances, larger than the anatomic area of interest. Therefore, it is crucial for the radiographer to appropriately collimate for the imaging procedure so that the patient is not unnecessarily exposed to radiation.

RADIOGRAPHIC GRIDS

The radiographic grid was invented in 1913 by Gustave Bucky and continues to be the most effective means for limiting the amount of scatter radiation that reaches the IR. Approximately ¼ inch thick and ranging from 8 × 10 inches (20 × 25 cm) to 17 × 17 inches (43 × 43 cm), a **grid** is a device consisting of very thin lead strips with radiolucent interspaces intended to absorb scatter radiation emitted from the patient. Placed between the patient and the IR, grids are invaluable in the practice of radiography. They work well to improve radiographic contrast; however, they possess certain drawbacks. As discussed later in this chapter, using a grid requires additional mAs, resulting in a higher patient dose. Therefore, grids are typically used only when the anatomic part is 10 cm (4 inches) or greater in thickness and more than 60 kVp is needed for the examination.

As scatter radiation leaves the patient, a significant amount is directed toward the IR. As previously stated, scatter radiation is detrimental to image quality because it adds unwanted exposure (fog) to the IR without adding any radiographic information. Scatter radiation decreases radiographic contrast. Ideally, grids would absorb, or clean up, all scattered photons directed toward

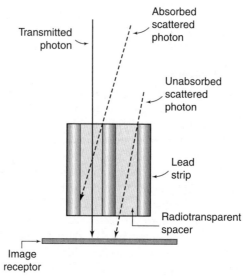

FIG. 7-12 Ideally, grids would absorb all scattered radiation and allow all transmitted photons to reach the image receptor (IR). In reality, however, some scattered photons pass through to the IR, and some transmitted photons are absorbed.

the IR and would allow all transmitted photons emitted from the patient to pass to the IR. Unfortunately, this does not happen (Fig. 7-12). When used properly, however, grids can greatly increase the contrast of the radiographic image.

IMPORTANT RELATIONSHIP

Scatter Radiation and Image Quality

Scatter radiation adds unwanted exposure (fog) to the IR and decreases image quality.

Grid Construction

Grids contain thin lead strips or lines that have a precise height, thickness, and space between them. Radiolucent **interspace material** separates the lead lines. Interspace material typically is made of aluminum. An aluminum front and back panel cover the lead lines and interspace material of the grid. Grid construction can be described by grid frequency and grid ratio. **Grid frequency** expresses the number of lead lines per unit length, in inches, centimeters, or both. Grid frequencies can range in value from 25 to 80 lines/cm (63–200 lines/inch). A typical value for grid frequency might be 40 lines/cm (100 lines/inch). Another way of describing grid construction is by its grid ratio. **Grid ratio** is defined as the ratio of the height of the lead strips to the distance between them (Fig. 7-13). Grid ratio can also be mathematically expressed as follows:

$$\text{Grid ratio} = h / D,$$

in which h is the height of the lead strips and D is the distance between them.

FIG. 7-13 Grid ratio is the ratio of the height of the lead strips to the distance between them.

▶▶ MATHEMATICAL APPLICATION

Calculating Grid Ratio

What is the grid ratio when the lead strips are 2.4 mm high and separated by 0.2 mm?

$$\text{Grid ratio} = h / D$$

$$\text{Grid ratio} = \frac{2.4}{0.2} = 12 \text{ or } 12:1$$

Grid ratios range from 4:1 to 16:1. High-ratio grids remove, or clean up, more scatter radiation than lower-ratio grids having the same grid frequency, thereby further increasing radiographic contrast.

There is a relationship among grid ratio, grid frequency, and the amount of lead content (measured in mass per unit area). Increasing the grid ratio for the same grid frequency increases the amount of lead content and therefore increases scatter absorption.

⚙ IMPORTANT RELATIONSHIP

Grid Ratio and Radiographic Contrast

As the grid ratio increases for the same grid frequency, scatter cleanup improves and radiographic contrast increases; as grid ratio decreases for the same grid frequency, scatter cleanup becomes less effective and radiographic contrast decreases.

Information about a grid's construction is contained on a label placed on the tube side of the grid. This label usually states the type of interspace material used, grid frequency, grid ratio, grid size, and information about the range of SIDs that can be used with the grid. The radiographer should read this information before using the grid because these factors influence grid performance, exposure technique selection, grid alignment, and image quality.

Grid Pattern

Grid pattern refers to the linear pattern of the lead lines of a grid. Two types of grid patterns exist: linear and crossed or crosshatched. A **linear grid** has lead lines that run in only one direction (Fig. 7-14). Linear grids are the most popular grid pattern because they allow angulation of the x-ray tube along the length of the lead lines. A **crossed grid** or **crosshatched grid** has lead lines

FIG. 7-14 Linear grid pattern.

FIG. 7-15 Crossed or crosshatched grid pattern.

FIG. 7-16 Parallel, or nonfocused, type of grid.

FIG. 7-17 Focused type of grid.

that run at right angles to one another (Fig. 7-15). Crossed grids remove more scattered photons than linear grids because they contain more lead strips, oriented in two directions. However, applications are limited with a crossed grid because the x-ray tube cannot be angled in any direction without producing grid cutoff (i.e., absorption of the transmitted x-rays). Grid cutoff is undesirable and is discussed later in this chapter.

Grid Focus

Grid focus refers to the orientation of the lead lines relative to one another. A **parallel grid** or **nonfocused grid** has lead lines that run parallel to one another (Fig. 7-16). Parallel grids are used primarily in fluoroscopy and mobile imaging. A **focused grid** has lead lines that are angled, or canted, to approximately match the angle of divergence of the primary beam (Fig. 7-17). The advantage of focused grids compared with parallel grids is that focused grids allow more transmitted photons to reach the IR. As seen in Fig. 7-18, transmitted photons are more likely to pass through a focused grid to reach the IR than they are to pass through a parallel grid.

 IMPORTANT RELATIONSHIP

Focused versus Parallel Grids

Focused grids have lead lines that are angled to approximately match the divergence of the primary beam. Thus, focused grids allow more transmitted photons to reach the IR than parallel grids.

As seen in Fig. 7-19, if imaginary lines were drawn from each of the lead lines in a linearly focused grid, these lines would meet to form an imaginary point called the **convergent point**. If points were connected along the length of the grid, they would form an imaginary line called the **convergent line**. Both the convergent line and the convergent point are important because

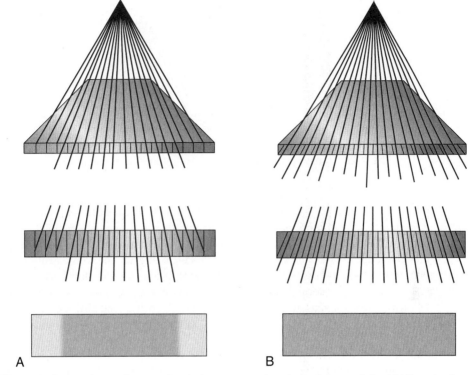

FIG. 7-18 Comparison of transmitted photons passing through a parallel grid (**A**) and a focused grid (**B**).

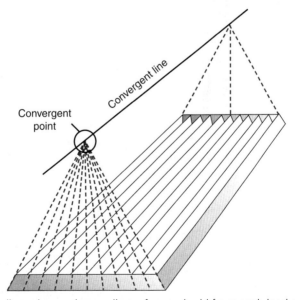

FIG. 7-19 Imaginary lines drawn above a linear focused grid from each lead strip meet to form a convergent point; the points form a convergent line.

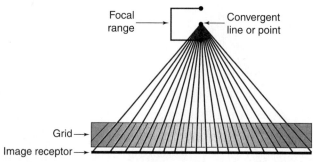

FIG. 7-20 The convergent line or point of a focused grid falls within a focal range.

they determine the focal distance of a focused grid. The **focal distance** (sometimes referred to as *grid radius*) is the distance between the grid and the convergent line or point, and it is important because it is used to determine the focal range of a focused grid. The **focal range** is the recommended range of SIDs that can be used with a focused grid. The convergent line or point always falls within the focal range (Fig. 7-20). For example, a common focal range is 36 to 42 inches (90–105 cm), with a focal distance of 40 inches (100 cm). Another common focal range is 66 to 74 inches (165–185 cm), with a focal distance of 72 inches (180 cm). Because the lead lines in a parallel grid are not angled, they have a focal range extending from a minimum SID to infinity.

Types of Grids

Grids are available for use by the radiographer in several forms and can be stationary or moving. Stationary, nonmoving grids include the wafer grid, grid cassette, and grid cap. A **wafer grid** matches the size of the cassette and is used by placing it on top of the IR. Wafer grids typically are taped to the IR to prevent them from sliding during the radiographic procedure. A **grid cassette** is an IR that has a grid permanently mounted on its front surface. A **grid cap** contains a permanently mounted grid and allows the IR to slide in behind it; this is useful because the grid is secure, and many IRs can be interchanged behind the grid before processing the CR images.

Stationary and Reciprocating Grids

When grids are stationary, it is possible to examine them closely and see the grid lines on the radiographic image. Slightly moving the grid during the x-ray exposure blurs the grid lines (motion unsharpness), rendering them less visible.

Moving or reciprocating grids are part of the **Bucky**, more accurately called the *Potter–Bucky diaphragm*. Located directly below the radiographic tabletop, the grid is found just above the tray that holds the IR. Grid motion is electrically controlled by the x-ray exposure switch. The grid moves slightly back and forth in a lateral direction over the IR during the entire exposure. These grids typically have dimensions of 17 × 17 inches (43 × 43 cm) so that a 14 × 17 inches (35 × 43 cm) IR can be positioned under the grid either lengthwise or crosswise, depending on the examination requirements.

Long-Dimension versus Short-Dimension Grids

Linear grids can be constructed with either long dimension or short dimension. A **long-dimension** linear grid has lead strips running parallel to its long axis, whereas a **short-dimension** linear grid has lead strips running perpendicular to its long axis (Fig. 7-21). For example, whereas a 14 × 17-inch (35 × 43-cm) long-dimension grid has 17-inch (43-cm)-long lead strips, a short-dimension grid has 14-inch (35-cm)-long lead strips. A short-dimension grid may be useful

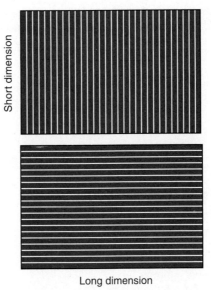

FIG. 7-21 A long-dimension grid has lead strips running parallel to the long axis of the grid. A short-dimension grid has lead strips running perpendicular to the long axis of the grid. (From Johnston JN, Fauber TL: *Essentials of Radiographic Physics and Imaging*, ed 2, St. Louis, 2016, Mosby.)

for examinations when it is difficult to correctly center or angle the central ray for the long-dimension grid (e.g., imaging a decubitus or stretcher chest in the crosswise IR direction).

Grid Performance

The purpose of using grids in radiography is to increase radiographic contrast. In addition to improving contrast by cleaning up scatter, grids reduce the total amount of x-rays reaching the IR. The better the grid is at absorbing scattered photons, such as with a higher-ratio grid, the fewer the photons reach the IR. To compensate for this reduction, additional mAs must be used to maintain exposure to the IR. The **grid conversion factor (GCF)**, or **Bucky factor**, can be used to determine the required adjustment in mAs when changing from using a grid to nongrid (or vice versa) or for changing to grids with different grid ratios.

The GCF can be mathematically expressed as follows:

$$GCF = \frac{mAs\ with\ the\ grid}{mAs\ without\ the\ grid}$$

IMPORTANT RELATIONSHIP

Grid Ratio and Exposure to Image Receptor

As the grid ratio increases, exposure to the IR decreases; as the grid ratio decreases, exposure to the IR increases.

Table 7-2 presents specific grid ratios and grid conversion factors. When a grid is added to the IR, mAs must be increased by the factor indicated to maintain the same number of x-ray photons reaching the IR. This calculation requires multiplication by the GCF for the particular grid ratio.

TABLE 7-2   Grid Conversion Factor (GCF)/Bucky Factor

Grid Ratio	GCF/Bucky Factor
No grid	1
5:1	2
6:1	3
8:1	4
12:1	5
16:1	6

≫ **MATHEMATICAL APPLICATION**

Adding a Grid

If a radiographer produced a shoulder radiograph with nongrid exposure using 3 mAs and then wanted to use a 12:1 ratio grid, what mAs should be used to produce the same exposure to the IR?

Nongrid exposure = 3 mAs

GCF (for 12:1 grid) = 5 (from Table 7-2)

$$GCF = \frac{mAs \text{ with the grid}}{mAs \text{ without the grid}}$$

$$5 = \frac{mAs \text{ with the grid}}{3}$$

$$15 = mAs \text{ with the grid}$$

When adding a 12:1 ratio grid, mAs must be increased by a factor of 5 (in this case to 15 mAs).

Likewise, if a radiographer chooses not to use a grid during a procedure but knows the appropriate mAs only for when a grid is used, the mAs must be decreased by the GCF. This calculation requires division by the GCF for the particular grid ratio.

≫ **MATHEMATICAL APPLICATION**

Removing a Grid

If a radiographer produced a knee radiograph using an 8:1 ratio grid and 10 mAs and on the next exposure wanted to use nongrid exposure, what mAs should be used to produce the same exposure to the IR?

Grid exposure = 10 mAs

GCF (for 8:1 grid) = 4 (from Table 7-2)

$$GCF = \frac{mAs \text{ with the grid}}{mAs \text{ without the grid}}$$

$$4 = \frac{10 \text{ mAs}}{mAs \text{ without the grid}}$$

$$2.5 = mAs \text{ without the grid}$$

When removing an 8:1 ratio grid, mAs must be decreased by a factor of 4 (in this case to 2.5 mAs).

The GCF is also useful when changing between grids with different grid ratios. When changing from one grid ratio to another, the following formula should be used to adjust the mAs:

$$\frac{mAs_1}{mAs_2} = \frac{GCF_1}{GCF_2}$$

⟩⟩ MATHEMATICAL APPLICATION

Decreasing the Grid Ratio

If a radiographer used 40 mAs with a 12:1 ratio grid, what mAs should be used with a 6:1 ratio grid to produce the same exposure to the IR?

Exposure 1: 40 mAs, 12:1 grid, GCF = 5

Exposure 2: _____ mAs, 6:1 grid, GCF = 3

$$\frac{mAs_1}{mAs_2} = \frac{GCF_1}{GCF_2}$$

$$\frac{40}{mAs_2} = \frac{5}{3}$$

$$mAs_2 = 24$$

Decreasing the grid ratio requires less mAs.

⟩⟩ MATHEMATICAL APPLICATION

Increasing the Grid Ratio

If a radiographer performed a routine portable pelvic examination using 40 mAs with an 8:1 ratio grid, what mAs should be used if a 12:1 ratio grid is substituted?

Exposure 1: 40 mAs, 8:1 grid, GCF = 4

Exposure 2: _____ mAs, 12:1 grid, GCF = 5

$$\frac{mAs_1}{mAs_2} = \frac{GCF_1}{GCF_2}$$

$$\frac{40}{mAs_2} = \frac{4}{5}$$

$$mAs_2 = 50$$

Increasing the grid ratio requires additional mAs.

The increase in mAs required to maintain the exposure to the IR results in an increase in patient dose. This increase is significant, as the GCF numbers indicate. It is important to remember that patient dose is increased by the following factors:

- Using a grid compared with not using a grid
- Using a higher-ratio grid

◤ IMPORTANT RELATIONSHIP

Grid Ratio and Patient Dose

As the grid ratio increases, patient dose increases because of the increase in mAs; as the grid ratio decreases, patient dose decreases because of the decrease in mAs.

❗ RADIATION PROTECTION ALERT

Grid Selection

Decisions regarding the use of a grid and grid ratio should be made by balancing image quality and patient protection. To minimize patient exposure, grids should be used only when appropriate, and the grid ratio selected should be the lowest capable of providing sufficient contrast improvement. In exams in which the anatomic part does not produce excessive scatter, a grid may not be necessary because the computer can vary contrast in the displayed image.

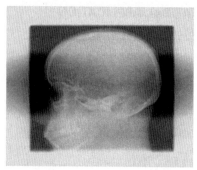

FIG. 7-22 Radiographic image produced with an upside-down focused grid.

Grid Cutoff

In addition to the disadvantage of increased patient dose associated with grid use, another disadvantage is the possibility of grid cutoff. **Grid cutoff** refers to a decrease in the number of transmitted photons that reach the IR because of some misalignment of the grid. The primary radiographic effect of grid cutoff is a further reduction in the number of photons reaching the IR. Grid cutoff may require the radiographer to repeat the radiographic image, increasing patient dose yet again. Grid ratio has a significant impact on grid cutoff, with higher grid ratios resulting in more potential cutoff.

Types of Grid Cutoff Errors

Grid cutoff can occur because of four types of errors in grid use. To reduce or eliminate grid cutoff, the radiographer must have a thorough understanding of the importance of proper grid alignment in relation to the IR and x-ray tube.

Upside-Down Focused. Upside-down focused grid cutoff occurs when a focused grid is placed upsidedown on the IR, resulting in the grid lines going opposite the angle of divergence of the x-ray beam resulting in a significant loss of exposure along the edges of the image (Fig. 7-22). Photons easily pass through the center of the grid because the lead lines are perpendicular to the IR surface. Lead lines that are more peripheral to the center have steeper angles and absorb the transmitted photons. Upside-down focused grid error is easily avoided because every focused grid should have a label indicating the tube side. This side of the grid should always face the tube, away from the IR.

 IMPORTANT RELATIONSHIP

Upside-Down Focused Grids and Grid Cutoff

Placing a focused grid upsidedown on the IR causes the edges of the IR to be significantly underexposed.

Off-Level. Off-level grid cutoff results when the x-ray beam is angled across the lead strips. It is the most common type of cutoff and can occur from either the tube or the grid being angled (Fig. 7-23). Off-level grid cutoff can often occur with mobile radiographic studies or horizontal beam examinations and is visualized as a loss of exposure across the entire IR. This type of grid cutoff is the only type that occurs with both focused and parallel grids.

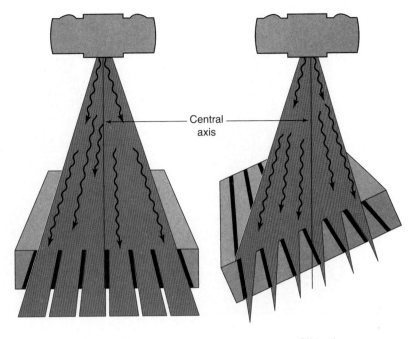

Central axis

Proper position   Off-level

FIG. 7-23 An off-level grid can cause grid cutoff.

 IMPORTANT RELATIONSHIP

Off-Level Error and Grid Cutoff

Angling the x-ray tube across the grid lines or angling the grid itself during exposure produces an overall decrease in exposure across the entire IR.

Off-Center. Also called *lateral decentering,* off-center grid cutoff occurs when the central ray of the x-ray beam is not aligned from side to side with the center of a focused grid. Because of the arrangement of the lead lines of the focused grid, the divergence of the primary beam does not match the angle of these lead strips when not centered (Fig. 7-24). Off-center grid cutoff may cause an overall loss of exposure across the entire IR.

IMPORTANT RELATIONSHIP

Off-Center Error and Grid Cutoff

If the center of the x-ray beam is not aligned from side to side with the center of a focused grid, grid cutoff can occur as a loss of exposure across the entire IR.

Off-Focus. Off-focus grid cutoff occurs when using an SID outside the recommended focal range. Grid cutoff occurs if the SID is less than or greater than the focal range and results in a loss of exposure at the periphery of the IR.

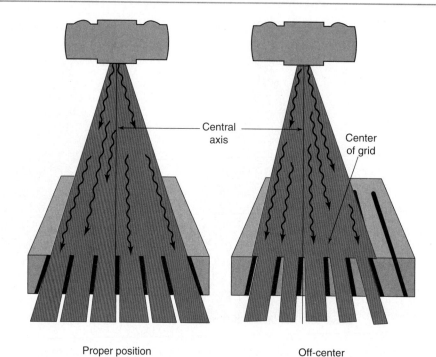

Proper position   Off-center

FIG. 7-24 Centering to one side of a focused grid can cause off-center grid cutoff.

> ### ◤ IMPORTANT RELATIONSHIP
> #### *Off-Focus Error and Grid Cutoff*
>
> Using an SID outside the focal range creates a loss of exposure at the periphery of the IR.

Grid alignment errors may be difficult to identify because the computer will adjust for exposure errors to the IR. However, adjusting the brightness during computer processing may not overcome a grid alignment error and still produce a poor-quality image (Fig. 7-25). When using a grid, the radiographer should pay close attention to the alignment of the grid to the x-ray tube and IR.

Table 7-3 summarizes important relationships regarding the use of radiographic grids.

Moiré Effect

The **moiré effect** or zebra pattern is an artifact that can occur when a stationary grid is used during computed radiography (CR) imaging (Fig. 7-26). If the grid frequency is similar to the laser scanning frequency or scans parallel to the grid strips during CR image processing, a zebra pattern can result on the digital image. The use of a higher grid frequency or a moving grid with CR digital imaging eliminates this type of grid error. In addition, if a grid cassette is placed in a Bucky, imaging the double grids creates a zebra pattern on the radiograph.

Grid Usage

The radiographer needs to consider several factors when deciding the type of grid, if any, to be used for an examination. Although quite efficient at preventing scatter radiation from reaching the IR, grids are not appropriate for all examinations. When appropriate, selection of a grid involves consideration of contrast improvement, patient dose, and the likelihood of grid cutoff.

FIG. 7-25 Grid cutoff. **A**, Image created with proper alignment of computed radiography and no grid cutoff. **B**, Image created with off-level grid cutoff. The overall brightness was maintained, but the image quality is poor. (From Johnston JN, Fauber TL: *Essentials of Radiographic Physics and Imaging*, ed 3, St. Louis, 2020, Elsevier.)

TABLE 7-3 **Radiographic Grids**	
Increased Factor	**Result**
Grid ratio[a]	Contrast *increases*
	Patient dose *increases*
	The likelihood of grid cutoff *increases*

[a]Milliamperage-seconds adjusted to maintain exposure to the image receptor.

Radiographers typically choose between parallel and focused grids, high- and low-ratio grids, grids with different focal ranges, and whether to use a grid at all.

As indicated earlier, the choice of whether to use a grid is based on the kVp necessary for the examination and the thickness of the anatomic part being examined. Parts 10 cm (4 inches) or larger, together with kVp values higher than 60, produce enough scatter to necessitate the use of a grid. The next question is which grid to use. There is no single best grid for all situations. A 16:1 focused grid provides excellent contrast improvement, but the patient's dose is high, and the radiographer must ensure that the grid and x-ray tube are perfectly aligned to prevent grid cutoff. The 5:1 parallel grid does a mediocre job of scatter cleanup, especially at kVp values greater than 80. However, the patient dose is significantly lower, and the radiographer need not be concerned with the cutoff caused by being off center, the SID

FIG. 7-26 Moiré effect. Radiographic image demonstrating the zebra pattern as a result of the moiré effect. (Courtesy of Andrew Woodward.)

used, or having the grid upside down. Selection between grids with different focal ranges depends on the radiographic examination. Supine abdomen studies should use a grid that includes 40 inches (100 cm) in the focal range; upright chest studies should have grids that include 72 inches (180 cm). In general, most radiographic rooms use a 10:1 or 12:1 focused grid, which provides a compromise between contrast improvement and patient dose. Stationary grids, for mobile examinations, may have a lower ratio, be a parallel type, or both to allow the radiographer greater positioning latitude.

Grids differ from one another in performance, especially in the areas of grid ratio and focal distance. Before using a grid, the radiographer must determine the grid ratio so that the appropriate exposure factors can be selected. Also, the radiographer must be aware of the focal range of focused grids so that an appropriate SID is selected.

Box 7-2 lists the attributes of the grid typically used in radiography. Box 7-3 summarizes grid errors and their radiographic effects. Box 7-4 provides information on quality-control checks for grid uniformity and alignment.

BOX 7-2   Typical Grid

- Is linear instead of crossed
- Is focused instead of parallel
- Is of mid-ratio (8:1 to 12:1)
- Has a focal range that includes an SID of 40 inches (100 cm) or 72 inches (180 cm)

BOX 7-3 Grid Cutoff Errors and Their Radiographic Effects

Grid Error	Radiographic Effect
Upside-down focused grid: placing a focused grid upside down on the IR	Significant underexposure to the lateral edges of the IR
Off-level error: angling the x-ray tube across the grid lines or angling the grid itself during exposure	Decrease in radiation exposure to the entire IR
Off-center error: the center of the x-ray beam is not aligned from side to side with the center of a focused grid	Decrease in radiation exposure to the entire IR
Off-focus error: using an SID outside the focal range	A loss of exposure at the periphery of the IR

BOX 7-4 Quality-Control Check: Grid Uniformity and Alignment

- Non-uniformity of a grid (lack of uniform lead strips) may create artifacts on the image. Grid uniformity can be easily evaluated by imaging a grid and measuring pixel brightness throughout the image. Pixel brightness level readings should be within ±0.20 for proper uniformity.
- Misalignment of a focused grid (off-center) can reduce exposure to the IR as a result of grid cutoff. A grid alignment tool made of radiopaque material with cut-out holes in a line can be imaged to evaluate correct alignment of the grid with the x-ray field.

Radiation Protection

Limiting the size of the x-ray field to the anatomic area of interest will decrease scatter production and reduce patient exposure. Although the mAs may be increased to compensate for decreasing the size of the x-ray field, the tissues located closest to the lateral edge or outside the collimated x-ray beam will receive the least amount of radiation exposure. Tissues that lie inside the collimated edge of the x-ray beam will receive the greatest amount of radiation exposure. Collimating to the anatomic area of interest is an important radiation protection practice that should be routinely performed.

The use of grids requires an increase in mAs to maintain exposure to the IR. As a result, patient radiation exposure is increased when using grids. The higher the grid ratio, the greater the mAs needed to maintain exposure to the IR, and therefore, patient radiation exposure is increased. Limiting the use of grids or using a grid with a lower grid ratio decreases the radiation exposure to the patient.

AIR GAP TECHNIQUE

Although the radiographer may use the grid most often to prevent scatter from reaching the IR, the grid is not the only available tool. The air gap technique, although limited in its usefulness, provides another method for limiting the scatter reaching the IR. The **air gap technique** is based on the simple concept that much of the scatter will miss the IR if there is increased distance between the patient and the IR (increased object-to-image-receptor distance [OID]) (Fig. 7-27). The greater the gap, the greater the reduction in scatter reaching the IR. Like when using a grid, contrast is increased, the number of photons reaching the IR is reduced because less scatter reaches the IR, and the mAs must be increased to compensate. There may be slightly less exposure because a grid absorbs some of the transmitted photons (grid cutoff), but the air gap technique does not.

FIG. 7-27 The air gap technique used in magnification radiography of the lateral skull.

The air gap technique is limited in its usefulness because the necessary OID results in decreased spatial resolution. To overcome this increase in unsharpness, an increase in SID is required, which may not always be feasible. The most common use for air gap technique is a trauma lateral cervical spine. Lateral cervical spine positioning creates a natural increase in OID because of the positions of the shoulders.

IMPORTANT RELATIONSHIP

Air Gap Technique and Scatter Control

The air gap technique is an alternative to using a grid to control the scatter reaching the IR. By moving the IR away from the patient, more scatter radiation will miss the IR. The greater the gap, the lesser the scatter reaches the IR.

SCATTER CONTROL AND DIGITAL IMAGING

Computer processing during digital imaging typically produces an image with appropriate brightness. If the amount of x-ray exposure reaching the IR is low, computer processing functions to produce the appropriate brightness, which may result in an image with increased quantum noise. This can occur with all forms of grid cutoff or if the mAs is not increased to compensate for adding a grid or changing to a higher-ratio grid. Excessive noise in a digital image is one of the primary reasons for repeating the image.

If the digital IR receives too much exposure, computer processing produces appropriate brightness; however, image contrast is decreased because of excessive scatter. This may occur when a grid is removed and mAs is not decreased or by not making adjustments in mAs when a change is made to a lower-ratio grid.

Grid errors during digital imaging can easily be masked by computer processing. The radiographer should evaluate the exposure indicator value along with the overall quality of the digital image to determine whether any exposure errors exist.

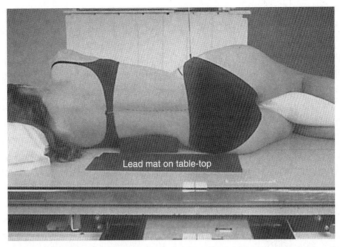

FIG. 7-28 Shielding accessory: lead shield placed to absorb scatter radiation from the patient. (From Bontrager KL, Lampignano JP: *Textbook of Radiographic Positioning and Related Anatomy*, ed 7, St. Louis, 2010, Mosby.)

SHIELDING ACCESSORIES

Efforts to control the amount of scatter radiation produced within the patient and reaching the IR are important considerations during radiography. Restricting the size of the x-ray beam to the anatomic area of interest reduces the radiation exposure to the patient and improves image quality. There are situations in which it is beneficial to use shielding devices to absorb the scatter radiation exiting the patient; placing a lead shield on the x-ray table close to the collimated edge of the area of interest absorbs scatter exiting the patient that could degrade image quality. The lateral lumbar spine projection and the lateral (L5-S1) spot are projections in which a significant amount of scatter exits the patient. Placing a lead shield behind the patient's lower back absorbs the scatter and reduces the amount striking the IR (Fig. 7-28). Accurate placement of the lead shield is important so it does not impact the processing of the digital image. It is important to note that placing a lead shield on the table to limit the scatter radiation reaching the IR does not reduce the exposure to the patient.

Because the patient is the greatest source of scatter radiation, all persons remaining in the radiographic room during an exposure must wear a lead apron. This, together with standing as far from the patient as possible, decreases the amount of occupational exposure to scatter radiation.

It is the radiographer's responsibility to reduce the amount of scatter radiation produced and reaching the IR. Reducing the amount of scatter produced through beam restriction and the amount reaching the IR using a grid, avoiding grid cutoff errors, and making appropriate exposure adjustments as needed help to produce good-quality radiographic images.

CHAPTER SUMMARY

- Scatter radiation, the result of Compton interactions, is detrimental to radiographic image quality. Excessive scatter results in additional unwanted exposure (fog) and reduced contrast.
- The effect of scatter radiation can be reduced by limiting the amount produced and by absorbing the scatter before it reaches the IR.
- The amount of scatter produced increases as the volume of irradiated tissue increases, and the proportion and energy of scatter exiting the patient increase as kVp increases.

- Beam restriction limits the area exposed to radiation, the patient dose, and the amount of scatter produced in the patient. Aperture diaphragms, cones and cylinders, and collimators are types of beam restrictors.
- Radiographic grids are devices placed between the patient and the IR to absorb scatter radiation. Consisting of a series of lead strips and radiolucent interspaces, grids allow transmitted radiation to pass through while scatter radiation is absorbed.
- Grid designs include linear parallel, focused parallel, crossed, short dimension, and long dimension, each with advantages and disadvantages.
- The use of a grid in a radiographic examination results in fewer photons reaching the IR. The grid conversion (or Bucky) factor is used to calculate the change in exposure (mAs) needed when grids are used.
- Adding a grid requires an increase in mAs to maintain exposure to the IR, therefore increasing radiation exposure to the patient.
- Grid alignment errors, producing grid cutoff, include using an upside-down focused grid and errors caused by off-level, off-center, and off-focus equipment alignment.
- The use and type of a grid depends on the thickness of the part, kVp, patient dose, contrast improvement, and likelihood of grid errors.
- Grid errors during digital imaging can easily be masked by computer processing.
- The air gap technique is another method, although seldom used, for reducing the amount of scatter reaching the IR.
- Placing a lead shield behind the patient's lower back when performing a lateral lumbar spine absorbs the scatter and reduces the amount striking the IR.
- Because the patient is the greatest source of scatter radiation, all persons remaining in the radiographic room during an exposure must wear a lead apron.

REVIEW QUESTIONS

1. The projected shape of the unrestricted primary beam is _____.
   A. square
   B. rectangular
   C. circular
   D. elliptical
2. One purpose of beam-restricting devices is to _____ by changing the size and shape of the primary beam.
   A. increase patient dose
   B. decrease scatter radiation produced
   C. increase exposure to the IR
   D. decrease image contrast
3. The most effective type of beam-restricting device is the _____.
   A. cone
   B. aperture diaphragm
   C. cylinder
   D. collimator
4. Of the beam-restricting devices listed in question 3, which two are most similar to one another?
   A. A and B
   B. A and C
   C. B and C
   D. B and D

5. The purpose of automatic collimation is to ensure that _____.
   A. the quantity of scatter production is minimal
   B. the field size does not exceed the IR size
   C. maximal spatial resolution and contrast are achieved
   D. exposure to the IR is maintained
6. When making a significant increase in collimation, _____.
   A. mAs should be increased
   B. kVp should be increased
   C. mAs should be decreased
   D. kVp should be decreased
7. Which one of the following increases as collimation increases?
   A. Patient exposure
   B. Scatter production
   C. Fog
   D. Contrast
8. Which of the following statements is true for positive beam-limiting devices?
   A. They are required on all radiographic installations.
   B. They are required on all new radiographic installations.
   C. They have never been required on radiographic installations.
   D. They were once required on new radiographic installations.
9. The purpose of a grid in radiography is to _____.
   A. increase exposure to the IR
   B. increase image contrast
   C. decrease patient dose
   D. increase spatial resolution
10. Grid ratio is defined as the ratio of the _____.
    A. height of the lead strips to the distance between them
    B. width of the lead strips to their height
    C. number of lead strips to their width
    D. width of the lead strips to the width of the interspace material
11. Compared with parallel grids, focused grids _____.
    A. have a greater grid frequency and lead content
    B. can be used with either side facing the tube
    C. have a wider range of grid ratios and frequencies
    D. allow more transmitted photons to reach the IR
12. With which one of the following grids would a convergent line be formed if imaginary lines from its grid lines were drawn in space above it?
    A. Linear focused
    B. Crossed focused
    C. Linear parallel
    D. Crossed parallel
13. If 15 mAs is used to produce a particular level of exposure to the IR without a grid, what value of mAs would be needed to produce that same level of exposure using a 16:1 grid?
    A. 45
    B. 60
    C. 90
    D. 105

14. With exposure technique compensation, which of the following would result in the greatest radiation exposure to the patient?
    A. 14 × 17 x-ray field size
    B. Air gap technique
    C. Cylinder beam restrictor
    D. 12:1 grid ratio

15. Off-focus grid cutoff occurs by using an SID that is not _____.
    A. within the focal range of the grid
    B. equal to the focal distance of the grid
    C. at the level of the convergent line of the grid
    D. at the level of the convergent point of the grid

16. The type of motion most often used for moving grids today is _____.
    A. longitudinal
    B. reciprocating
    C. circular
    D. single stroke

17. A grid should be used whenever the anatomic part size exceeds _____.
    A. 3 cm
    B. 6 cm
    C. 10 cm
    D. 12 cm

18. The air gap technique uses an increased _____ instead of a grid.
    A. kVp
    B. mAs
    C. SID
    D. OID

Exposure Technique Selection

OBJECTIVES

After completing this chapter, the reader will be able to perform the following:

1. Define all the key terms in this chapter.
2. State all the important relationships in this chapter.
3. State the purpose of automatic exposure control (AEC) in radiography.
4. Differentiate among the types of radiation detectors used in AEC systems.
5. Recognize how detector size and configuration affect the response of an AEC device.
6. Explain how alignment and positioning affect the response of an AEC device.
7. Discuss patient and exposure technique factors and their effects on the response of an AEC device.
8. Analyze poor-quality images produced using AEC and identify possible causes.
9. Describe the patient radiation protection issues associated with AEC.
10. State the importance of calibration of the AEC system to the type of image receptor used.
11. Define anatomically programmed techniques.
12. Differentiate between the types of exposure technique charts.
13. State exposure technique modifications for the following considerations: pediatric, geriatric, and bariatric patients and varying projections and positions, soft tissue, casts and splints, contrast media, and pathological conditions.

KEY TERMS

anatomically programmed
  technique
automatic exposure control
  (AEC)

backup time
body mass index (BMI)
calipers
comparative anatomy

contrast medium
density controls
detectors
exposure adjustment

The radiographer is responsible for selecting exposure factor techniques to produce quality radiographic images for a wide variety of equipment and patients. There are many thousands of possible combinations of kilovoltage peak (kVp), milliamperage (mA), source-to-image-receptor distance (SID), exposure time, image receptors (IRs), and grid ratios. When patients of various sizes and with various pathological conditions are considered, the selection of proper exposure factors becomes a formidable task. Tools are available to assist the radiographer in selecting appropriate exposure techniques: **automatic exposure control (AEC)** devices, anatomically programmed techniques, and exposure technique charts. Knowledge about the performance of these tools and their operation assists radiographers in producing quality radiographic images.

AUTOMATIC EXPOSURE CONTROL

An AEC system is a tool available on most modern radiographic units to assist the radiographer in determining the amount of radiation exposure to produce a quality image. AEC is a system used to consistently control the amount of radiation reaching the IR by terminating the length of exposure. AEC systems also are called *automatic exposure devices,* and sometimes they are erroneously referred to as *phototiming.* When using AEC systems, the radiographer must still use individual discretion to select an appropriate kVp, mA, IR, and grid. However, the AEC device determines the exposure time (and total exposure) that is used.

 IMPORTANT RELATIONSHIP

Principle of AEC Operation

Once a predetermined amount of radiation is transmitted through a patient, the x-ray exposure is terminated. This determines the exposure time and therefore the total amount of radiation exposure to the IR.

AEC systems are excellent at producing consistent levels of exposure when used properly; however, radiographers must also be aware of the limitations of using an AEC system in patient positioning and centering, detector size and selection, collimation, and IR variation.

AEC Radiation Detectors

All AEC devices work by the same principle of operation: radiation is transmitted through the patient and converted into an electrical signal, terminating the exposure time; this occurs when a predetermined amount of radiation has been detected, as indicated by the charge of the electrical signal produced. Service personnel calibrate the predetermined level of radiation to meet the departmental standards of image quality.

The difference in AEC systems lies in the type of device that is used to convert radiation into electricity. Two types of AEC systems have been used: phototimers and ionization chambers. Phototimers

FIG. 8-1 The size and arrangement of the three automatic exposure control (AEC) detectors are clear on this upright chest unit. (From Johnston JN, Fauber TL: *Essentials of Radiographic Physics and Imaging*, ed 2, St. Louis, 2016, Mosby.)

represent the first generation of AEC systems used in radiography, and it is from this type of system that the term *phototiming* has evolved. *Phototiming* specifically refers to the use of an AEC device that uses photomultiplier tubes or photodiodes, even though these systems are uncommon today. Therefore, the use of the term *phototiming* is usually incorrect. The more common type of AEC system uses ionization chambers. Regardless of the specific type of AEC system used, almost all systems use a set of three radiation-measuring detectors, arranged in a specific manner (Fig. 8-1). The radiographer selects the configuration of these devices, determining which one (or more) of the three measures radiation exposure reaching the IR. These devices are variously referred to as *sensors*, *chambers*, *cells*, or *detectors*. These radiation-measuring devices are referred to here for the remainder of the discussion as **detectors**. In this chapter, AEC detectors are differentiated from flat-panel detector type IRs.

> ### IMPORTANT RELATIONSHIP
> #### Radiation-Measuring Devices
>
> Detectors are the AEC devices that measure the amount of radiation transmitted. The radiographer selects the combination of the detectors to use.

Phototimers

Phototimers used a fluorescent (light-producing) screen and a device that converts light into electricity. A **photomultiplier tube** is an electronic device that converts visible light energy into electrical energy. A photodiode is a solid-state device that performs the same function. Phototimer AEC devices were considered as exit-type devices because the detectors are positioned behind the IR (Fig. 8-2) so that radiation must exit the IR before it is measured by the detectors. Light paddles, coated with a fluorescent material, served as the detectors; radiation interacts with these paddles, producing visible light. This light was then transmitted to remote photomultiplier tubes or photodiodes that convert it into electricity. The timer is tripped, and the radiographic exposure was terminated when a sufficiently large charge had been received. This electrical charge was in proportion to the radiation to which the light paddles had been exposed. Phototimers have largely been replaced with ionization chamber systems.

Light paddles, together with photomultiplier
tubes, measure radiation exposure after
it passes through the image receptor.

FIG. 8-2 The phototimer AEC system has the light paddles (detectors) located directly below the image receptor (IR). This is an exit-type device in that the x-rays must exit the IR before they are measured by the detectors.

Ionization Chamber Systems

An **ionization or ion chamber**, is a hollow cell that contains air and is connected to the timer circuit via an electrical wire. Ionization chamber AEC devices are considered to be entrance-type devices because the detectors are positioned in front of the IR (Fig. 8-3) so that radiation can interact with the detectors just before interacting with the IR. When the ionization chamber is exposed to radiation from a radiographic exposure, the air inside the chamber becomes ionized, creating an electrical charge. This charge travels along the wire to the timer circuit. The timer is tripped, and the radiographic exposure is terminated when a sufficiently large charge has been received. This electrical charge is in proportion to the radiation to which the ionization chamber has been exposed. Compared with phototimers, ion chambers are less sophisticated and less accurate, but they are less prone to failure. Most AEC systems today use ionization chambers.

IMPORTANT RELATIONSHIP

Function of the Ionization Chamber

The ionization chamber interacts with exit radiation before it reaches the IR. Air in the chamber is ionized, an electrical charge proportional to the amount of radiation is created, and this charge travels to the timer circuit where the exposure is terminated.

mAs Readout

When a radiographic study is performed using an AEC device, the total amount of radiation (milliamperage-seconds [mAs]) required to produce the appropriate exposure to the IR is determined by the system. Many radiographic units include an **mAs readout** display, where

Ionization chamber

Image receptor

Ionization chamber measures radiation
exposure before it reaches the image receptor.

FIG. 8-3 The ionization chamber AEC system has the detectors located directly in front of the IR. This system is termed *entrance type* because the x-ray exposure is measured just before entering the IR.

the actual amount of mAs used for that image is displayed immediately after the exposure, sometimes for only a few seconds. It is critical for the radiographer to take note of this information when it is available. Knowledge of the mAs readout has numerous advantages. It allows the radiographer to become more familiar with manual exposure technique factors. If the image is unacceptable, knowing the mAs readout provides a basis from which the radiographer can make exposure adjustments by switching to a manual technique. There may be procedures with different positions where AEC and the manual technique are combined because of difficulty with accurate centering. For example, knowing the mAs readout for the anteroposterior (AP) lumbar spine gives the radiographer an option to switch to manual techniques for the oblique exposures, making technique adjustments based on reliable mAs information.

IMPORTANT RELATIONSHIP
AEC and mAs Readout

If the radiographic unit has an mAs readout display, the radiographer should take note of the reading after an exposure is made. This information can be invaluable.

kVp and mA Selections

AEC controls only the quantity of radiation reaching the IR and has no effect on other image characteristics, such as contrast. The kVp for a particular examination should be selected without regard to whether an AEC device is used. The radiographer must select the kVp level that provides an appropriate level of subject contrast and is at least the minimum kVp needed to penetrate the part. Although contrast can be computer manipulated in digital imaging, the kVp should still be selected to best visualize the area of interest. High kVp is used for chest imaging with a grid to

FIG. 8-4 Kilovoltage. **A,** Radiographic image created using a high kilovoltage peak (kVp) (109) and the outer two AEC detectors. The image demonstrates low subject contrast typical for chest imaging. **B,** Radiographic image created using a low kVp (60) and the outer two AEC detectors. The image demonstrates high subject contrast not typical for chest imaging. The milliampere-seconds (mAs) readout indicated significantly more radiation than *A* as a result of using a low kVp. (From Johnston JN, Fauber TL: *Essentials of Radiographic Physics and Imaging*, ed 3, St. Louis, 2020, Elsevier.)

best visualize the widely varying tissues (Fig. 8-4). In addition, the higher the kVp value used, the shorter is the exposure time needed by the AEC device. Because high kVp radiation is more penetrating (reducing the total amount of x-ray exposure to the patient because more x-ray photons exit the patient) and the detectors are measuring the quantity of radiation, the preset amount of radiation exposure is reached sooner with a higher kVp.

⚑ IMPORTANT RELATIONSHIP
kVp and AEC Response

The radiographer must set the kVp as needed to ensure adequate penetration while producing the appropriate level of subject contrast. The kVp selected determines the length of exposure time when using AEC. A low kVp requires more exposure time to reach the predetermined amount of exposure. A high kVp decreases the exposure time to reach the predetermined amount of exposure and reduces the overall radiation exposure to the patient.

❗ RADIATION PROTECTION ALERT
Kilovoltage Selection

Using a higher kVp with AEC decreases the exposure time and the overall mAs needed to produce a diagnostic image, significantly reducing patient exposure. The kVp selected for an examination should produce the desired subject contrast for the part examined while being as high as possible to minimize the patient's radiation exposure.

When the radiographer uses a control panel that allows the mA and time to be set independently, he or she should select the mA without regard to whether an AEC device is used. The mA selected has an inverse effect on the exposure time needed by the AEC device, as it does when using a manual exposure technique to maintain exposure to the IR. Therefore, if the radiographer wants to decrease the exposure time for a particular examination, he or she may easily do so by increasing the mA value. For a given procedure, increasing the mA on the control panel decreases the exposure time, and decreasing the mA selected on the control panel increases the exposure time.

IMPORTANT RELATIONSHIP

mA and AEC Response

If the radiographer can set the mA when using AEC, it will inversely affect the time of exposure for a given procedure. Increasing the mA decreases the exposure time to reach the predetermined amount of exposure. Decreasing the mA increases the exposure time to reach the predetermined amount of exposure.

Minimum Response Time

The term **minimum response time** refers to the shortest exposure time that the system can produce. Minimum response time (1 ms with modern AEC systems) is usually longer with AEC systems than with other types of radiographic timers (i.e., other types of radiographic timers usually are able to produce shorter exposure times than AEC devices). This can be a problem with some segments of the patient population, such as pediatric or uncooperative patients. Typically, the radiographer increases the mA so that the time of exposure terminates more quickly. If the minimum response time is longer than the amount of time needed to terminate the preset exposure, it results in an increased amount of radiation reaching the IR. With pediatric patients and other patients who cannot or will not cooperate with the radiographer by holding still or holding their breath during the exposure, AEC devices may not be the technology of choice.

Backup Time

Backup time refers to the maximum length of time for which the x-ray exposure will continue when using an AEC system. The backup time may be set by the radiographer or automatically controlled by the radiographic unit. It may be set as backup exposure time or as backup mAs (the product of mA and exposure time). The backup time acts as a safety mechanism when an AEC system fails or the equipment is not used properly. In either case, the backup time protects the patient from receiving unnecessary exposure and protects the x-ray tube from reaching or exceeding its heat-loading capacity. If the backup time is automatically controlled, it should terminate at a maximum of 600 mAs when equipment is operated at or above 50 kVp.

IMPORTANT RELATIONSHIP

Function of Backup Time

Backup time, the maximum exposure time allowed during an AEC examination, serves as a safety mechanism when AEC is not used properly or is not functioning properly.

The backup time might be reached as a result of operator oversight when an AEC examination, such as a chest x-ray, is conducted at the upright Bucky and the radiographer has set the control panel for a table Bucky. The table detectors are forced to wait for an excessively long time to measure enough radiation to terminate the exposure. The backup time is reached, and the exposure is terminated, limiting patient exposure and preventing the tube from overloading. However, newer x-ray units with AEC include a sensor in the Bucky tray for the IR and do not allow an exposure to activate if the table Bucky detectors are selected but the x-ray tube is centered to the upright Bucky.

When controlled by the radiographer, the backup time should be set high enough to exceed the exposure needed but low enough to protect the patient from excessive exposure in case of a problem. Setting the backup time at 150% to 200% of the expected exposure time is appropriate.

 IMPORTANT RELATIONSHIP

Setting Backup Time

The backup time should be set to 150% to 200% of the expected exposure time. This allows the properly used AEC system to appropriately terminate the exposure but protects the patient and tube from excessive exposure if a problem occurs.

! RADIATION PROTECTION ALERT

Monitoring Backup Time

To minimize patient exposure, the backup time should be neither too long nor too short. Backup time that is too short results in the exposure being stopped prematurely, and the image may need to be repeated because of poor quality. Backup time that is too long results in the patient receiving unnecessary radiation if a problem occurs and the exposure does not end until the backup time is reached. In addition, the image may have to be repeated because of poor quality.

Similar to using a manual technique, overexposure may not be visually apparent when using the AEC device because the computer will adjust image brightness. It is therefore important for the radiographer to monitor the exposure indicator along with image quality to determine whether over or under exposure has occurred.

Exposure Adjustment

AEC devices are equipped with a mechanism (**exposure adjustment**) that allows the radiographer to adjust the amount of preset radiation detection values (also known as **density controls**). These are generally in the form of buttons on the control panel that are numbered −2, −1, +1, +2, and +3. The actual numbers presented on exposure adjustment vary, but each button changes exposure time by some predetermined amount or increment expressed as a percentage. A common increment is 25%, meaning that the predetermined exposure level needed to terminate the timer can be either increased or decreased from normal in one increment (+25% or −25%) or two increments (+50% or −50%).

A diagnostic quality image (Fig. 8-5A) was produced using 81 kVp and the center detector with 0 exposure adjustment, Fig. 8-5B was produced using 81 kVp and the center detector with +3 exposure adjustment, and Fig. 8-5C was produced using 81 kVp and the center detector with −3 exposure adjustment. Although the brightness was adjusted by the computer, the actual mAs applied and exposure indicator for each of the images varied greatly and reflected the exposure to the IR.

Manufacturers usually provide information for their equipment on how these exposure adjustments should be used. Common sense and practical experience should also serve as guidelines for

FIG. 8-5 Exposure adjustment. **A**, Radiographic image of the hip using 81 kVp, the center AEC detector, and 0 exposure adjustment. **B**, Radiographic image of the hip using 81 kVp, the center AEC detector, and +3 exposure adjustment. The image demonstrates less quantum noise than image *A*. **C**, Radiographic image of the hip using 81 kVp, the center AEC detector, and −3 exposure adjustment. The image demonstrates more quantum noise than *B*. The mAs readout for *B* and *C* reflect the exposure adjustment accordingly. (From Johnston JN, Fauber TL: *Essentials of Radiographic Physics and Imaging*, ed 3, St. Louis, 2020, Elsevier.)

the radiographer. Routinely using plus or minus exposure adjustments to produce an acceptable image indicates that a problem exists, possibly a problem with the AEC calibration.

Alignment and Positioning Considerations
Detector Selection
Selection of the detectors to be used for a specific examination is critical when using an AEC system. AEC systems with multiple detectors typically allow the radiographer to select any combination of one, two, or three detectors. Radiographic equipment can also be purchased with five AEC detectors (Fig. 8-6), which provide greater flexibility in imaging a wide variety of patients. The selected detectors actively measure radiation during exposure, and the electrical signals are averaged. Typically, the detector that receives the greatest amount of exposure has the greatest impact on the total exposure.

Measuring radiation that passes through the anatomic area of interest is important. The general guideline is to select the detectors that would be superimposed by the anatomic structures that are of greatest interest and need to be visualized on the radiographic image. Failure to select the proper detector(s) could result in either underexposure or overexposure to the IR. In the case of a posteroanterior (PA) chest radiograph, the area of radiographic interest includes the lungs and heart; therefore, one or two outside detectors should be selected to place the detectors directly beneath the critical anatomic area. If the center detector were mistakenly selected, the anatomy superimposing this detector includes the thoracic spine. If the exposure is made, the resultant image shows sufficient exposure in the spine, with the lungs overexposed (Fig. 8-7). Although brightness was adjusted by the computer, the actual mAs applied and exposure indicator reflect the image overexposure. It is important for radiographers to evaluate image quality, the applied mAs, and the exposure indicator when using the AEC device. AEC device manufacturers provide recommendations for which detectors to use for specific examinations. Recommendations for detector combination also can be found in many radiographic procedure textbooks.

FIG. 8-6 Multiple detectors. Illustration of radiographic equipment with five AEC detectors.

Many radiographic units have AEC devices in both a table Bucky and an upright Bucky. If more than one Bucky per radiographic unit uses AEC, the radiographer must be certain to select the correct Bucky before making an exposure. Failure to do so may result in the patient and IR being exposed to excessive radiation. If the backup time is reached, the exposure is prematurely terminated, and a repeat radiographic study may need to be done, increasing patient dose.

A similar problem can occur in some systems when not using a Bucky, such as with cross-table, tabletop or stretcher, or wheelchair studies. If the AEC system is activated with these types of examinations, an unusually long exposure results because the detectors are not being exposed to radiation. Again, the backup time will likely be reached, and the patient's dose will be excessive. Some radiographic units are designed so that an exposure does not occur if the AEC device has been selected and there is no IR detected in the Bucky.

IMPORTANT RELATIONSHIP

Detector Selection

The combination of detectors affects the amount of exposure reaching the IR. If the area of radiographic interest is not directly over the selected detectors, that area will likely be over-exposed or underexposed. When performing a radiographic study in which the IR is located outside the Bucky, the AEC system should be deactivated, and a manual technique should be used.

FIG. 8-7 Detector selection. **A,** Radiographic image created using the outer two AEC detectors appropriate for chest imaging. **B,** Radiographic image created when the center detector was inappropriately selected for a chest image, placing the thoracic spine directly over the detector. The resulting chest image has increased radiation exposure in the area of the spine, and therefore the lungs are overexposed. Although the brightness in the area of interest was computer adjusted, the mAs readout reflected the overexposure of the IR for chest image. (From Johnston JN, Fauber TL: *Essentials of Radiographic Physics and Imaging*, ed 3, St. Louis, 2020, Elsevier.)

Patient Centering

Proper centering of the part being examined is crucial when using an AEC system. The anatomic area of interest must be properly centered over the detectors that the radiographer has selected; improper centering of the part over the selected detectors may underexpose or overexpose the IR. For example, when an AEC device is used for a thoracic spine image, if the central ray is positioned over the right lung and the center detector is selected (as appropriate), the soft tissue and ribs superimpose the detector rather than the spine. In this case, the soft tissue and ribs demonstrate sufficient exposure, but the spine itself is underexposed (Fig. 8-8).

> **⚡ IMPORTANT RELATIONSHIP**
>
> *Patient Centering*
>
> Accurate centering of the area of interest over the detectors is critical to ensure proper exposure to the IR. If the area of interest is not properly centered to the detectors, overexposure or underexposure may occur.

When the anatomy of interest is not centered directly over the detector, the image is underexposed or overexposed, possibly requiring the image to be repeated and the patient to receive more radiation than necessary.

If the digital IR is underexposed or overexposed, the computer adjusts the exposure error, but the image quality, patient exposure, or both are compromised. Underexposure may result in the visibility of quantum noise, and overexposure increases patient exposure and may decrease contrast. It is important for radiographers to evaluate image quality, the applied mAs, and the exposure indicator when using the AEC device. Errors in selecting the appropriate combination

FIG. 8-8 Centering. **A,** The center detector was selected for this thoracic spine and the central ray (CR) midpoint to the thoracic spine. **B,** The CR was centered over the right lung field. The resulting image demonstrates appropriate brightness levels in the right lung and ribs, but the thoracic vertebral bodies are underexposed. (From Johnston JN, Fauber TL: *Essentials of Radiographic Physics and Imaging,* ed 3, St. Louis, 2020, Elsevier.)

of AEC detectors, detector size, or positioning errors may not be visually apparent because of computer adjustment of image brightness.

Detector Size

The size of the detectors manufactured within an AEC system is fixed and cannot be adjusted. Therefore, it is important for the radiographer to determine whether AEC should be used during the radiographic procedure. The radiographer must first determine whether the patient's anatomic area of interest can adequately cover the detector combination. For example, if the patient for a procedure is very small, such as a toddler, his or her chest may not adequately cover the outer two detectors. In this case, the patient's chest is smaller than the dimensions of the selected detectors. If a portion of the detector is directly exposed to the primary beam, the radiation exposure level necessary to terminate the exposure is reached almost immediately, resulting in underexposure of the area of interest.

It is critical for the radiographer to determine whether the anatomic area of interest can adequately superimpose the dimension of the detector combination. If the detector combination is larger in size than the area of interest, the use of a manual exposure technique would be necessitated.

> ⚠ **RADIATION PROTECTION ALERT**
>
> ### Errors in AEC Use
>
> It is important for radiographers to evaluate image quality, the applied mAs, and the exposure indicator when using the AEC device. Errors in selecting the appropriate combination of AEC detectors, detector size, or positioning errors may not be visually apparent because of computer adjustment.

Compensating Issues
Patient Considerations

The AEC system is designed to compensate for changes in patient thickness. If the area of interest is thicker because of an increase in the patient's size, the exposure time will lengthen to reach the preset exposure to the detectors. AEC systems that do not adequately compensate for changes in patient thickness may need to be calibrated.

Some patients may require greater technical consideration when AEC is used for radiographic procedures. For example, abdominal examinations using AEC can be compromised if a patient has an excessive amount of bowel gas. If a detector is superimposed by an area of the abdomen with excessive gas, the timer will prematurely terminate the exposure, resulting in underexposure to the IR. Likewise, destructive pathological conditions can cause underexposure of the area of radiographic interest. The presence of positive contrast media, an additive pathological condition, or a prosthetic device superimposing the detector can cause excessive exposure.

If the anatomic area directly over the detector does not represent the anatomic area of interest, inappropriate exposure to the IR may result. This can happen when the anatomic area over the detector contains a foreign object, a pocket of air, or contrast media. The radiographer must consider these circumstances individually and determine how to best image the patient or part. Using the exposure adjustment buttons may work in some cases, but in others, it may be necessary to recenter the patient or part. Sometimes the best solution is a manual technique determined through use of a technique chart. AEC is not a replacement for a knowledgeable radiographer using critical thinking skills.

> ⚠ **RADIATION PROTECTION ALERT**
>
> ### Patient Variability
>
> Factors related to the patient affect the time of exposure reaching the IR and ultimately the image quality; such factors include pathology, contrast media, foreign objects, and pockets of gas. Increases or decreases in patient thickness result in changes in the time of exposure if the AEC system is functioning properly.

Collimation

The size of the x-ray field is a factor when AEC systems are used because the additional scatter radiation produced by failure to accurately restrict the beam may cause the detector to prematurely terminate the exposure. The detector is unable to distinguish transmitted radiation from scattered radiation and, as always, ends the exposure when a preset amount of exposure has been reached. Because the detector is measuring both types of radiation exiting the patient, the timer is turned off too soon when scatter is excessive, resulting in underexposure of the area of interest.

In addition, if the x-ray field size is collimated too closely, the detector does not initially receive sufficient exposure and may prolong the exposure time, which could result in overexposure.

The radiographer should open the collimator to the extent that the part being radiographed is appropriately imaged but not so much as to cause the AEC device to terminate the exposure before the area being imaged is properly exposed.

 IMPORTANT RELATIONSHIP

Collimation and AEC Response

Excessive or insufficient collimation may affect the amount of exposure reaching the IR. Insufficient collimation may result in excessive scatter reaching the detectors, causing the exposure time to terminate too quickly. Excessive collimation may result in an extremely long exposure time.

Image Receptor Variations

Different types of IRs cannot be interchanged easily after an AEC device is calibrated to terminate exposures at a preset level. When calibration is performed, it is done for a specific type of IR.

 IMPORTANT RELATIONSHIP

Type of IR and AEC Response

The AEC system is calibrated based on the type of IR used. If an IR of a different type is used, the detectors will not sense the difference, and the exposure time will terminate at the preset value, which may jeopardize image quality.

The AEC device cannot sense when the radiographer uses a different type of IR and instead produces an exposure based on the system for which it was calibrated, resulting in either too much or too little exposure for that IR.

Calibration

As with any radiographic unit, it is imperative that systematic equipment testing be performed to ensure proper system performance. Calibration and quality-control testing are essential procedures to maintain the proper functioning of the AEC system (Box 8-1).

For an AEC device to function properly, the radiographic unit, including the type of IR, and the AEC device must be calibrated to meet departmental standards. When a radiographic unit with AEC is first installed, the AEC device is calibrated (and at intervals thereafter). The purpose of this calibration is to ensure that consistent and appropriate exposures to the IR are produced.

BOX 8-1   Quality-Control Check: AEC

- The AEC device should provide consistent exposures to the IR for variations in technique factors, patient thicknesses, and detector selection. Several aspects of the AEC performance can be monitored by imaging a homogeneous patient equivalent phantom plus additional thickness plates.
- Consistency of exposures with varying mA, kVp, part thicknesses, and detector selection can each be evaluated individually and in combination by imaging a patient equivalent phantom and measuring the resultant milliroentgen (mR) exposure and pixel brightness levels. Reproducibility of exposures for a given set of exposure factors and selected detector should result in mR readings within 5% and pixel brightness levels for areas within the displayed image should be within 30%

Failure to maintain regular calibration of the unit results in a lack of consistent and reproducible exposures to the detectors and could affect image quality. This situation ultimately leads to overexposure of the patient, poor efficiency of the imaging department, and the possibility of improper interpretation of radiographs.

The radiographer must use AEC accurately, regardless of the type of IR used. Failure to do so can result in overexposure of the patient to ionizing radiation or production of a poor-quality image. It cannot be overstated that when using digital IRs, the radiographer must be very conscientious about excessive radiation exposure to the patient. If a high amount of radiation reaches the digital IR, the image may appear diagnostic while the patient receives unnecessary exposure. During computer processing, image brightness can be adjusted after underexposure; however, there may be an increase in the visibility of quantum noise. The radiographer must monitor the exposure indicator as a means of detecting AEC malfunctions for digital IRs.

The response of the AEC device when changing exposure variables and their effect on exposure time and brightness in the area of interest are presented in Table 8-1.

ANATOMICALLY PROGRAMMED TECHNIQUE

Anatomic programming, or **anatomically programmed technique,** refers to a radiographic system that allows the radiographer to select a particular button on the control panel that represents an anatomic area for which a preprogrammed set of exposure factors are displayed and can be selected. The appearance of these controls varies depending on the unit (Fig. 8-9), but the operation of all anatomically programmed systems is based on the same principle. Anatomically programmed techniques are controlled by an integrated circuit or computer chip that has been programmed with exposure factors for different projections and positions of different anatomic parts. After an anatomic part and projection or position has been selected, the radiographer can adjust the exposure factors that are displayed.

Anatomically programmed technique systems and AEC are not related in their functions, other than as systems for making exposures. However, these two different systems are commonly combined in radiographic units because of their similar dependence on integrated computer circuitry and often are used in conjunction with one another. A radiographer can use an anatomically programmed technique to select a projection or position for a specific anatomic part and view the kVp, mA, and exposure time for a manual technique. When anatomically programmed techniques are used in conjunction with AEC on some radiographic units, the system not only selects and displays manual exposure factors but also selects and displays the AEC detectors to be used for a specific radiographic examination. For example, pressing the "Lungs PA" button results in selection of 120 kVp, the upright Bucky, and the two outside AEC detectors. As with AEC, the anatomically programmed technique is a system that automates some of the work of radiography. However, the individual judgment and discretion of the radiographer is still required to use the anatomically programmed technique system correctly for the production of diagnostic quality images (see Box 8-2 "Manual Techniques versus AEC").

! RADIATION PROTECTION ALERT

Anatomically Programmed Technique and Patient Exposure

When using a preprogrammed set of exposure factors, the radiographer must evaluate the appropriateness of the selected exposure technique factors. Adjustment of the preprogrammed exposure factors may be necessary for that patient or procedure.

TABLE 8-1 Digital Imaging and Automatic Exposure Control

An upright PA chest exam performed using the following factors produce a diagnostic image:

Flat-panel detector	AEC with two outer detectors
120 kVp	Upright Bucky
400 mA	0 (normal) exposure adjustment

Assuming all other factors remain the same, unless indicated, how would the following changes affect the response of the AEC device and image quality?

Change	Effect on Exposure Time	Effect on Brightness in Area of Interest	Explanation
CR IR	No effect	No effect	The AEC is calibrated to the flat-panel detector. The exposure ends when the exposure is sufficient for the IR, which is suboptimal for the CR image receptor. The computer maintains the brightness, but quantum noise is apparent because of underexposure of the imaging plate.
Center detector selected	Increased	No effect	Because the thoracic spine lies over the center detector, the IR receives more exposure than is needed. The mAs and exposure indicator will reflect an increase in exposure to the image receptor. The computer maintains the brightness, but the image contrast is decreased because of excessive scatter, and the patient is overexposed.
70 kVp	Increased	No effect	The length of exposure to the IR will be increased, resulting in an increase in the actual mAs to maintain the exposure to the IR. However, the subject contrast is increased because of the lower kVp.
100 mA	Increased	No effect	The length of exposure is increased to maintain exposure to the IR.
−2 exposure adjustment	Decreased	No effect	Changing the exposure adjustment button changes the setting of the AEC so it turns off the exposure much sooner. The mAs and exposure indicator will reflect a decrease in exposure to the IR. The computer maintains the brightness, but quantum noise is apparent because of underexposure of the IR.
Selecting the table Bucky setting but still using the upright Bucky	Increased	No effect	Excessive radiation reaches the IR because the detectors in the table Bucky are unable to terminate the exposure. The mAs and exposure indicator will reflect an increase in exposure to the IR. The computer maintains the brightness, but the image contrast is decreased because of excessive scatter, and the patient is overexposed.
Patient has a cardiac pacemaker positioned over the detector	Increased	No effect	The detector that is behind the pacemaker takes a long time to turn off the exposure because the radiation must pass through the pacemaker. The mAs and exposure indicator will reflect an increase in exposure to the IR. The computer maintains the brightness, but the image contrast is decreased because of excessive scatter, and the patient is overexposed.

AEC, Automatic exposure control; *CR,* computed radiography; *IR,* imaging receptor; *kVp,* kilovoltage peak; *mA,* milliamperage; *mAs,* milliamperage-second; *PA,* posteroanterior.

FIG. 8-9 Anatomically programmed technique selections are displayed on this console. The radiographer can choose from posteroanterior lungs, lateral skull, knee, and hand, among others. Each selection displays the preprogrammed technical factors that the radiographer can decide to use or adjust. (Courtesy of Philips Healthcare, Andover, Massachusetts.)

BOX 8-2   Manual Techniques versus AEC

- Manual exposure techniques require the radiographer to select the kVp and mAs necessary for the radiographic procedure. This requires the radiographer to consider the procedure, primary and secondary exposure variables, and patient considerations. Different from manual exposure techniques, the use of AEC systems terminates the radiation exposure exiting the patient based on the preset calibration of the radiation detectors; therefore, the actual mAs is not set by the radiographer. The decision to select manual exposure techniques or use the AEC device requires the radiographer to consider many variables.
- As previously discussed, the detector(s) selected must be adequately covered by the patient's anatomic area of interest. In the case of a pediatric patient or distal extremities, the area of interest may be too small to adequately cover the detector(s), and therefore the use of a manual exposure technique would be more appropriate.
- Patient factors, such as pathology, contrast media, or a foreign object, may cause the AEC device to terminate prematurely or result in an excessive exposure. The radiographer must consider these patient variations individually and determine whether the use of a manual exposure technique would be best.
- A few anatomic regions may be more challenging for the radiographer when using the AEC device. For example, centering for the axial clavicle to ensure the proper radiation exposure may be more difficult than selecting a manual exposure technique. In addition, any slight movement of the patient before the activation of the radiation exposure could result in the area of interest not being adequately centered to the central ray, such as a lateral cervical spine. In these situations, the radiographer could evaluate the mAs readout for an AP projection and then change to a manual exposure technique for the axial, lateral, or oblique positions.
- For radiographic procedures best suited, routine use of AEC is recommended. Proper use and calibration of the AEC system will lessen the potential for overexposures. This is especially important during digital imaging because computer processing will rescale image brightness, and an excessive radiation exposure would not be easily apparent to the radiographer.

EXPOSURE TECHNIQUE CHARTS

Exposure technique charts are useful tools that assist the radiographer in selecting a manual exposure technique or when using AEC, regardless of the type of IR. **Exposure technique charts** are pre-established guidelines used by the radiographer to select standardized manual or AEC exposure factors for each type of radiographic examination. Technique charts standardize the selection of exposure factors for the typical patient so that the quality of radiographic images is consistent. Additional information, such as collimation, AEC detector selection, and patient shielding, can be included in the technique chart.

For each radiographic procedure, the radiographer consults the technique chart for the recommended exposure variables—kVp, mAs, type of IR, grid, and SID. Based on the thickness of the anatomic part to be imaged, the radiographer selects the exposure factors presented in the technique chart. For example, if a patient is scheduled for a routine abdominal examination, the radiographer positions the patient and aligns the central ray to the patient and IR, measures the abdomen for a manual technique, and consults the chart for the pre-determined standardized exposure variables.

Because many factors have an impact on the selection of appropriate exposure factors, technique charts are instrumental in the production of consistent quality radiographic images, reduction in repeat radiographic studies, and reduction in patient exposure. The proper development and use of technique charts are keys to the selection of appropriate exposure factors.

IMPORTANT RELATIONSHIP
Exposure Technique Charts and Radiographic Quality

Exposure technique charts are important for digital imaging because digital systems have a wide dynamic range and can compensate for exposure technique errors. Technique charts should be developed and used with all types of radiographic imaging systems to maintain patient radiation exposure *as low as reasonably achievable* (ALARA).

Conditions

A technique chart presents the exposure factors that are to be used for a specific examination on the basis of the type of radiographic equipment. Technique charts help to ensure that consistent image quality is achieved throughout the entire radiology department; they also decrease the number of repeat radiographic studies needed and therefore decrease patient exposure.

Technique charts do not replace the critical thinking skills required of the radiographer. The radiographer must continue to use individual judgment and discretion in properly selecting exposure factors for each patient and type of examination. The primary task of the radiographer is to produce diagnostic quality images while delivering the least amount of radiation exposure. Technique charts are designed for an average or typical patient and do not account for unusual circumstances. Patient variability in terms of body build or physical condition or the presence of a pathological condition requires the radiographer to problem solve when selecting exposure factors. These atypical conditions require accurate patient assessment and appropriate exposure technique adjustment by the radiographer.

A technique chart should be established for each x-ray tube, even if a single generator is used for more than one tube. For example, if a radiographic room has two x-ray tubes, one for a radiographic table and one for an upright Bucky unit, each tube should have its own technique chart because of possible inherent differences in the radiation output produced by each tube. Furthermore, a portable radiographic unit must also have its own technique chart.

For technique charts to be effective tools in producing images of consistent quality, departmental standards for radiographic quality should be established. In addition, the standardization of exposure factors and the use of accessory devices are needed. For example, an average adult knee can be adequately radiographed with or without the use of a grid. Although both images might be acceptable, departmental standards may specify that the knee be radiographed with the use of a grid. These types of decisions should be made before technique chart development takes

FIG. 8-10 A caliper is used to measure part thickness. (From Johnston JN, Fauber TL: *Essentials of Radiographic Physics and Imaging*, ed 2, St. Louis, 2016, Mosby.)

place so that the departmental standards can be clarified. Technique charts are then constructed using these standards, to which radiographers should adhere.

For technique charts to be effective, the radiographic system should be operating properly. A good-quality control program for all radiographic equipment ensures monitoring of any variability in the performance of the equipment.

Accurate measurement of part thickness is a critical condition for the effective use of technique charts. The measured part thickness determines the selected kVp and mAs values for the radiographic examination. If the part is measured inaccurately, incorrect exposure factors may be selected. Measurement of part thickness must be standardized throughout the radiology department.

Calipers are devices that measure part thickness and should be readily accessible in every radiographic room (Fig. 8-10). In addition, the technique chart should specify the exact location for measuring part thickness. Part measurement may be performed at the location of the central ray midpoint or the thickest portion of the area to be radiographed. Errors in part thickness measurement are common mistakes made when one is consulting technique charts.

Because the range of exposures needed to produce a quality digital image is wider (wide exposure latitude), precise measurement of the anatomic part is not as critical. Although the technique charts discussed in this chapter use patient measurement to determine the exposure factors to be selected, categorizing the typical patient according to size (small, medium, and large) may be sufficient when using digital IRs.

Types of Technique Charts

Technique charts can vary widely in terms of their design, but they share some common characteristics. The primary exposure factors of kVp and mA and common accessory devices used,

TABLE 8-2   Variable kVp/Fixed mAs Technique Chart

Anatomic part: knee	IR: flat-panel detector
Projection: AP	Tabletop/Bucky: Bucky
Measuring point: midpatella	Grid ratio: 12:1
SID: 40 inches	Focal spot size: small

cm	kVp	mAs
10	63	8
11	65	8
12	67	8
13	69	8
14	71	8
15	73	8
16	75	8
17	77	8
18	79	8

AP, Anteroposterior; *IR*, image receptor; *kVp*, kilovoltage peak; milliamperage-second; *SID*, source-to-image-receptor distance.

such as IRs of various types and grid ratios, are included regardless of the type of technique chart used. Two primary types of exposure technique charts exist: fixed kVp/variable mAs and variable kVp/fixed mAs. Each type of chart has different characteristics, and both have advantages and disadvantages.

Variable kVp/Fixed mAs Technique Chart

The **variable kVp/fixed mAs technique chart** is based on the concept that kVp can be increased as the anatomic part size increases. Specifically, the baseline kVp is increased by 2 for every 1-cm (0.4-inch) increase in part thickness, whereas mAs is maintained (Table 8-2). The baseline kVp is the original kVp value predetermined for the anatomic area to be radiographed. The baseline kVp is then adjusted for changes in part thickness.

Accurate measurement of part thickness is critical to the effective use of this type of technique chart. Part thickness must be accurately measured to ensure that the 2-kVp adjustment is appropriately applied. The radiographer consults the technique chart and prepares the exposure factors specified for the type of radiographic examination (i.e., mAs, SID, grid use, and type of IR). The anatomic part is accurately measured, and the kVp is appropriately adjusted. For example, a standard exposure technique for a patient's knee measuring 10 cm (4 inches) is 63 kVp at 8 mAs, flat-panel IR, and the use of a 12:1 table Bucky grid. A patient with a knee measuring 15 cm (6 inches) would require a change only in the kVp from 63 to 73 (2-kVp change for every 1-cm [~0.5-inch] change in part thickness).

IMPORTANT RELATIONSHIP

Variable kVp/Fixed mAs Technique Chart

The variable kVp chart adjusts the kVp for changes in part thickness while maintaining a fixed mAs (2-kVp change for every 1-cm [~0.5-inch] change in part thickness).

TABLE 8-3 **Fixed kVp/Variable mAs Technique Chart**		
Anatomic part: knee	IR: flat-panel detector	
Projection: AP	Tabletop/Bucky: Bucky	
Measuring point: midpatella	Grid ratio: 12:1	
SID: 40 inches	Focal spot size: small	
cm	**kVp**	**mAs**
10–13	73	4
14–17	73	8
18–21	73	16

AP, Anteroposterior; *IR,* image receptor; *kVp,* kilovoltage peak; milliamperage-second; *SID,* source-to-image-receptor distance.

Determination of the baseline kilovoltage for each anatomic area has not been standardized. Historically, various methods have been used to determine the baseline kVp value. The goal is to determine a kVp value that adequately penetrates the anatomic part when using a 2-kVp adjustment for every 1-cm (~0.5-inch) change in tissue thickness. The baseline kVp value can be experimentally determined with the use of radiographic phantoms (patient-equivalent devices).

Developing a variable kVp technique chart that can be used effectively throughout the kilovoltage range has proved to be problematic. In addition, technology advances in IRs may challenge the applicability of the variable kVp/fixed mAs-type technique chart.

In general, changing the kVp values for variations in part thickness may be ineffective throughout the entire range of radiographic examinations. A variable kVp/fixed mAs chart may be most effective with pediatric patients or when small extremities, such as hands, toes, and feet, are being imaged. At low kVp levels, small changes in kVp may be more effective than changing the mAs.

This type of chart has the advantage of being easy to formulate because making kVp changes to compensate for different part sizes is simple. However, because kVp is variable, subject contrast may also vary, and these types of charts tend to be less accurate for part-size extremes. In addition, adequate penetration of the part is not assured.

Fixed kVp/Variable mAs Technique Chart

The **fixed kVp/variable mAs technique chart** (Table 8-3) uses the concept of selecting an optimal kVp value that is required for the radiographic examination and adjusting the mAs for variations in part thickness. **Optimal kVp** can be described as the kVp value that is high enough to ensure penetration of the part but not too high to diminish subject contrast. For this type of chart, the optimal kVp value for each part is indicated and mAs is varied as a function of part thickness.

IMPORTANT RELATIONSHIP

Fixed kVp/Variable mAs Technique Chart

The fixed kVp/variable mAs technique chart identifies optimal kVp values and alters the mAs for variations in part thickness (every 4- to 5-cm [1.6- to 2-inch] change in part thickness, the mAs should be adjusted by a factor of 2).

Optimal kVp values required for each anatomic area have not been standardized. Although charts identifying common kVp values for different anatomic areas can be found, experienced radiographers tend to develop their own optimal kVp values. The goal is to determine the kVp that penetrates the part without compromising subject contrast; however, digital computer processing provides the opportunity to vary the image contrast displayed. Specifying the optimal kVp value used in a fixed kVp/variable mAs technique chart encourages all radiographers to adhere to the departmental standards.

After optimal kVp values are established, fixed kVp/variable mAs technique charts alter the mAs for variations in the thickness of the anatomic part. Because x-rays are attenuated exponentially, a general guideline is that for every 4- to 5-cm (1.6- to 2-inch) change in part thickness, the mAs should be adjusted by a factor of 2. Using the previous example for a patient's knee measuring 10 cm (4 inches) and an optimal kVp, the exposure technique would be 73 kVp at 4 mAs, flat-panel IR with a 12:1 table Bucky grid. A patient with a knee measuring 15 cm (6 inches) would require a change only in the mAs from 4 to 8 (a 5-cm [2-inch] increase in part thickness requires a doubling of the mAs).

Accurate measurement of the anatomic part is important but is less critical compared with the precision needed with variable kVp charts. An advantage of fixed kVp/variable mAs technique charts is that patient groups can be formed for around 4- to 5-cm (1.6- to 2-in) changes. Alternatively, patients can be grouped by size (e.g., small, medium, large, extra large) or actual weight ranges in pounds (e.g., 100–130 pounds), and therefore measuring the thickness would not be required. In addition, using consistently higher "optimal" kVp ranges with digital imaging systems can reduce the variability among exposure techniques for the same or similar anatomic region.

The fixed kVp/variable mAs technique chart has the advantages of easier use, more consistency in the production of quality images, greater assurance of adequate penetration of all anatomic parts, uniform subject contrast, and increased accuracy with extreme variation in the size of the anatomic part.

Exposure Technique Chart Development

Radiographers can develop effective technique charts that assist in exposure technique selection. The steps involved in technique chart development are similar, regardless of the design of the technique chart. The primary tools needed are radiographic phantoms, calipers for accurate measurement, and a calculator. After diagnostic images are produced using these phantoms, exposure techniques can be **extrapolated** (mathematically estimated) for imaging other similar anatomic areas.

A critical component in technique chart development is to determine the minimal kVp value that adequately penetrates the anatomic part being radiographed. One available method is to use the concept of **comparative anatomy**, which can assist the radiographer in determining minimal kVp values. This concept states that different parts of the same size can be radiographed by use of the same exposure factors, provided that the minimal kVp value needed to penetrate the part is used in each case. For example, a radiographer knows what exposure factors to use with a particular radiographic unit for a knee that measures 10 cm (4 inches) for the AP projection, but he or she now needs to radiograph a shoulder; the radiographer measures the shoulder for the AP projection and determines that it measures 10 cm (4 inches). The radiographer does not have a technique for a shoulder for this radiographic unit. The concept of comparative anatomy states that the shoulder in this case can be successfully radiographed using the same technique that the radiographer has used for the 10-cm (4-inch) knee as long as the minimal kVp to penetrate the part has been used for the shoulder or knee.

BOX 8-3   How to Develop an Exposure Technique Chart

- Select a kVp value appropriate to the anatomic area to be imaged. Determine the mAs value that produces the desired exposure to the IR.
- Using a patient-equivalent phantom, produce several images by varying the kVp and mAs values. Use the general rules for exposure technique adjustment (i.e., the 15% rule). Exposures to the IR should be similar.
- Evaluate the quality of the images and eliminate those deemed unacceptable.
- Of the remaining acceptable images, select those having a kVp value appropriate for the type of technique chart desired and according to departmental standards.
- Extrapolate the exposure techniques (variable kVp or variable mAs) for changes in part thickness.
- Use the concept of comparative anatomy to develop technique charts for similar anatomic areas.
- Test the technique chart for accuracy and revise if needed.

The stages for development of exposure technique charts are similar, regardless of the type of chart (Box 8-3). Patient-equivalent phantoms for sample anatomic areas provide a means for establishing standardized exposure factors. Using the concept of comparative anatomy assists the radiographer in extrapolating exposure techniques for similar anatomic areas. After the initial development of an exposure technique chart, the chart must be tested for accuracy and revised if necessary.

Poor radiographic quality may result when the exposure technique chart is not used properly. Radiographers need to problem solve by evaluating the numerous exposure variables that could have contributed to a poor-quality radiograph before assuming that the chart is ineffective.

A commitment by management and staff to use exposure technique charts is critical to the consistent production of quality images. Well-developed technique charts are of little use if radiographers choose not to consult them.

 IMPORTANT RELATIONSHIP

Exposure Technique Charts

A commitment by management and staff to use exposure technique charts is critical to the consistent production of quality radiographic images. Well-developed technique charts are of little use if radiographers choose not to consult them.

SPECIAL CONSIDERATIONS

Appropriate exposure factor selection and its modification for variability in the patient are critical to the production of a quality image. The radiographer must be able to recognize a multitude of patient and equipment variables and have a thorough understanding of how these variables affect the resulting image to make adjustments to produce a quality radiographic image.

Pediatric Patients

Pediatric patients are a technical challenge for radiographers for many reasons. Because of their smaller size, they require lower kVp and mAs values than adults.

Pediatric chest radiography requires the radiographer to choose fast exposure times to stop diaphragm motion in patients who cannot or will not voluntarily suspend their breathing. A fast exposure time may eliminate the possibility of using AEC systems for pediatric chest radiography.

Owing to their small size, pediatric patients may not adequately cover AEC detectors, and therefore, a manual exposure technique should be used.

Exposure factors used for the adult skull can be used for pediatric patients aged 6 years and older, because the bone density of these children has developed to an adult level. However, exposure factors must be modified for patients younger than 6 years. It is recommended for the radiographer to decrease the kVp by at least 15% to compensate for this lack of bone density. In addition, one should limit the use of grids whenever possible. Radiographic examination of all other parts of pediatric patients' anatomy requires an adjustment in exposure techniques.

Because pediatric patients are more sensitive to ionizing radiation and have a longer life span than adults, it is even more critical to monitor the exposure indicator during digital imaging in an effort to minimize unnecessary radiation exposure.

Geriatric Patients

Aging patients may experience physical changes such as limitations in hearing, vision, and balance. Additionally, their skin is thinner and more easily torn or bruised. Psychological changes in the mental state of geriatric patients may impact their ability to follow instructions during imaging procedures. Radiographers should be prepared to provide enhanced patient care in terms of additional time for imaging procedures; sensitivity to patient comfort by using a table pad, positioning sponges, and blankets for warmth; and attention to the safety of geriatric patients during transport on and off of the table and positioning during the procedure.

Exposure techniques may need to be decreased for patients who appear thin and frail. Tissues may be lower in subject contrast and therefore require decreased kVp, which results in higher subject contrast. To eliminate motion, it is recommended for the radiographer to accordingly adjust the mA and exposure time.

Bariatric Patients

Body mass index (BMI) is a person's weight in kilograms divided by the square of height in meters. A high BMI (>30) can be an indicator of obesity. Imaging patients who are categorized as obese are more commonplace in radiology. Bariatric surgery is becoming more routine, and therefore imaging procedures may be needed both before and after surgery. Bariatric patients bring unique challenges in terms of their weight and body diameter.

Important issues to consider when imaging bariatric patients include the table weight limit and the size (aperture) diameter of fluoroscopic imaging equipment. Bariatric patients need an increase in both kVp and mAs values to produce diagnostic images. In addition, the use of a grid is important to reduce the scatter radiation from reaching the IR, which would decrease image contrast. Depending on the imaging procedure performed, bariatric patients may need to be imaged in quadrants owing to the size limitation of the IR.

Projections and Positions

Different radiographic projections and patient positions of the same anatomic part often require modification of exposure factors. For example, an oblique position of the lumbar spine requires more exposure than an AP projection because of an increase in the amount of tissue through which the primary beam must pass. However, an oblique ankle image requires slightly less exposure than the AP for comparable exposure to the IR.

General guidelines, based on variations in radiographic projection or patient position, can be followed to change exposure factors. Compared with an AP projection, an increase or a decrease in the amount of tissue should determine any changes in exposure factors for oblique and lateral patient positions.

Casts and Splints

Casts and splints can be produced from materials that attenuate x-rays differently. Selecting appropriate exposure factors can be challenging because of the wide variety of materials used for these devices. The radiographer should pay close attention to both the type of material and how the cast or splint is used.

Casts

Casts can be made of either fiberglass or plaster. Fiberglass generally requires no change in exposure factors from the values used for the same anatomic part without a cast.

Plaster presents a problem in terms of exposure factors. Plaster casts require an increase in exposure factors compared with that needed to image the same part without a cast. However, the method and amount of increase in exposure have not been standardized.

Exposure factor adjustments for cast materials may be based on the part thickness using a technique chart. For example, if an AP ankle measured through the CR is 4 inches (10 cm) without the cast and 8 inches (20 cm) with the cast, the radiographer simply increases the exposure technique to that of an ankle measuring 8 inches (20 cm) to obtain an acceptable image.

Splints

Splints present less of a challenge for the determination of appropriate exposure factors than casts. Inflatable (air) and fiberglass splints do not require any increase in exposure. Wood, aluminum, and solid plastic splints may require that exposure factors be increased but only if they are in the path of the primary beam. For example, if two pieces of wood are bound to the sides of a lower leg, no increase in exposure is necessary for an AP projection because the splint is not in the path of the primary beam and does not interfere with the radiographic image. Using the same example, if a lateral projection is produced, the splint is in the path of the primary beam and interferes with the imaging of the part. An increase in the exposure technique is required to produce a properly exposed radiographic image.

Pathologic Conditions

Pathological conditions that can alter the absorption characteristics of the anatomic part being examined are divided into two categories. *Additive diseases* are diseases or conditions that increase the absorption characteristics of the part, making the part more difficult to penetrate. *Destructive diseases* are diseases or conditions that decrease the absorption characteristics of the part, making the part less difficult to penetrate. Table 8-4 lists additive and destructive diseases. Generally, it is necessary to increase the kVp when radiographing parts that have been affected by additive diseases and to decrease the kVp when radiographing parts affected by destructive diseases.

However, it is not necessary to compensate for all additive and destructive diseases. It is often desirable to image diseases with exposure factors that would normally be used for a specific anatomic part so that the effect of that disease on that part can be clearly visualized.

When it is necessary or desirable to compensate for additive or destructive diseases or conditions, it is best to make changes in the kVp. Changing the kVp is fundamentally correct because the kVp affects the penetrating ability of the primary beam, and it is the penetrability of the anatomic part that is affected by these specific diseases and conditions. It is impossible to state an exact amount or percentage by which the kVp should be changed, because the state or severity of the disease or condition differs with each patient; however, a minimum change of 15% in kVp is recommended. There are some instances in which a change in mAs may be more appropriate to the type of pathological condition. For example, if the anatomic area has a significant increase in gas, such as in bowel obstruction, a large decrease in mAs is best.

TABLE 8-4	**Common Additive and Destructive Diseases and Conditions by Anatomic Area**
Additive Conditions	**Destructive Conditions**
Abdomen	
Aortic aneurysm	Bowel obstruction
Ascites	Free air
Cirrhosis	
Hypertrophy of some organs (e.g., splenomegaly)	
Chest	
Atelectasis	Emphysema
Congestive heart failure	Pneumothorax
Malignancy	
Pleural effusion	
Pneumonia	
Skeleton	
Hydrocephalus	Gout
Metastases (osteoblastic)	Metastases (osteolytic)
Osteochondroma (exostoses)	Multiple myeloma
Paget's disease (late stage)	Paget's disease (early stage)
Osteoporosis	
Nonspecific Sites	
Abscess	Atrophy
Edema	Emaciation
Sclerosis	Malnutrition

Soft Tissue

Objects such as small pieces of wood, glass, or swallowed bones are difficult to radiographically visualize using the normal exposure factors for a specific anatomic part. Several situations in which a soft tissue technique (decreased mAs) may be needed are visualization of the larynx in a young child with croup, possible foreign body obstruction in the throat, and foreign body location in the extremities (Fig. 8-11). However, digital imaging systems allow visualization of soft tissues without changing the exposure technique.

Contrast Media

A contrast medium (also called *contrast agent*) is used when imaging anatomic tissues that have low subject contrast. A **contrast medium** is a substance that can be instilled into the body by injection or ingestion. The type of contrast medium used changes the absorption characteristics of the area of interest by either increasing or decreasing the attenuation of the x-ray beam. Positive contrast agents, such as barium (atomic # 56) and iodine (atomic # 53), have a high atomic number and absorb more x-rays (increase attenuation) than the surrounding tissue (Fig. 8-12). Negative contrast agents, such as air (atomic # 8), decrease the attenuation of the x-ray beam and transmit more radiation than the surrounding tissue (Fig. 8-13). Positive contrast agents produce more brightness on the image than the adjacent tissues; negative contrast agents produce less brightness on the image than the adjacent tissues.

FIG. 8-11 Soft tissue imaging. Lateral soft tissue neck radiographic image. (From Frank E: *Merrill's Atlas of Radiographic Positioning and Procedures*, ed 12, St. Louis, 2012, Mosby.)

FIG. 8-12 Positive contrast agents. Radiographic image showing increased brightness because of the increase in x-ray beam attenuation by use of a positive contrast agent.

FIG. 8-13 Negative contrast agents. Radiographic image showing decreased brightness because of the decrease in x-ray beam attenuation by use of a negative contrast agent.

Although negative contrast agents decrease the attenuation characteristics of the part being examined, their use does not require a change in exposure factors. Negative contrast agents can also be used in conjunction with positive contrast agents. Positive contrast media studies require an increase in exposure factors compared with imaging the same part without a positive contrast medium. The use of a contrast agent is an effective method of increasing the subject contrast when imaging areas of low subject contrast.

The quality of the radiographic image depends on a multitude of variables. Knowledge of these variables and their radiographic effect assists the radiographer in selecting exposure techniques to produce quality radiographic images.

CHAPTER SUMMARY

- AEC systems are designed to produce sufficient radiation exposure to the IR to produce a quality image.
- AEC uses detectors (typically ionization type) that measure the amount of radiation exiting the patient and terminate the exposure when it reaches a preset amount; this amount corresponds to the amount of radiation needed to produce diagnostic image quality.
- The kVp selected must penetrate the part and produce the desired subject contrast. Increasing or decreasing the kVp causes the exposure time to be decreased or increased accordingly when using AEC.
- Changing the mA, when available, causes the exposure time to be decreased or increased accordingly when using AEC.
- The mAs readout displayed after the AEC exposure informs the radiographer of the total radiation exposure used for the procedure.

- For AEC to work accurately, the x-ray beam must be centered precisely to the anatomic area of interest, the correct detectors must be selected, and the anatomic part must cover the dimension of the detectors.
- Other AEC features that can be manipulated include exposure adjustment controls that allow increased or decreased exposure to the IR and the backup time (or mAs) provides a safety mechanism that prevents the exposure from exceeding a set amount.
- Limitations of AEC systems include that they typically allow only one type of IR and that the minimum response time may be longer than the exposure needed.
- Anatomically programmed technique is another exposure system that allows the selection of a specific body part and position, resulting in display of preprogrammed exposure factors. These may include AEC information.
- Quality control is important in monitoring the performance of the AEC system. Reproducibility of exposures for a given set of exposure factors and selected detector should result in mR readings within 5% and pixel brightness levels for areas within the displayed image should be within 30%.
- Exposure technique charts standardize the selection of exposure factors for a typical patient so that the quality of radiographic images is consistent.
- The variable kVp/fixed mAs technique chart is based on the concept that kVp can be increased as the anatomic part size increases. The baseline kVp is adjusted for changes in part thickness.
- The fixed kVp/variable mAs technique chart uses the concept of selecting an optimal kVp value that is required for the radiographic examination and adjusting the mAs for variations in part thickness.
- Exposure factors may need to be modified for pediatric, geriatric, and bariatric patients and varying projections and positions, casts and splints, pathological conditions, soft tissue, and contrast media.

REVIEW QUESTIONS

1. AEC devices work by measuring _____.
   A. radiation leaving the tube
   B. radiation that exits the patient
   C. radiation that is absorbed by the patient
   D. attenuation of primary radiation by the patient
2. How many detectors are typically found in an AEC system?
   A. One
   B. Two
   C. Three
   D. Four
3. Minimum response time refers to _____.
   A. the proper exposure time needed for an optimal exposure when an AEC device is used
   B. exposure time minus the amount of time the AEC detectors spend measuring the radiation
   C. the difference in exposure times between AEC systems and electronic timers
   D. the shortest exposure time possible when an AEC device is used
4. Which of the following statements about using AEC during digital imaging is true?
   A. Adjusting the mA value affects image brightness.
   B. Adjusting the kVp value affects image brightness.
   C. Adjusting the backup time affects image brightness.
   D. Adjusting the exposure adjustment control affects the exposure to the IR.

5. Which one of the following statements comparing ionization chamber AEC systems with phototimers is true?
   A. Ionization chamber systems are accurately called phototimers.
   B. Ionization chamber systems measure radiation before it interacts with the IR.
   C. Phototimers are more modern.
   D. Phototimers measure radiation before it interacts with the IR.

6. The purpose of the backup timer is to _____.
   A. ensure a diagnostic exposure each time AEC is used
   B. produce consistent levels of exposure on all images
   C. determine the exposure time that is used
   D. limit unnecessary x-ray exposure

7. What detector(s) should be selected for a right AP shoulder when the patient is supine on the x-ray table?
   A. Right detector only
   B. Center detector only
   C. Right and left detectors only
   D. Right, center, and left detectors

8. The purpose of anatomically programmed techniques is to _____.
   A. present the radiographer with a preselected set of exposure factors
   B. override AEC when the radiographer has made a mistake in its use
   C. determine which AEC detectors should be used for a specific examination
   D. prevent overexposure and underexposure of images, which sometimes happen when AEC is used

9. Which statement concerning both AEC and anatomically programmed techniques is true?
   A. The skilled use of both requires less knowledge of exposure factors on the part of the radiographer.
   B. The use of both requires the radiographer to be less responsible for accurate centering of the anatomic part.
   C. The individual judgment and discretion of the radiographer is still necessary when using these systems.
   D. The tasks involved with practicing radiography generally are made more difficult with these systems.

10. When using AEC with digital imaging systems, assuming all other factors are correct, selecting the center detector on a PA chest image results in _____.
    A. decreased exposure in the lung area
    B. increased exposure in the lung area
    C. appropriate exposure in the lung area
    D. increased quantum noise in the image

11. When using AEC with digital imaging systems, assuming all other factors are correct, selecting the −2 exposure adjustment on a PA chest image results in _____.
    A. increased quantum noise
    B. increased brightness in the lung area
    C. appropriate brightness in the lung area
    D. A and C

12. Which of the following special considerations may require an increase in mAs?
    A. contrast media
    B. bariatric patient
    C. plaster cast
    D. all of the above

13. What type of exposure technique system uses a fixed mAs regardless of part thickness?
    A. Fixed kVp
    B. Variable kVp
    C. Manual
    D. AEC
14. A primary goal of an exposure technique chart is to _____.
    A. extend the life of the x-ray tube
    B. improve the radiographer's accuracy
    C. produce quality images consistently
    D. increase the patient workflow
15. Which of the following is an important condition required for technique charts to be effective?
    A. Equipment must be calibrated to perform properly.
    B. One technique chart should be used for all radiographic units.
    C. All technologists should use the same mAs setting.
    D. The chart should not be revised once it has been used.
16. Instilling a negative contrast agent in the gastrointestinal tract has what effect in the area of interest on the digital image?
    A. Increased brightness
    B. Decreased contrast
    C. Decreased brightness
    D. No effect

Film-Screen Imaging

CHAPTER OUTLINE

Film Image Quality
Radiographic Film
    Latent Image Formation
    Film Characteristics
Intensifying Screens
    Screen Speed
Automatic Film Processing
    Processing Stages

Processing Systems
Quality Control
Silver Recovery
Film-Screen Characteristics
    Density
    Contrast
Sensitometry
    Equipment

Sensitometric Curve
Film Characteristics
Clinical Considerations
Image Display

OBJECTIVES

*After completing this chapter, the reader will be able
to perform the following:*

1. Define all the key terms in this chapter.
2. State all the important relationships in this
   chapter.
3. Describe the characteristics of a quality film
   radiograph.
4. Explain how latent images are formed on film.
5. State the purpose of intensifying screens in
   film-screen imaging.
6. Explain how intensifying screens can be
   characterized based on the type of phosphor,
   spectral emission, spectral sensitivity, and
   screen speed.
7. Recognize the effect intensifying screens have on
   image quality and patient radiation exposure.
8. Explain how latent images are converted
   to manifest images during automatic film
   processing.

9. State the developing and fixing agents used in
   chemical processing.
10. List the sequential stages and systems needed
    to process a quality radiographic film image.
11. State methods to maintain the archival quality
    of film radiographs.
12. Discuss the role of chemical replenishment,
    temperature control, and silver recovery during
    film processing.
13. State the requirements for darkroom safelights,
    temperature, and humidity control.
14. Describe how optical density is measured and
    its role in film image quality.
15. Differentiate short-scale from long-scale
    contrast.
16. Define sensitometry and discuss film speed,
    contrast, and latitude.

KEY TERMS

automatic film processor
average gradient
base plus fog (B + F)

cassette
D_{max}
D_{min}

densitometer
developing agents
diagnostic densities

KEY TERMS—cont'd

double-emulsion film	long-scale contrast	sensitometric curve
dynamic range	low contrast	sensitometric strip
emulsion layer	luminescence	sensitometry
exposure latitude	maximum contrast	short-scale contrast
feed tray	optical density (OD)	shoulder region
film contrast	optimal density	silver halide
film-screen contact	penetrometer	silver recovery
film speed	phosphor layer	slope
fixing agent	radiographic density	spectral emission
fluorescence	rare earth elements	spectral matching
gradient point	recirculation system	spectral sensitivity
high contrast	reducing agents	speed
illuminators	relative speed (RS)	speed exposure point
immersion heater	replenishment	speed point
intensifying screen	scale of contrast	standby control
intensity of radiation exposure	screen film	step-wedge densities
latent image centers	screen speed	straight-line region
latent image formation	sensitometer	toe region

Before the development of digital IRs, radiographic images were acquired, processed, and displayed on film. Film is placed in a cassette housing two intensifying screens to reduce patient exposure. To create and display a radiographic image, an active layer or emulsion is adhered to a sheet of polyester plastic. The emulsion contains crystals suspended in gelatin that serve as the latent imaging centers. To reduce patient exposure, radiographic film is placed between two intensifying screens. The intensifying screens convert the exit radiation intensities into visible light, and the light exposes the crystals in the emulsion.

The film must be chemically processed in an automatic processor before it is visualized on the sheet of polyester plastic. After it is chemically processed, the film image displays densities ranging from dark to light that correspond to the variations in the intensities of radiation exiting the anatomic tissues. The dark densities are created when the exposed crystals are converted to black metallic silver. The light or clear areas on the film result from the removal of unexposed crystals during chemical processing. The resulting image represents a range of densities created as a result of the x-ray attenuation characteristics of the anatomic structures. Anatomic tissues through which radiation is transmitted are visualized as dark densities and those in which radiation is absorbed are visualized as light or clear areas on the film.

FILM IMAGE QUALITY

The visibility of the anatomic structures and the accuracy of their structural lines recorded (sharpness) determine the overall quality of the radiographic image (Fig. 9.1). Visibility of the anatomic details refers to the density and contrast of the image. The accuracy of the structural lines (sharpness) is achieved by maximizing the amount of recorded detail and minimizing the amount of distortion. Visibility of the anatomic tissues is achieved by the proper balance of density and contrast. In addition, the anatomic details must be recorded accurately and with the greatness amount of sharpness (Fig. 9.2).

Film Image Quality

FIG. 9-1 Film image quality: factors affecting the quality of a film image. Photographic properties (visibility) include density and contrast. Geometric properties (sharpness) include recorded detail and distortion. (From Johnston JN, Fauber TL: *Essentials of Radiographic Physics and Imaging*, ed 3, St. Louis, 2020, Elsevier.)

FIG. 9-2 Quality film image. Radiograph demonstrating the proper balance of density and contrast, maximum recorded detail, and minimal distortion. (From Johnston JN, Fauber TL: *Essentials of Radiographic Physics and Imaging*, ed 3, St. Louis, 2020, Elsevier.)

The following sections of this chapter focus on construction of radiographic film and intensifying screens, automatic film processing to convert the latent image into a manifest image, density and contrast, sensitometry, and displaying the radiographic image.

RADIOGRAPHIC FILM

Radiographic film acquires a latent image and must be chemically processed before it is visible. Consequently, film serves as the medium for image acquisition, processing, and display. Several types of radiographic film may be used in medical imaging departments. Depending on the specific application, film manufacturers produce film in a variety of sizes ranging from 20 × 25 cm (8 × 10 inches) to 35 × 43 cm (14 × 17 inches). The composition of film can be described in layers (Box 9.1). The most important layer for creating the image is the **emulsion layer**. This is a radiation- and light-sensitive layer of the film. The emulsion of film consists of silver halide crystals suspended in gelatin. **Silver halide** is a material that is sensitive to radiation and light. The emulsion layer is fragile and must have a layer composed of a polyester base so that the film can be handled and processed while remaining physically strong after processing. Most film used in radiographic procedures has a dye or tint added to the base layer to decrease eye strain when viewed on a view (illuminator) box.

Screen film is the most widely used radiographic film. As its name implies, it is intended to be used with one or two intensifying screens. Screen film is more sensitive to light and less sensitive to x-rays. Screen film can have either a single- or double-emulsion coating. **Double-emulsion film** has an emulsion coating on both sides of the base. Film-screen imaging typically uses double-emulsion film with two intensifying screens.

BOX 9-1   Composition of Radiographic Film

- *Supercoat:* durable protection layer
- *Emulsion:* radiation- and light-sensitive layer
- *Adhesive:* adheres layers together
- *Film base:* polyester layer that gives the film physical stability

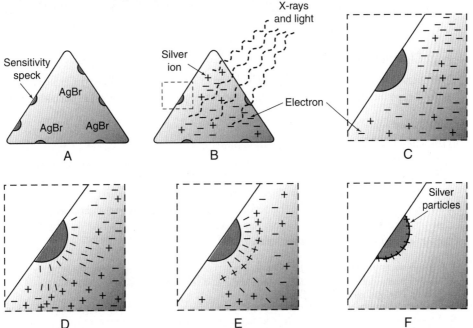

FIG. 9-3 Latent image formation theory. **A,** Before exposure, silver halide (AgBr and AgI) is suspended in gelatin in the emulsion layer. Sensitivity specks exist as physical imperfections in the film lattice. **B,** Exposure to x-rays and light ionizes the silver halide. **C,** Negatively charged electrons and positively charged silver ions float freely in the emulsion gelatin. **D,** Sensitivity specks trap electrons. **E,** Each trapped electron attracts a silver ion. **F,** Metallic silver clumps around the sensitivity specks.

Latent Image Formation

The specific way in which latent images are formed is unknown, but the Gurney–Mott theory of **latent image formation** is most widely believed to explain best the manner in which this process occurs. To explain latent image formation, it is necessary to describe what happens at the molecular level in the emulsion layer of the film—specifically, what happens to silver halide crystals when exposed to x-rays and light.

Physical imperfections, known as *sensitivity specks,* in the silver halide crystals are the sites of the latent image formation (Fig. 9.3). Exposure to x-rays and light ionizes the silver halide crystals, and the freed electrons become trapped at the sensitivity specks. The negatively charged sensitivity specks attract the freed silver ions. Every silver ion that combines with an electron is neutralized by that electron, thereby becoming metallic silver. Several sensitivity specks with many silver ions attracted to them become **latent image centers**. These latent image centers appear as areas of **radiographic density** on the manifest image after processing. It is believed that for a latent image center to appear, it must contain at least three sensitivity specks with at least three silver atoms each. With more exposure to the film, more metallic silver is visualized as radiographic density.

 IMPORTANT RELATIONSHIP

Sensitivity Specks and Latent Image Centers

Sensitivity specks serve as the focal points for the development of latent image centers. After exposure, these specks trap the free electrons and then attract and neutralize the positive silver ions. After enough silver is neutralized, the specks become a latent image center and are converted into metallic silver after chemical processing.

Film Characteristics

Manufacturers of radiographic film offer a wide variety of films. These differ not only in size and general type but also in film speed, film contrast, exposure latitude, and spectral sensitivity.

Film Speed

Film speed is the degree to which the emulsion is sensitive to x-rays or light. The greater the speed of a film, the more sensitive it is. Because sensitivity increases, less exposure is necessary to produce a specific density. Two primary factors, both relating to the silver halide crystals found in the emulsion layers, affect the speed of radiographic film. The first factor is the number of silver halide crystals present, and the second factor is the size of these crystals. Radiographic film manufacturers control film speed by manipulating both of these factors during the production of radiographic films with specific speeds.

 IMPORTANT RELATIONSHIP

Silver Halide and Film Sensitivity

As the number and/or size of silver halide crystals increase, film sensitivity or speed increases. A faster film speed requires less radiation exposure to produce a specific density.

Film Contrast and Latitude

Film contrast refers to the ability of radiographic film to provide a certain level of image contrast (density differences). High-contrast film accentuates more black and white areas, whereas low-contrast film primarily shows shades of gray. The latitude of film affects the range of radiation exposures that can provide **diagnostic densities**. A radiographic film capable of responding to a wide range of exposures to produce diagnostic densities is considered to be a *wide-latitude film*.

Spectral Sensitivity

Spectral sensitivity refers to the color of light to which a particular film is most sensitive. In radiography, there are generally two categories of spectral sensitivity films: blue sensitive and green sensitive (orthochromatic). When radiographic film is used with intensifying screens, it is important to match the spectral sensitivity of the film with the spectral emission of the screens. **Spectral emission** refers to the color of light produced by a particular intensifying screen. In radiography, two categories of spectral emission generally exist: blue light–emitting screens and green light–emitting screens. It is critical to use blue-sensitive film with blue light–emitting screens and green-sensitive film with green light–emitting screens. **Spectral matching** refers to correctly matching the color sensitivity of the film to the color emission of the intensifying screen. An incorrect match of film and screens based on spectral emission and sensitivity results in radiographs that display inappropriate levels of radiographic density.

INTENSIFYING SCREENS

An **intensifying screen** is a device found in radiographic cassettes that contains phosphors to convert x-ray energy into light, which then exposes the radiographic film (Fig. 9.4). The purpose of this device is to intensify the action of the x-rays and permit much lower x-ray exposures compared with film alone.

As with radiographic film, the construction of screens can be described in layers (Box 9.2). The **phosphor layer**, or active layer, is the most important screen component because it contains the phosphor material that absorbs the transmitted x-rays and converts them to visible light. The

FIG. 9-4 Typical set of intensifying screens inside a cassette.

BOX 9-2 **Composition of Intensifying Screen**

- *Protective layer:* plastic that protects the phosphor
- *Phosphor layer:* absorbs radiation and converts it to light
- *Reflecting layer:* reflects light toward the film or *absorbing layer:* absorbs light directed toward it
- *Base:* provides support and stability for the phosphor layer

most common phosphor materials consist of chemical compounds of elements from the rare earth group. **Rare earth elements** are elements that range in atomic number from 57 to 71 on the periodic table; they are referred to as *rare earth elements* because they are relatively difficult and expensive to extract from the Earth.

Intensifying screen systems used in cassettes generally include two screens. The screen that is mounted on the side of the cassette facing the x-ray tube is called the *front screen*, and the screen that is mounted on the opposite side is called the *back screen*. With two screens, the film (double-emulsion) is exposed to approximately twice as much light as that in a single-screen system because the film is exposed to light from both sides. Some screen systems use only a single screen and are used with single-emulsion film. When a single screen is used, it is mounted as a back screen on the side of the cassette that is opposite from the tube side. When loading a single-emulsion film into the appropriate cassette with a single screen, the emulsion side of the film must be placed against the intensifying screen.

Film is much more sensitive to visible light than to x-rays. By converting each absorbed high-energy x-ray photon into thousands of visible light photons, intensifying screens amplify film density. Without screens, the total amount of energy to which the film is exposed comprises only x-rays. With screens, the total amount of energy to which the film is exposed is divided between x-rays and light. When intensifying screens are used, approximately 90% to 99% of the total energy to which the film is exposed is light. X-rays account for the remaining 1% to 10% of the energy.

Intensifying screens operate by a process known as *luminescence*. **Luminescence** is the emission of light from the screen when stimulated by radiation. The desired type of luminescence in imaging is *fluorescence*. **Fluorescence** refers to the ability of phosphors to emit visible light only while exposed to x-rays (with little or no afterglow). An undesired type of luminescence is phosphorescence. *Phosphorescence* is the emission of light after x-ray exposure has terminated. Phosphorescence or afterglow causes unwanted exposure to the film.

Screen Speed

The purpose of intensifying screens is to decrease the radiation dose to the patient. Because screen phosphors can intensify the action of x-rays by converting them to visible light, the use of such screens allows the radiographer to use considerably lower milliamperage-seconds (mAs) values. The disadvantage of using screens is the reduction in recorded detail. The reason for the reduction is that visible light photons created within the screen tend to disperse before reaching the film emulsion; this blurs the image.

 IMPORTANT RELATIONSHIP

Screen Speed and Recorded Detail

As screen speed increases, recorded detail decreases; as screen speed decreases, recorded detail increases.

Screen manufacturers produce a variety of intensifying screens that differ in how well they intensify the action of the x-rays and therefore differ in their capacity to produce accurate recorded detail.

The capability of a screen to produce visible light is called **screen speed**. A faster screen produces more light than a slower screen for the same exposure. Although very fast screens reduce patient exposure, they also degrade recorded detail and increase quantum mottle (noise), and hence, a balance must be chosen.

IMPORTANT RELATIONSHIP

Screen Speed, Light Emission, and Patient Dose

> The faster an intensifying screen, the more light is emitted for the same intensity of x-ray exposure. As the screen speed increases, less radiation is necessary, and the radiation dose to the patient is decreased; as screen speed decreases, more radiation is necessary, and the radiation dose to the patient is increased.

Several factors affect how fast or slow an intensifying screen is, including absorption efficiency, conversion efficiency, thickness of the phosphor layer, and size of the phosphor crystal (Table 9.1). The presence of a reflecting layer, an absorbing layer, or dye in the phosphor layer also affects screen speed.

Absorption efficiency refers to the ability of the screen to absorb the incident x-ray photons. A rare earth phosphor screen absorbs approximately 60% of the incident photons. *Conversion efficiency* describes how well the screen phosphor takes these x-ray photons and converts them to visible light. Increased absorption and conversion efficiency mean that rare earth phosphors have increased speed compared with a previously used screen phosphor, calcium tungstate. This increased speed allows the radiographer to substantially reduce the x-ray exposure required to produce images with the appropriate amount of density.

In addition, the thickness of the phosphor layer and the size of the crystal affect the screen speed. A thicker phosphor layer contains more phosphor material than a thinner one. Phosphor converts x-rays into light; hence, if more phosphor material is present in a screen, more light is produced, increasing the screen speed. The size of the phosphor material crystals also affects screen speed. Larger phosphor crystals produce more light than smaller phosphor crystals. Again, more light being produced means that the screen is faster.

The final factors that affect screen speed are the presence or absence of a reflecting layer, a light-absorbing layer, or light-absorbing dyes in the phosphor layer. When present, a reflecting layer increases screen speed (at the expense of decreased recorded detail) by redirecting retrograde light back toward the film emulsion. Conversely, a light-absorbing layer or light-absorbing dyes present in the phosphor layer are used to decrease screen speed (and increase recorded detail) by absorbing light that would otherwise reach and expose the film.

The ability of the screen to produce visible light can also be described in terms of its **relative speed (RS)**. RS results from comparing film-screen systems on the basis of the amount of light produced for a given exposure. Film-screen RSs range from 50 to 800 RS. Most radiology departments that use film-screen technology have at least two different speeds of intensifying screen systems. A fast system is usually available with an RS of approximately 400. A 400-RS system is a good compromise between the beneficial effect of decreasing the patient dose and the detrimental effect of decreasing the recorded detail. A slower system is usually available, and it is sometimes labeled on the outside

TABLE 9-1 Summary of Effects of Screen Factors on Screen Speed, Recorded Detail, and Patient Dose

Screen Factor	Screen Speed	Recorded Detail	Patient Dose
Thicker phosphor layer	↑	↓	↓
Larger phosphor crystal size	↑	↓	↓
Reflective layer	↑	↓	↓
Absorbing layer	↓	↑	↑
Dye in phosphor layer	↓	↑	↑

of the cassette as *detail* or *extremity*. Typically, the RS of this system is 100. Detail or extremity screen systems are relatively slow and require greater exposure and result in higher patient doses. However, the anatomic parts imaged with detail or extremity screen systems are generally small; therefore, they do not require large exposures. Detail or extremity screen systems produce excellent recorded detail. The radiographer must be careful in selecting the appropriate screen system for the ordered examination. Cassettes with extremity and detail screens should be used only for tabletop examinations. They should never be used in the Bucky tray because of the excessive amount of exposure required.

Because the film-screen system speed affects radiographic density, the mAs should be adjusted if the film-screen speed is changed. Increasing the film-screen system speed requires a decrease in the mAs to maintain radiographic density. A decrease in the film-screen system speed requires an increase in the mAs to maintain density.

 IMPORTANT RELATIONSHIP

Film-Screen System Speed and mAs

> Increasing the film-screen speed requires a decrease in the mAs to maintain density. Decreasing the film-screen speed requires an increase in the mAs to maintain density.

The RS classification of film-screen systems provides a method whereby exposure techniques can be adjusted for changes in film-screen speed. The relative film-screen speed conversion formula is a mathematical formula for adjusting the mAs for changes in the film-screen system speed:

$$\frac{mAs_1}{mAs_2} = \frac{RS_2}{RS_1}$$

The correct relative film-screen speed factors must be used to calculate the new mAs required to compensate for the change in density. The new mAs then produces an exposure comparable with that of the original exposure technique.

 MATHEMATICAL APPLICATION

Adjusting mAs for Changes in Film-Screen System Speed

> A quality radiograph is obtained using 10 mAs at 65 kVp and a 100-speed film-screen system. What new mAs is used to maintain radiographic density when changing to a 400-speed film-screen system?
>
> $$\frac{10\,mAs}{X} = \frac{400\ speed}{100\ speed}$$
>
> $$10\,mAs \times 100; 1000 = 400X;\ \frac{1000}{400} = 2.5\,mAs = X$$

Screen Maintenance

The maintenance of intensifying screens is significant because radiographic quality depends in large part on how well the screens are continuously maintained. Two important maintenance procedures should be performed on intensifying screens. The first is regular cleaning. The outside surface of screens comes into contact with the environment and with the hands of those unloading and loading cassettes, which results in the natural oils on fingers and hands being deposited on the screen surface. These oils tend to attract dust and dirt, which can build up to the point at which they are actually imaged on radiographs as artifacts. Screen cleaning should be done routinely. The cleaning is accomplished with commercially available antistatic intensifying screen cleaner fluid and gauze pads.

The second important maintenance procedure is to check cassettes for **film-screen contact**. Good film-screen contact exists when the screen or screens are in direct contact with the film. Poor film-screen contact greatly degrades recorded detail and is usually seen as a localized area of unsharpness somewhere on the radiographic image. Rarely is film-screen contact so poor that unsharpness can be seen across the entire radiograph. A major part of testing for film-screen contact is identifying problem cassettes.

The film-screen contact test is easily accomplished, but it requires a special wire mesh test tool. The wire mesh tool is placed on the cassette in question and radiographed with an appropriate technique. The resultant radiograph (Fig. 9.5) is then viewed from approximately 6 feet to determine any areas of unsharpness, which indicate poor recorded detail. Areas of poor contact appear darker than areas of good contact because of the increased spreading of the light photons. See Box 9.3 for additional quality-control checks on intensifying screens.

The remaining component in the film-screen IR is the **cassette**. Serving as a container for both the intensifying screens and the film, the cassette must be light-proof, lightweight for portability, and rigid enough not to bend under a patient's weight, all while allowing the maximum amount of radiation to pass through and reach the screens. Low x-ray-absorbing materials, such as thermo-set plastic, magnesium, or even graphite carbon fiber, can be found inside the fronts of cassettes. Inside the backs of cassettes may be found thin sheets of lead foil designed to absorb backscatter before it exposes the film.

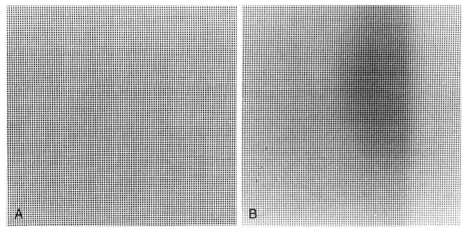

FIG. 9-5 Wire mesh test images. Image produced with a wire mesh test tool. **A**, Proper film-screen contact. **B**, Poor film-screen contact. (Part A courtesy of Fluke Biomedical. Part B courtesy of Barbara Smith Pruner.)

BOX 9-3   Quality-Control Check: Intensifying Screens

- Intensifying screens should produce an image with uniform density, provide uniform resolution, and not create image artifacts. Several simple quality-control procedures can be performed to monitor the performance of intensifying screens.
- A step-wedge or homogeneous phantom can be imaged to evaluate the uniformity of optical densities (ODs) within one screen and compare ODs for screens of the same speed. ODs should be within ±0.05 throughout each image and within ±0.20 among screens of the same speed.
- A resolution test tool can be imaged to measure the spatial resolution of each screen. Intensifying screens with the same speed should visualize the same number of line pairs per millimeter.
- An ultraviolet lamp can be used to evaluate the condition of the surface of the screen. The surface should be free of dirt, stains, and defects.

AUTOMATIC FILM PROCESSING

After the exposure of the film to radiant energy from x-rays and the light from intensifying screens, the film must be chemically processed to view the radiographic image.

The purpose of radiographic film processing is to convert the latent image into a manifest (visible) image. According to the Gurney–Mott theory, exposure of the silver bromide crystals in the film emulsion by light or x-ray photons creates the latent image and initiates the conversion process. Chemical processing of the exposed film completes the conversion process and transforms the image into a permanent visible image.

Processing Stages

An **automatic film processor** (Fig. 9.6) is a device that includes chemical tanks, a roller transport system, and a dryer system for the processing of radiographic film. The processing of a radiograph occurs in four stages: developing, fixing, washing, and drying. Each stage has its specific function and implementation method (Table 9.2).

Developing

The primary function of developing is to convert the latent image into a manifest (or visible) image. The purpose of the **developing agents**, or **reducing agents**, is to reduce exposed silver halide to metallic silver and to add electrons to the exposed silver halide. Two chemicals are used to accomplish this purpose: phenidone and hydroquinone. *Phenidone* is said to be a fast reducer, producing gray (lower) densities. *Hydroquinone* is said to be a slow reducer, producing black (higher) densities. The developer solution needs an alkaline pH environment for the chemicals to properly function.

FIG. 9-6 Type of automatic film processors used in radiography. (From Johnston JN, Fauber TL: *Essentials of Radiographic Physics and Imaging*, ed 2, St. Louis, 2016, Mosby.)

TABLE 9-2   Automatic Film Processing Stages

Developing
Converts latent image to a manifest or visible image
- Developing or reducing agents
  - Phenidone: faster and produces gray densities
  - Hydroquinone: slower and produces black densities

Fixing
Removes unexposed silver halide from film; stops the development process; hardens the emulsion

- Fixing agent: ammonium thiosulfate

Washing
Removes fixing solution from surface of film

Drying
Removes 85%–90% of moisture from film

 IMPORTANT RELATIONSHIP

Developing or Reducing Agents

The developing agents are responsible for reducing the exposed silver halide crystals to metallic silver, visualized as radiographic densities. Phenidone is responsible for creating the lower densities, and hydroquinone is responsible for creating the higher densities. Their combined effect results in a range of visible densities on the radiograph.

During the development process, a developer solution donates additional electrons to the sensitivity specks, or electron traps, in the emulsion layers of the film. These additional electrons attract more silver to these areas, amplifying the amount of atomic silver at each latent image center. Exposed silver halide is reduced to metallic silver when bromide and iodide ions are removed from the emulsion. The atomic silver that was exposed to radiant energy (light and x-rays) is converted to metallic silver and presented as radiographic densities. Unexposed silver halide does not immediately react to the developer because it has not been ionized and does not accept electrons from the developer. Given extended exposure to developing solution or exposure to excessively heated developing solution, however, even unexposed areas of film can react to developing solution.

Fixing

The primary functions of the fixing stage are to remove unexposed silver halide from the film and to make the remaining image permanent. In addition, there are two secondary functions of fixing. One is to stop the development process; the other is to harden the emulsion further. Fixing solution must function to remove all undeveloped silver halide while not affecting the metallic silver image.

The purpose of the **fixing agent** is to clear undeveloped silver halide from the film. A thiosulfate (sometimes referred to as *hypo*), such as ammonium thiosulfate, is the chemical used as this agent. The fixer solution needs an acidic pH environment for the chemicals to properly function.

 IMPORTANT RELATIONSHIP

Clearing the Unexposed Crystals

The fixing agent, ammonium thiosulfate, is responsible for removing the unexposed crystals from the emulsion.

Washing

The purpose of the washing process is to remove fixing solution from the surface of the film. This is a further step in making the manifest image permanent. If not properly washed, the resulting radiograph will show a brown staining of the image, resulting in image loss and a decrease in its diagnostic value. This staining is caused by thiosulfate (fixing agent) that remains in the emulsion layers. A certain amount of thiosulfate always remains within the film, but the goal of washing is to remove enough so the radiograph can be used for an extended period.

 IMPORTANT RELATIONSHIP

Archival Quality of Radiographs

Maintaining the archival (long-term) quality of radiographs requires most of the fixing agent to be removed (washed) from the film. Staining or fading of the permanent image results when too much thiosulfate remains on the film.

The process by which washing works is referred to as *diffusion*. Diffusion exposes the film to water, which has a lower concentration of thiosulfate than the film; thus, the fixing agent diffuses into the water.

Eventually, thiosulfate concentrations in the wash water can become greater than the concentrations in the films being processed; therefore, the wash water must be frequently replaced. Water flows freely from the input water supply through the wash tank and down the drain while the roller transport system is operating. This type of system provides a constant supply of fresh wash water to aid in the diffusion process. The moving water also causes agitation and increases diffusion.

Drying

The final process in automatic processing is drying. The purpose of drying films is to remove 85% to 90% of the moisture from the film so that it can be easily handled and stored while maintaining the quality of the diagnostic image. As a result, finished radiographs should retain 10% to 15% of their moisture when processing is complete. If films are excessively dried, the emulsion layers can crack, decreasing the diagnostic quality of the radiograph.

 IMPORTANT RELATIONSHIP

Archival Quality of Radiographs

Permanent radiographs must retain a moisture content of 10% to 15% to maintain archival quality. Excessive drying can cause the emulsion layers to crack.

Increased relative humidity decreases the efficiency of dryers in processors, so an increased drying temperature is necessary. Processors are equipped with thermostatic controls to allow selection of a wide range of dryer temperatures.

To chemically process a radiographic image, specialized equipment and systems must perform concurrently to move the film through the processing stages according to the manufacturer's specifications.

Processing Systems

Automatic processors use a vertical transport system of rollers that advance the film through the various stages of film processing (Fig. 9.7). A film is introduced into the processor on the feed tray. The **feed tray** is a flat metal surface with an edge on either side that permits the film to easily

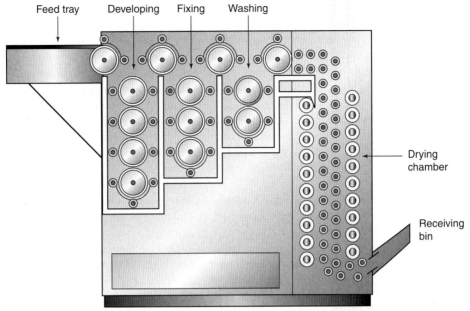

Feed tray   Developing   Fixing   Washing

Drying
chamber

Receiving
bin

FIG. 9-7 Cross-section of an automatic processor showing the vertical transport system of rollers.

enter the processor while remaining correctly aligned. Automatic processors use different types of rollers to move the film through the processor. Transport and crossover rollers ensure that the film is moved into and through the tanks at a constant speed.

An electric motor provides power for the roller assemblies to transport the film through the processor. The on–off switch that provides electrical power to the processor activates this motor. Most processors are also equipped with a **standby control**, which is an electrical circuit that shuts off power to the roller assemblies when the processor is not being used. Pushing the standby control switch when one is ready to process a film can reactivate the roller assemblies and water intake.

Replenishment refers to the replacement of fresh chemicals (specifically, developer solution and fixer solution) after chemical losses during processing. The replenishment of the chemicals used in the automatic processor is necessary because these chemicals eventually become exhausted or inactive, and their ability to perform their functions decreases. Developing solution becomes exhausted from both use and exposure to air, which reduces its chemical strength.

Fixer solution becomes exhausted for several reasons: it becomes weakened from use as a result of accumulations of silver halide removed from the film during the fixing process and because developer solution remains in the film, which decreases the strength and activity of the fixer solution.

▶ IMPORTANT RELATIONSHIP
Replenishment and Solution Performance

The replenishment system provides fresh chemicals for the developing and fixing solutions to maintain their chemical activity and volume when they become depleted during processing.

The amount of solution that is replenished is preset and based on the size of the film or occurs at timed intervals. Replenishment systems are usually adjusted so that more fixer solution is replenished per film compared with developer solution.

Automatic processors have a recirculation system for the developer and fixer tanks. Each tank has a separate system that consists of a pump and connecting tubing. The **recirculation system** acts to circulate the solutions in each of these tanks by pumping solution out of one portion of the tank and returning it to a different location within the same tank from which it was removed. The recirculation system keeps the chemicals mixed, which helps to maintain solution activity and provides agitation of the chemicals around the film to facilitate fast processing.

Recirculation also helps to maintain the proper temperature of the developer solution. The developer recirculation system includes an in-line filter that removes impurities as recirculation takes place.

Temperature control of the developer solution is important because the activity of this solution depends directly on its temperature. An increase or decrease in developer temperature can adversely affect the quality of the radiographic image.

In most 90-s automatic processors, the developer temperature must be maintained at 93° to 95°F (33.8°–35°C). An **immersion heater** is a heating coil that is immersed in the bottoms of the developer and fixer tanks. Most automatic processors are thermostatically controlled to heat the developer solution to its proper temperature and maintain that temperature as long as the processor is turned on.

 IMPORTANT RELATIONSHIP

Developer Temperature and Radiographic Quality

Variations in developer temperature can adversely affect the quality of the radiographic image. Increasing the developer temperature increases the density, and decreasing it decreases the density. Furthermore, radiographic contrast may be adversely affected by changes in the developer temperature.

Radiographs must be properly dried to be viewed and stored. The film is dried by hot air that is blown onto both surfaces of the film as it moves through the dryer. This air is forced through the dryer by a blower and is directed onto the film by air tubes. The temperature of the air that is used for drying films is thermostatically monitored for accurate control of moisture removal from the film.

Inadequate processing is evidenced by certain appearances of the finished radiograph. Particular problems can be pinpointed by analyzing the radiographs. These problems and the radiographic appearances that indicate them are summarized in Table 9.3.

Quality Control

Unexposed film should be stored in its original packaging so that important information about it, such as its expiration date and lot number, can be retained. Film boxes should be vertically and not horizontally stored to prevent pressure artifacts from forming on the film. Film should be stored away from heat sources and ionizing radiation. Both heat and radiation can cause the silver halide in the film emulsion to break down, resulting in fogged film. The shelf life of film, as expressed by its expiration date, must be observed. Film should not be used beyond its expiration date.

The manner in which film is handled in the darkroom can have a profound effect on radiographs. Common hazards to radiographic quality that can be found in darkrooms are white-light exposure, safelight exposure, ionizing radiation exposure, and other potential hazards.

Darkrooms must be free from all outside white-light exposure. A white-light source may be located inside the darkroom, but it should be connected to an interlock system whereby the film

TABLE 9-3 Indicators of Inadequate Processing

Radiographic Appearance	Processing Problem
Decrease in density	Developer exhausted Developer underreplenishment Processor running too fast Low developer temperature Developer improperly mixed
Increase in density	Developer overreplenishment High developer temperature Light leak in processor Developer improperly mixed
Pinkish stain (dichroic fog)	Contamination of developer by fixer Developer or fixer underreplenishment
Brown stain (thiosulfate stain)	Inadequate washing
Emulsion removed by developer	Insufficient hardener in developer
Milky appearance	Fixer exhausted Inadequate washing
Streaks	Dirty processor rollers Inadequate washing Inadequate drying
Water spots	Inadequate drying
Minus-density scratches	Scratches from guide plates caused by roller or plate misalignment

bin may not be opened as long as the darkroom white-light source is on. In addition, temperature and humidity can adversely affect the film. Film should be stored and handled at temperatures ranging from 55° to 75°F (14°–24°C) with a relative humidity of 30% to 60%. Without moisture in the air (low humidity), any build-up of static charges can expose the film.

Countertops must be clean and static free to avoid the formation of radiographic artifacts on the films. Several brands of commercial cleaning fluids contain an antistatic component ideal for cleaning darkroom countertops and processor feed trays.

Other potential hazards to film in darkrooms include heat and chemical exposure. Film stored within the darkroom should not be near any heat source. Processing chemicals must be kept away from film and film-handling areas to prevent exposure and contamination of these areas.

Ionizing radiation exposure to film in the darkroom is a potential hazard because many darkrooms share common walls with radiographic rooms. The walls that are common between the darkroom and a radiographic room must be lined with lead as required by law for standard protection from radiographic exposures. The bin where film is stored and available for immediate use should also be lined with lead to prevent fog that may result from radiation exposure.

Safelights used in the darkroom must be equipped with a safelight filter appropriate for the type of film being handled. Commonly used filters include Kodak Wratten 6B for blue-sensitive film and Kodak GBX for orthochromatic film, which is sensitive to both blue-violet and green visible light. Safelight filters must be free of cracks, because white light that leaks from the safelight could expose the film. The power rating of the light bulbs used in safelights should be no greater than that recommended by film manufacturers (generally 7.5–15 W), which is indicated on the outside of the box of radiographic film.

Good radiographic quality cannot be achieved when film is improperly stored, mishandled before or after exposure, or incorrectly processed. Common film artifacts resulting from improper storage, darkroom handling, or improper processing are shown in Fig. 9.8. Furthermore, a quality-control program must be implemented and systematically followed to ensure proper processing of radiographic film. Box 9.4 describes quality-control methods for evaluating the darkroom and film processor.

Silver Recovery

Because fixer solution is used to remove unexposed silver halide from the film, used fixer solution contains a high concentration of accumulated silver. Some type of silver recovery must be used under such conditions. **Silver recovery** refers to the removal of silver from used fixer solution. For some facilities that regularly process large volumes of radiographs, the financial rewards of silver recovery may be an added incentive.

Silver-recovery units are available for on-site silver recovery and generally require servicing by an outside contractor familiar with the equipment and its method of removing silver. These silver-recovery units are directly connected to the drain system of the fixer tank to remove silver as used fixer solution passes through the unit. After the silver has been recovered, the used fixer is drained.

Silver-recovery units work by one of two methods. The first is called *metallic replacement*. There are two types of metallic replacement silver-recovery units: one uses steel wool, and the other uses a silver-extraction filter. A steel wool metallic replacement unit uses steel wool to filter the used fixer solution. Silver replaces the iron in the steel wool and can then be easily removed after significant accumulation in a canister or replacement cartridge occurs. A silver-extraction unit uses a foam filter that is impregnated with steel wool. Again, the silver from used fixer solution replaces the iron in the steel wool. A silver-extraction filter is more efficient at removing silver from used fixer and lasts longer than a simple steel wool metallic replacement unit.

FIG. 9-8 Film artifacts. **A,** Plus-density half-moon artifacts can be caused by bending or kinking the film *(arrow)*. **B,** Plus-density static discharge artifact can be caused by sliding a film over a flat surface.

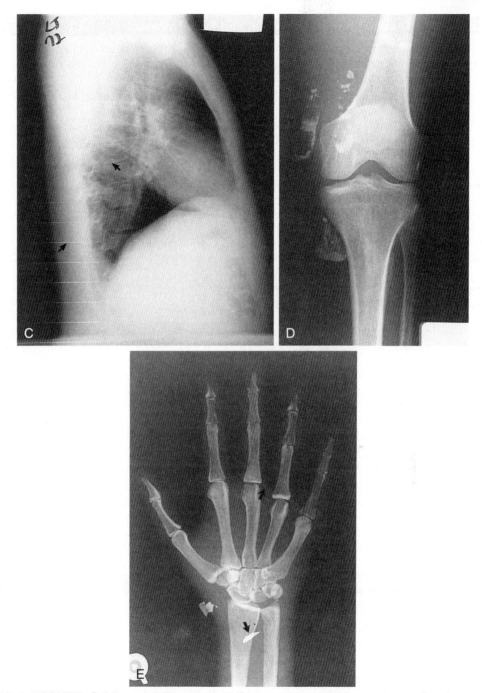

FIG. 9-8 CONT'D C, Minus-density scratch artifacts can be caused by transport rollers *(arrows).*
D, Minus-density caused by moisture on a finger. **E,** Dirty screens or cassettes can cause non-specific minus-density artifacts.

BOX 9-4   Quality Control: Darkroom and Film Processor

A quality-control program must be implemented and systematically followed to ensure proper processing of radiographic film. A good quality-control program should include steps for monitoring all the equipment and activities required for the production of quality radiographic images, including (but not limited to) the following:

- Sensitometric monitoring of the film processor should be done to provide valuable information about the daily functioning of the processor.
- Following the establishment of baseline measurements, daily exposure and processing of a sensitometric strip, measurement of the appropriate OD points with a densitometer, and plotting them on a control chart with predetermined upper and lower acceptable limits. The graph provides a visual indicator of any acute or evolving processor malfunction.
- Typically, a processor control chart should monitor B + F, medium OD or speed, and upper and lower density differences to evaluate contrast.
- Speed and contrast indicators should not have an OD value that varies more than ±0.15 from baseline measurements.
- B + F should not have an OD value greater than +0.05 from the baseline measurement.
- Developer temperature should be measured daily with a digital thermometer and should not vary by more than ±0.5°F (0.3°C).
- The darkroom environment should be well ventilated, clean, organized, and safe.
- A safelight fog test should be performed semiannually and result in an OD of less than +0.05 because of added fog.
- Replenishment rates should be checked weekly and fall within ±5% of the manufacturer's specification.
- Recommended quarterly quality-control checks include the following:
  - Developer solution pH should be maintained between 10 and 11.5.
  - Fixer pH should be maintained between 4 and 4.5.
  - Developer specific gravity should not vary by more than ±0.004 from the manufacturer's specifications.

The second method of silver recovery is the *electrolytic method*, and it is the most efficient one; however, the units needed for this process are more expensive than metallic replacement units. Electrolytic units have an electrically charged drum or disc that attracts silver. The silver plates onto the drum or disc and can be removed when a substantial amount of silver has been collected.

Silver is considered a heavy metal, and its disposal is regulated by local and state agencies. In many locales, strict limits are placed on the concentrations of silver in used fixer that can be disposed of via the sewer system. Silver recovery is an important process in radiology because silver is a natural resource that can be toxic to the environment and has monetary value.

 IMPORTANT RELATIONSHIP

Silver Recovery

Silver is a natural resource and is a heavy metal that can be toxic to the environment, and it must be removed from the used fixer.

FILM-SCREEN CHARACTERISTICS

Film-screen imaging has several limitations that were overcome with digital imaging. One major deficiency is the limited **dynamic range** of film screen. This limitation renders film-screen image receptors very sensitive to under- or overexposure, which may necessitate image retakes. A limited dynamic range also restricts visibility of structures that differ greatly in x-ray attenuation. An example is the difficulty of optimally visualizing both soft tissue and bony structures within a given film image.

> ### ◆ IMPORTANT RELATIONSHIP
> #### *Dynamic Range*
>
> The range of exposure intensities an image receptor can accurately detect determines its dynamic range. Film-screen image receptors have a narrow dynamic range when compared with digital image receptors.

Factors that affect the quality of the film-screen image are presented in Table 9.4. These factors are discussed thoroughly in Chapter 6. Unlike digital imaging, the intensity of exposure reaching

TABLE 9-4 Film-Screen Image Receptors

Factors	Exposure to IR	Density	Contrast[a]	Recorded Detail	Distortion
mAs					
• Increase	Increase	Increase	No effect[b]	No effect	No effect
• Decrease	Decrease	Decrease	No effect[b]	No effect	No effect
kVp					
• Increase	Increase	Increase	Decrease	No effect	No effect
• Decrease	Decrease	Decrease	Increase	No effect	No effect
OID					
• Increase	Decrease	Decrease	Increase[c]	Decrease	Increase
SID					
• Increase	Decrease	Decrease	No effect	Increase	Decrease
• Decrease	Increase	Increase	No effect	Decrease	Increase
Focal Spot Size					
• Increase	No effect	No effect	No effect	Decrease	No effect
• Decrease	No effect	No effect	No effect	Increase	No effect
Grid					
• Increase ratio	Decrease	Decrease	Increase	No effect	No effect
• Decrease ratio	Increase	Increase	Decrease	No effect	No effect
Beam Restriction					
• Increase	Decrease	Decrease	Increase	No effect	No effect
• Decrease	Increase	Increase	Decrease	No effect	No effect
Film-Screen Speed					
• Increase	No effect	Increase	No effect	Decrease	No effect
• Decrease	No effect	Decrease	No effect	Increase	No effect
Patient Thickness					
• Increase	Decrease	Decrease	Decrease	Decrease	Increase
• Decrease	Increase	Increase	Increase	Increase	Decrease
Patient Motion	No effect	No effect	No effect	Decrease	No effect
Central Ray					
• Increase angle	Decrease	Decrease	No effect	Decrease	Increase

[a] Increase is higher contrast, and decrease is lower contrast.
[b] Contrast is not affected unless the density is insufficient or excessive.
[c] Increased (higher) contrast because of less scatter reaching the image receptor (IR); this effect is dependent on the anatomic region, thickness, and amount of object-to-image-receptor distance. *kVp,* Kilovoltage peak; *mAs,* milliamperage-seconds; *OID,* object-to-image-receptor distance; *SID,* source-to-image-receptor distance.

FIG. 9-9 Density. **A,** Film image that was exposed to insufficient radiation. **B,** Film image that was exposed to excessive radiation. (From Johnston JN, Fauber TL: *Essentials of Radiographic Physics and Imaging*, ed 3, St. Louis, 2020, Elsevier.)

the film-screen image receptor has a direct effect on the amount of density produced in the processed image (Fig. 9.9).

Density

Radiographic film that has been exposed to radiant energy and chemically processed is composed of minute deposits of black metallic silver visualized as density. The varying densities on the processed film represent the attenuation properties of the anatomic part imaged. Radiographic density is the amount of overall blackness produced on the processed image. If a radiograph is deemed unacceptable, the radiographer must determine what factors contributed to the density error. Knowledge about the factors that affect the density on a radiographic image is critical to developing effective problem-solving skills.

Optical Density

Density on the radiograph can be quantified and is therefore an objective measure that can be used for comparison. A **densitometer** is a device used to numerically determine the amount of blackness on the radiograph (i.e., it measures radiographic density).

This device is constructed to emit a constant intensity of light (incident) onto an area of the image and then measure the amount of light transmitted through the area (Fig. 9.10). The densitometer determines the amount of light transmitted and calculates a measurement known as **optical density (OD)**. OD is a numeric calculation that compares the intensity of light transmitted through an area on the film (I_t) with the amount of light originally striking (incident) the area (I_o). The ratio of these intensities is called *transmittance*. Box 9.5 shows the mathematical formula used for light transmittance. Because the range of radiographic densities is large, the calculation of radiographic densities is compressed into a logarithmic scale (Table 9.5) for easier management.

FIG. 9-10 A densitometer is used to measure optical densities (ODs). (Courtesy of Nuclear Associates.)

BOX 9-5   Light Transmittance Formula

$$\frac{I_t}{I_o} \times 100,$$

in which I_t represents the amount of light transmitted and I_o represents the original amount of light incident on the film.

This logarithmic value of light transmittance is termed *optical density*. The formula used to calculate OD is shown in Box 9.6. OD is defined as the logarithm (Log_{10}) of the inverse of transmittance For example, an area of the image that allows 10% of the original incident light to be transmitted has a transmittance of 1/10 or 0.1. The inverse of transmittance is therefore 10, and the logarithm of 10 (the OD) is 1. Similarly, an area that allows only 1% of the original incident light through has an OD of 2.

BOX 9-6   OD Formula

$$\text{Optical density} = Log_{10}\frac{I_o}{I_t}$$

in which I_o represents the original amount of light incident on the film and I_t represents the amount of transmitted light.

TABLE 9-5 Percentage of Light Transmittance and Calculated Optical Densities

Percentage of Light Transmitted ($I_t/I_o \times 100$)	Fraction of Light Transmitted (I_t/I_o)	Optical Density ($\log I_o/I_t$)
100	1	0
50	$\frac{1}{2}$	0.3
32	$\frac{8}{25}$	0.5
25	$\frac{1}{4}$	0.6
12.5	$\frac{1}{8}$	0.9
10	$\frac{1}{10}$	1
5	$\frac{1}{20}$	1.3
3.2	$\frac{4}{125}$	1.5
2.5	$\frac{1}{40}$	1.6
1.25	$\frac{1}{80}$	1.9
1	$\frac{1}{100}$	2
0.5	$\frac{1}{200}$	2.3
0.32	$\frac{2}{625}$	2.5
0.125	$\frac{1}{80}$	2.9
0.1	$\frac{1}{1000}$	3
0.05	$\frac{1}{2000}$	3.3
0.032	$\frac{2}{3125}$	3.5
0.01	$\frac{1}{10,000}$	4

IMPORTANT RELATIONSHIP

Light Transmittance and OD

> As the percentage of light transmitted decreases, the OD increases; as the percentage of light transmitted increases, the OD decreases.

Notice the relationship between light transmittance and OD (see Table 9.5). When 100% of the light is transmitted, the OD equals 0. When 50% of the light is transmitted, the OD is equal to 0.3, and when 25% of the light is transmitted, the OD equals 0.6. When a logarithmic scale base 10 is used, every 0.3 change in OD corresponds to a change in the percentage of light transmitted by a factor of 2 ($\log_{10}$ of 2 = 0.3).

 IMPORTANT RELATIONSHIP

OD and Light Transmittance

> For every 0.3 change in OD, the percentage of light transmitted has changed by a factor of 2. A 0.3 increase in OD results from a decrease in the percentage of light transmitted by half, whereas a 0.3 decrease in OD results from an increase in the percentage of light transmitted by a factor of 2.

Diagnostic Range

Optical densities can range from 0 to 4 OD. Because most radiographic film has a tint added to its base and processing adds a slight amount of fog, the lowest amount of OD is usually between 0.10 and 0.20. This minimum amount of density on the radiographic film is termed **base plus fog (B + F)**. However, the diagnostic range of optical densities for general radiography usually falls between 0.5 and 2 OD. This desired range of optical densities is found between the extreme low and high densities produced on the radiograph.

The radiation exposure to the film-screen image receptor primarily determines the amount of OD created on the film after processing. The **intensity of radiation exposure**, or exposure intensity, is a measurement of the amount and energy of the x-rays reaching an area of the film. When all other factors remain the same, increasing the exposure intensity increases the OD.

 IMPORTANT RELATIONSHIP

Exposure Intensity and OD

> Increasing the exposure intensity to the film-screen image receptor increases the OD, whereas decreasing the exposure intensity to the film-screen image receptor decreases the OD.

In film-screen imaging, the optical densities created on the processed radiograph cannot be altered. As a result, choosing the proper exposure intensity to create an appropriate range of optical densities (or diagnostic densities) during film-screen imaging is critical to producing a good-quality radiographic image. Diagnostic densities must be present in a radiographic image to visualize the anatomic area of interest.

FIG. 9-11 Contrast: radiograph demonstrating high contrast.

FIG. 9-12 Contrast: radiograph demonstrating low contrast.

Contrast

Radiographic film images are typically described by their **scale of contrast** or the range of densities visible. A radiograph with few densities but great differences among them is said to have **high contrast**. This is also described as **short-scale contrast** (Fig. 9.11). A radiograph with a large number of densities but little differences among them is said to have **low contrast**. This is also described as **long-scale contrast** (Fig. 9.12).

The inherent response of the film (receptor contrast) also affects radiographic contrast. Film can be manufactured to display different levels of contrast, such as medium or high. In addition, the quality of chemical processing affects the contrast displayed on the radiograph.

Radiographic contrast can be best evaluated when the radiographic density is adequate to visualize the density differences. When density is either too light or too dark, radiographic contrast cannot be adequately visualized. When radiographic density is unacceptable, radiographic contrast is decreased.

It is important to have a basic understanding of how radiographic film responds to radiation exposure and creates the optical densities visible after processing. This relationship demonstrates how inherent differences in the manufacturing of the film affect the visibility characteristics of the radiograph.

SENSITOMETRY

In film-screen imaging, **sensitometry** is the study of the relationship between the intensity of radiation exposure to a film and the amount of blackness produced after processing (density). The intensity of radiation exposure is the measure of the quantity of radiation reaching an area of the film. Sensitometry provides a method for evaluating the characteristics of film and film-screen combinations used in radiography. Radiographic film and intensifying screen manufacturers are capable of designing film and screens to respond differently to a given intensity of radiation exposure. In particular, film and screens designed for radiography of the chest or extremities respond differently to equal amounts of radiation exposure. The radiographer should understand how the selected film and film-screen system will respond to a given intensity of exposure.

Sensitometry is also a method of evaluating the performance of automatic film processors. Because automatic film processors affect a radiograph's density and contrast, the variability of their performance can be monitored by sensitometric methods.

Equipment

Several pieces of equipment are needed to evaluate the relationship between the intensity of radiation exposure and the density produced after processing. The radiographic film should be exposed to a range of radiation intensities to evaluate its response to low, middle, and high exposures. This can be accomplished easily by passing radiation through an object that varies in thickness using a radiographic x-ray unit. The resultant effect is an image of varying uniform densities that correspond to specific intensities of radiation exposure.

Penetrometer

A **penetrometer** is a device constructed of uniform absorbers of increasing thicknesses, such as aluminium or tissue-equivalent plastic (Fig. 9.13). When radiographed, the penetrometer produces a series of uniform densities that resemble a step wedge (Fig. 9.14). When **step-wedge densities** are produced with a penetrometer and a radiographic x-ray unit, the variability of the output of the equipment could affect the range of densities produced.

FIG. 9-13 Penetrometer. When radiographed, a penetrometer produces an image showing a series of uniform densities.

FIG. 9-14 Radiograph of a penetrometer showing step-wedge densities.

FIG. 9-15 A sensitometer is designed to produce consistent step-wedge densities. (Courtesy of Nuclear Associates.)

Sensitometer

A device known as a **sensitometer** is designed to produce consistent step-wedge densities by eliminating the variability of the x-ray unit (Fig. 9.15). It uses a controlled light source to expose an optical step-wedge template. The step-wedge template transmits light in varying intensities to expose the radiographic film. After the film has been processed, a density step-wedge image, or **sensitometric strip**, is produced. Penetrometers and sensitometers are available in 11-, 15-, and 21-step densities.

As discussed earlier, a densitometer is the device that measures the densities processed on the film. When the OD measurements from a sensitometric strip are graphed on semilogarithmic paper, the result is a curve characteristic of the radiographic film type.

Sensitometric Curve

This **sensitometric curve** visually demonstrates the relationship between the intensity of radiation exposure (x-axis) and the resultant optical densities (y-axis) (Fig. 9.16). The position of the curve on the x-axis and its shape can vary greatly and depends on the type of radiographic film used.

Log of Relative Exposure

When sensitometric methods are used to evaluate the characteristics of radiographic film, it is more useful to measure the intensity of radiation exposure in increments of a constant change, such as doubling or halving. For every doubling or halving change in the percentage of light transmitted, a change of 0.3 occurs in OD. Along the x-axis, for every change of 0.3 in log relative exposure, the intensity of radiation exposure changes by a factor of 2 (Fig. 9.17). When Fig. 9.17 is used as an example, the relative mAs (the product of milliamperage and exposure time) value

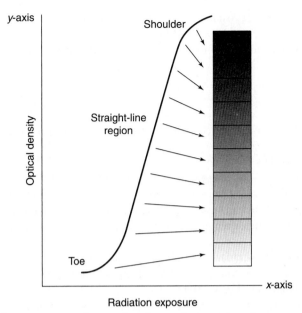

FIG. 9-16 Plotting ODs corresponding to the change in intensity of exposure results in a curve characteristic of the type of the film.

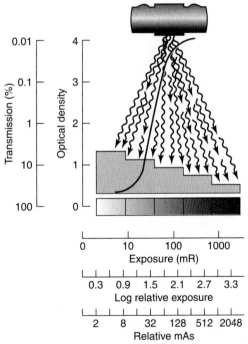

FIG. 9-17 A sensitometric curve is created by plotting the OD values obtained from the range of exposures that are used to create the step-wedge densities. The logarithmic relative exposure value representing the change in exposure by a factor of 2 is a more useful value than the milliroentgen (mR) exposure or relative milliamperage-seconds (mAs).

is 32 for a log of exposure of 1.5, and the relative mAs value is 64 for a log of exposure of 1.8. This relationship can be demonstrated throughout the log relative exposure scale on the sensitometric curve. Two exposures, one double the other, will always be separated by 0.3 on the logarithmic exposure scale.

Regions

A sensitometric curve demonstrates three distinct regions (Fig. 9.18). When the characteristics of different types of radiographic film are evaluated, differences will be demonstrated within any of these regions.

Toe Region.   The **toe region** of the sensitometric curve represents the area of low density. The point on the sensitometric curve where a minimum amount of radiation exposure produced a minimum OD is known as D_{min}. Generally, D_{min} is equal to B + F even though they represent two different measurements. Changes in exposure intensity in this region have little effect on the OD.

Straight-Line Region.   At a certain point along the x-axis, changes in exposure begin to have a much greater effect on the OD. This **straight-line region** is where the diagnostic or most useful range of densities is produced.

Shoulder Region.   There is a point on the sensitometric curve where changes in exposure intensity no longer affect the OD. In this **shoulder region**, the point on the curve where maximum density has been produced is known as D_{max}. When the maximum density achievable within the film has been reached (D_{max}), continued increases in exposure intensity begin to reverse the OD. This process is called *solarization*, and it is used in the design of duplicating film.

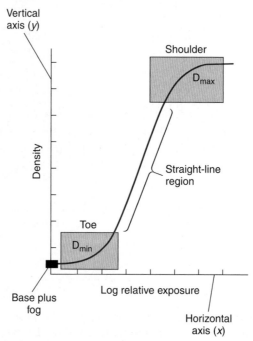

FIG. 9-18 The sensitometric curve demonstrates three distinct regions: toe, straight-line, and shoulder.

Film Characteristics

Comparing sensitometric curves in these regions provides information about three important characteristics of radiographic film. Each film characteristic plays an important role in radiographic imaging.

Speed

An important characteristic of radiographic film is its sensitivity to radiation exposure, which is referred to as its **speed**. The speed of a film indicates the amount of OD produced for a given amount of radiation exposure. It is a characteristic of the film's sensitivity to the intensity of radiation exposure.

Speed Point

Typically, the speed of radiographic film is determined by locating the point on a sensitometric curve that corresponds to the OD of 1.0 plus B + F. This point is called the **speed point** (Fig. 9.19). This OD point is used because it is within the straight-line portion of the sensitometric curve. The speed point serves as a standard method of indicating film speed.

Speed Exposure Point

When comparing film types, the radiographer must determine what log of exposure produces the speed point. This can be determined by drawing a line from the sensitometric curve speed point to the area on the x-axis (log of exposure) that produced the OD at 1.0 plus B + F (Fig. 9.20). This important point, called the **speed exposure point**, indicates the intensity of exposure needed to produce a density of 1.0 plus B + F (speed point). A film that has a speed exposure point of 0.9 is faster than a film having a speed exposure point of 1.2.

Fig. 9.21 presents two sensitometric curves and their respective speed and speed exposure points. A faster-speed film is positioned to the left (closer to the y-axis) of slower-speed film.

It is important to remember that the speed of the film is determined by the amount of exposure (log of exposure) needed to produce an OD of 1.0 plus B + F, regardless of the shape of the sensitometric curve (Fig. 9.22).

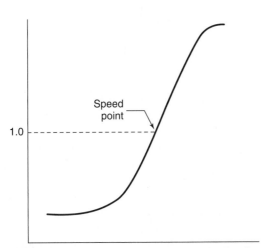

FIG. 9-19 The sensitometric curve speed point indicates the intensity of exposure needed to produce a density of 1.0 plus B + F.

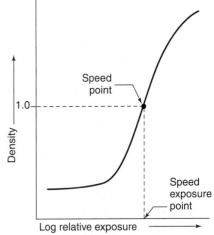

FIG. 9-20 The speed exposure point indicates the intensity of exposure needed to produce a density of 1.0 plus B + F (speed point).

FIG. 9-21 Obtaining the same speed point requires that film A has a log of exposure of 1.5 and film B has a log of exposure of 2.0. Faster-speed films are located to the left of slower-speed films.

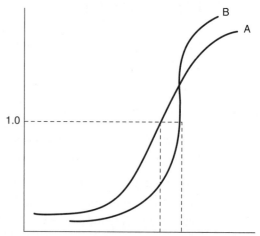

FIG. 9-22 As the shape of the sensitometric curve varies, the speed can also vary if it is measured at points other than the standard of 1.0 plus B + F.

BOX 9-7   Determining the Slope of a Line

$$\text{Slope} = \frac{Y\,(\text{rise})}{X\,(\text{run})}, \frac{y_2 - y_1}{x_2 - x_1}$$

The slope of a line mathematically indicates its tilt or slant. Comparisons of the slope (mathematical calculation) can be made among different lines. For radiography, the higher the number, the steeper the slope, and the lower the number, the lesser the slope.

Contrast

Radiographic contrast is a result of both the subject contrast and the **film contrast**. Film contrast is controlled by the design and manufacture of film components and the effects of processing. The ability of a radiographic film to provide a level of contrast can be evaluated by the steepness, or **slope**, of the sensitometric curve. The slope of this line mathematically indicates the ratio of the change in y (OD) for a unit change in x (log relative exposure) (Box 9.7).

Visually comparing the steepness (slope) of the straight-line region of the curve provides a method of evaluating the level of contrast produced by a film (Fig. 9.23). Radiographic film capable of producing higher contrast has a more vertical straight-line region (steeper slope). General-purpose radiographic film is categorized as either high contrast or medium contrast.

Gradient Point. Determining the slope along any portion of the sensitometric curve provides information about the contrast produced at that point, which is called the **gradient point**. Gradient points can be determined for any region of the sensitometric curve, such as the toe, middle, and shoulder. The gradient point can be determined by calculating the slope of the line (change in OD divided by the change in log exposure) at any portion of the curve.

Average Gradient. When comparing films, the radiographer typically determines contrast by calculating the sensitometric curve's **average gradient** of the slope of the straight-line region (Fig. 9.24). A standard used in sensitometry is to determine the film contrast between the optical densities of 0.25 and 2.0 plus B + F. Finding the difference between these two points and dividing

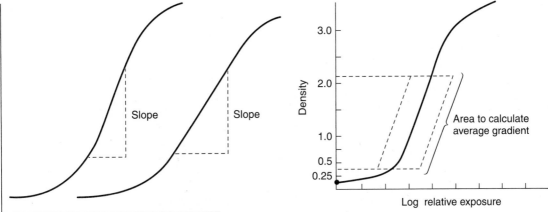

FIG. 9-23 The slope of the straight-line region determines the inherent film contrast. Steeper slopes indicate higher contrast.

FIG. 9-24 Film's average gradient is calculated between a low density (0.25 plus B + F) and a high density (2.0 plus B + F).

FIG. 9-25 A film's exposure latitude can be determined by finding the range of exposures that will produce densities within the straight-line region of the curve. The use of a low and high density similar to those used to calculate average gradient would provide ODs within the straight-line region of the sensitometric curve.

by the difference between their respective logarithms of exposure provides a numerical calculation for film contrast. Most radiographic films have an average gradient between 2.5 and 3.5; film contrast is higher for a film with an average gradient of 3.0 than one with an average gradient of 2.7.

Exposure Latitude

Exposure latitude refers to the range of exposures that produce optical densities within the straight-line region of the sensitometric curve (Fig. 9.25). Radiographic films that are capable of responding to a wide range of exposures to produce optical densities within the straight-line region are considered wide-latitude films. When comparing a film with narrow latitude with one

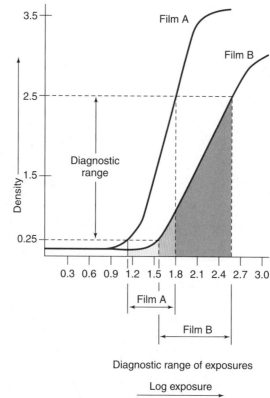

FIG. 9-26 A higher-contrast film, film A, has a narrower range of exposures available to produce ODs within the straight-line region compared with a lower-contrast film, film B.

with wide latitude, it is apparent that a film with narrow latitude is a higher-contrast film, and a film with wide latitude is a lower-contrast film (Fig. 9.26). A steep slope has a small range of exposures available to produce densities within the straight-line region, whereas a less steep slope has a greater range of such exposures.

When selecting what type of radiographic film to use, the radiographer should evaluate its characteristics in terms of speed, contrast, and latitude. Radiographic film used in chest radiography typically requires lower contrast and wider-exposure latitude, whereas film designed for use in extremity radiography requires higher contrast, resulting in a narrow exposure latitude. The speed of radiographic film is considered in combination with the intensifying screen speed to provide a film-screen system speed.

Clinical Considerations

To provide radiographic images of optimal quality, the radiographer must appropriately control the visibility factors of density and contrast. A relationship exists between density and contrast to maximize the amount of visible recorded detail.

Optimal Density

For a given anatomic area to be radiographed, the selected exposure techniques should produce radiographic densities that lie within the straight-line region of the sensitometric curve. Optical

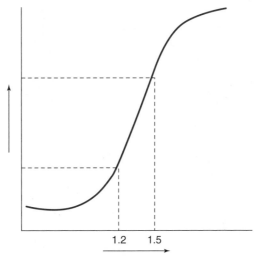

FIG. 9-27 When ODs lie within the straight-line region of the curve, a change in log exposure of 0.3 (change by a factor of 2) directly affects ODs.

within this range maximize the amount of information visible within the radiographic image, resulting in **optimal density**.

The challenge for radiographers is to determine the amount of radiation exposure necessary to produce optical densities within the straight-line region of a film's sensitometric curve. Different types of radiographic film may require different amounts of exposure to produce such densities. As previously demonstrated, it may take more or less radiation exposure to produce an OD of 1.0 plus B + F for film A compared with film B. Therefore, the relationship between radiation exposure and OD depends on the shape and position of a film's sensitometric curve.

For a given type of radiographic film, when optical densities lie within the straight-line region of the sensitometric curve, a change in the exposure technique has a direct effect on OD (Fig. 9.27). When optical densities lie outside the straight-line region, a greater or lesser change in exposure technique may be needed to move the optical densities back within the diagnostic range (0.5–2.0 OD); therefore, when evaluating a radiograph with a density error, the radiographer must determine the amount of change needed in the exposure technique.

In diagnostic radiology, one type of film is typically used for most procedures. Access to a film's sensitometric curve for the purpose of calculating exposure changes is not practical. Therefore, it is the radiographer's responsibility to use the standard guidelines regarding exposure changes to correct for density errors.

Maximum Film Contrast

Film contrast is the difference in OD between two points anywhere along the sensitometric curve (Fig. 9.28). If these differences in OD were to be plotted as points between the x- and y-axes, the result would be a film's contrast curve (Fig. 9.29). When the contrast curve is evaluated, it is apparent that **maximum contrast** (the greatest difference in optical densities) is achievable within the straight-line region of the sensitometric curve. When optical densities of the anatomic area of interest lie outside the straight-line region, film contrast is decreased. When optical densities lie within the straight-line region of the sensitometric curve, the film has reached its maximum capability in visualizing recorded detail.

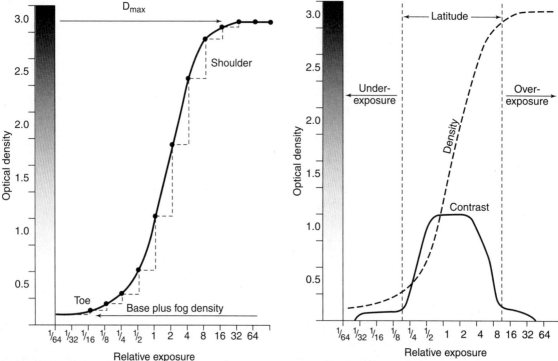

FIG. 9-28 Density differences calculated along the sensitometric curve can be used to evaluate film contrast.

FIG. 9-29 Plotting the density differences of a sensitometric curve results in a contrast curve. Maximum film contrast is achieved within the straight-line region.

BOX 9-8   Practical Tips

Sensitometric Curve Position Along the x-Axis
Sensitometric curves of faster-speed film are positioned to the left of slower-speed film, and sensitometric curves of slower-speed film are positioned to the right of faster-speed film.

Sensitometric Curve Slope
The slope of the straight-line portion of a sensitometric curve (average gradient) will indicate the film's level of contrast; the steeper the slope, the higher the contrast.

Changes in Exposure Technique to Correct for Density Errors
To correct for the density error, ODs that lie outside the straight-line region of the sensitometric curve (toe or shoulder region) require a greater or lesser change in exposure than those that lie within the straight-line region.

Achieving Maximum Film Contrast
To achieve the maximum contrast that the film is capable of producing, the radiographer must ensure that the ODs lie within the straight-line region of the sensitometric curve.

In summary, sufficient radiographic density is needed to visualize recorded detail. A film's maximum radiographic contrast can be visualized only when optical densities lie within the straight-line region of the sensitometric curve. When optical densities lie outside this region, film contrast is decreased. When both optimum density and maximum contrast have been achieved, the visibility of recorded details is of optimal radiographic quality. See Box 9.8 for practical tips.

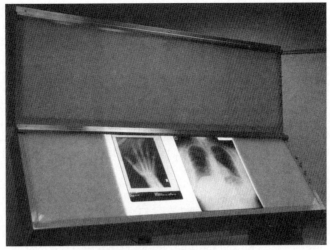

FIG. 9-30 Bank of illuminators.

IMAGE DISPLAY

To view a processed film image, it must be displayed on an illuminator. **Illuminators**, or view-boxes, are devices that provide light illumination so that the anatomy, displayed as various shades of optical densities, can be visualized.

The dimensions of an illuminator are typically 14 × 17 inches (35 × 43 cm) and can be individually arranged or combined in rows as a bank of illuminators (Fig. 9.30). The most important performance criterion of film illuminators is the uniformity of light intensity within and among viewboxes. Variations in light emission can affect the visibility of anatomic detail; therefore, maintaining clean and damage-free viewboxes along with proper bulb wattage is essential for quality control.

CHAPTER SUMMARY

- In film-screen imaging, film serves as the medium for image acquisition, processing, and display.
- A quality film image has the proper balance of density and contrast, maximum recorded detail, and minimal distortion.
- A film image is displayed on a polyester sheet of plastic composed of densities resulting from exposed crystals converted to black metallic silver after chemical processing.
- Silver halide crystals suspended in a film's emulsion layer absorb the radiant energy (x-rays and visible light) and form a latent image.
- Film is placed in a cassette between two intensifying screens, permitting lower x-ray exposures compared with film alone.
- The intensifying screen phosphors emit visible light (fluoresce) in proportion to the exit radiation to expose the film.
- Intensifying screens can be manufactured to have varying speeds. Increasing intensifying screen speed reduces not only the required radiation exposure but also the recorded detail in the image.
- Automatic film processing incorporates several chemical stages and systems to convert a latent image into a manifest image.
- Hydroquinone and phenidone are chemical reducing agents used during the developing stage to convert the exposed silver halide crystals to black metallic silver.

- Ammonium thiosulfate is the chemical fixing agent to clear undeveloped crystals from the film's emulsion.
- Maintaining the archival quality of radiographs requires that most of the fixing agent be washed from the film.
- During the drying stage, 85% to 90% of the moisture needs to be removed from the film for long-term storage.
- Important systems for processing films include replenishment, chemical recirculation, temperature control, and a transport system to move the film through the tanks at a constant speed.
- Film should be stored and handled in a darkroom at temperatures ranging from 55° to 75°F (14°–24°C) and with a relative humidity of 30% to 60%. Without moisture in the air (low humidity), any buildup of static charges can expose the film.
- Safelights used in the darkroom must be equipped with a safelight filter appropriate for the type of film being handled.
- Silver recovery can be accomplished by the electrolytic method or metallic replacement and is an important process because silver is a natural resource, is a heavy metal that can be toxic to the environment, and must be removed from the used fixer.
- OD is a measurement of the amount of light transmitted through an area on the film.
- Unlike digital imaging, the amount of radiation exposure reaching the film-screen IR has a direct effect on the amount of density produced in the processed image.
- Sensitometry is the study of the relationship between radiation exposure and the amount of density produced after a film is chemically processed.
- Radiographic film can be manufactured to differ in terms of speed, contrast, latitude, and spectral sensitivity.
- Speed is the sensitivity of film to radiation and has a direct relationship with OD. The location of the sensitometric curve along the x-axis indicates its speed.
- The slope of the straight-line portion of a sensitometric curve (average gradient) indicates the film's level of contrast; the steeper the slope, the higher is the contrast.
- Exposure latitude refers to the range of exposures that produce optical densities in the straight-line portion of the sensitometric curve and is inversely related to contrast. Higher-contrast films have narrower exposure latitudes.
- When both optimum density and maximum contrast have been achieved, the visibility of recorded detail is of optimal radiographic quality.
- Radiographic films are displayed on illuminators that emit uniform light intensity.

REVIEW QUESTIONS

1. Which of the following is the latent image center for radiographic film?
    A. Phosphor layer
    B. Polyester base
    C. Detector element
    D. Sensitivity speck
2. Which of the following describes a film's sensitivity to x-rays or light?
    A. Gamma
    B. Speed
    C. Contrast
    D. Latitude
3. Intensifying screens are used to _____.
    A. decrease patient exposure
    B. increase recorded detail

C. increase film latitude

D. decrease contrast

4. The ability to emit light only when stimulated by x-rays is known as _____.

  A. phosphorescence

  B. sensitometry

  C. conversion efficiency

  D. fluorescence

5. What reducing agent acts slowly to produce the higher densities on a film radiograph?

  A. Ammonium thiosulfate

  B. Hydroquinone

  C. Phenidone

  D. Cesium iodide

6. What chemical agent is responsible for clearing the unexposed silver halide crystals during film processing?

  A. Ammonium thiosulfate

  B. Hydroquinone

  C. Phenidone

  D. Cesium iodide

7. Which automatic processing system primarily maintains the chemical activity level?

  A. Replenishment

  B. Standby control

  C. Recirculation

  D. Quality control

8. Why is silver recovery necessary during film processing?

  A. It is a natural resource.

  B. It is toxic to the environment.

  C. It has monetary value.

  D. All of the above

9. What term is defined as a measure of the amount of light transmitted through the film?

  A. Sensitometry

  B. Film contrast

  C. Film speed

  D. OD

10. What is the diagnostic range of optical densities?

  A. 0.15 to 4.0

  B. 0.5 to 1.25

  C. 0.5 to 2.0

  D. 0.10 to 2.0

11. A change of_____ in OD results from a change in the percentage of light transmittance by a factor of 2.

  A. 0.03

  B. 0.3

  C. 3.0

  D. 30

12. Changes in radiation exposure have the greatest effect on optical densities in which sensito-metric region?

  A. Toe

  B. Shoulder

C. Straight-line

D. Toe and Shoulder

13. When the exposure technique used produces densities outside the straight-line portion of a sensitometric curve, how was contrast affected?

   A. Increased

   B. No effect

   C. Decreased

   D. Improved

14. Compare the sensitometric curves in Fig. 9.31. Which film is faster?

   A. Film A

   B. Film B

   C. Film C

   D. Film D

15. Compare the sensitometric curves in Fig. 9.31. Which film has lower contrast?

   A. Film A

   B. Film B

   C. Film C

   D. Film D

16. Film B has an exposure speed point of 1.5, and film A has an exposure speed point of 1.2. Is there a difference in speed?

   A. Film A is twice as fast as film B.

   B. Film A and B have equal speed.

   C. Film A is half as fast as film B.

   D. Film B is twice as fast as film A.

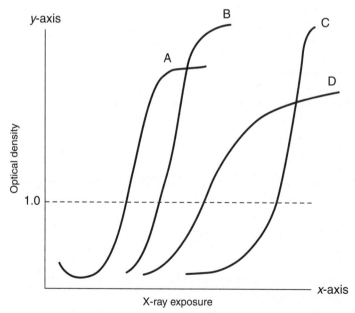

FIG. 9-31 Film types and sensitometric graphs (A–D). The shape and position of the graph along the x-axis display the differing characteristics of film speed, contrast, and latitude.

Dynamic Imaging: Fluoroscopy

CHAPTER OUTLINE

OBJECTIVES

After completing this chapter, the reader will be able to perform the following:

1. Define all the key terms in this chapter.
2. State all the important relationships in this chapter.
3. Differentiate between fluoroscopic and radiographic imaging.
4. Recognize the unique features of an image-intensified fluoroscopic unit and explain how the image is created and viewed.
5. Explain the process of brightness gain and the conversion factor during image intensification.
6. Define *automatic brightness* control and state its function.
7. Explain how using the magnification mode affects image quality and patient exposure.
8. Identify common types of image degradation resulting from image-intensified fluoroscopy.
9. Differentiate among the types of television cameras or electronic devices used to convert the output phosphor image for viewing on a display monitor.
10. List the types of recording devices available for image-intensified fluoroscopy.
11. Identify the unique features of flat-panel detector fluoroscopy and their effect on image quality and patient exposure.
12. Differentiate between continuous and pulsed fluoroscopy and their impacts on patient radiation dose.
13. Recognize the fluoroscopic features that impact image quality and patient radiation exposure.
14. Identify specialized fluoroscopic units and their use in radiology.
15. State radiation safety procedures used to reduce exposure to the patient and personnel.
16. Recognize the need for quality control on fluoroscopic units.

KEY TERMS

accelerating anode	continuous fluoroscopy	magnification mode
air kerma	conversion factor	mini C-arm
analog-to-digital converter (ADC)	dose-area product (DAP)	minification gain
automatic brightness control (ABC)	electronic magnification	mobile C-arm
	electrostatic focusing lenses	O-arm
automatic exposure rate control (AERC)	fluoro loop save	output phosphor
	fluoroscopy	photocathode
brightness gain	flux gain	photoemission
camera tube	frame averaging	pulse rate
charge-coupled device (CCD)	image intensifier	pulse width
complementary metal oxide semiconductor (CMOS)	input phosphor	pulsed fluoroscopy
	kerma area product (KAP)	spatial resolution
	last image hold (LIH)	virtual collimation

The previous chapters discussed radiographic imaging for producing static (stationary) images of anatomic tissues. However, imaging of the functioning or motion (dynamics) of anatomic structures is needed for evaluation and is accomplished by fluoroscopy. **Fluoroscopy** allows imaging of the movement of internal structures. It differs from radiographic imaging by its use of a continuous or pulsed beam of x-rays to create images of moving internal structures that can be viewed on a monitor. Internal structures, such as vascular or gastrointestinal systems, can be visualized in their normal state of motion with the aid of special liquid or gas substances (contrast media) that are either injected or instilled.

Traditional fluoroscopic units are designed with the x-ray tube underneath the table and the image-intensifier tube or digital detector located overtop of the patient. Radiology rooms can be designed solely for radiography or fluoroscopy but can also combine the two systems for radiography and fluoroscopy. These traditional units require the operator or radiographer to perform the procedures tableside. Remote-controlled fluoroscopy is an imaging system that is operated by a control console not located at the tableside. Modern remote-control units integrate or are configured with the table and tube in one system, allowing for both fluoroscopic and radiographic procedures. These remote-controlled systems have the x-ray tube located above the patient and the imaging detector located below the patient. Integrated remote-controlled fluoroscopic and radiographic systems are a more efficient use of imaging, especially for areas with low-volume fluoroscopic procedures.

This chapter discusses the components of traditional image-intensified and digital fluoroscopic units, viewing and recording systems, and important fluoroscopic features in use today.

IMAGE INTENSIFICATION

In image-intensified fluoroscopy, the milliamperage (mA) used during imaging is considerably lower (0.5–5 mA) than that in the radiographic mode, which is operated at a higher mA of 50 to 1200 mA. A low mA provides for the increased time the image intensifier is operated. Because the time of exposure is lengthened, the control panel includes a timer that buzzes audibly when 5 minutes of x-ray fluoroscopic time has been used. Another important feature of a fluoroscopic unit is the dead-man switch. The continuous x-ray beam is activated by either a hand switch on the unit or a foot pedal that must be continuously depressed for the x-rays to be produced. Releasing the pressure applied to the pedal or switch terminates the radiation exposure.

The **image intensifier** is an electronic vacuum tube that converts the remnant (exit) x-ray beam to light, then to electrons, then back to light, increasing the light intensity in the process. The entire intensifier tube is approximately 50 cm (20 inches) in length and 15 to 58 cm (6–23 inches) in diameter (diameter depends on manufacturer and intended use). Image intensification (Fig. 10-1) is the process in which the exit radiation from the anatomic area of interest interacts with the **input phosphor** for conversion to visible light. The input phosphor is made of cesium iodide and is bonded to the curved surface of the intensifier tube itself. Cesium iodide absorbs the remnant x-ray photon energy and emits light in response, proportional to the percentage of x-ray absorption. Thousands of light photons are created from just one x-ray photon. The light intensities are equal to the intensities of the exit radiation and are converted to electrons by a **photocathode** (photoemission). The photocathode is made of cesium and antimony compounds. These metals emit electrons in response to light stimulus in a process called **photoemission**. The ratio of light to electron emission is not one to one. It takes many light photons to result in the emission of one electron. The photocathode is bonded directly to the input phosphor using a very thin adhesive layer. These layers are curved so that all the electrons emitted from the photocathode travel the same distance to the output phosphor. As a result, the spatial resolution is maintained

FIG. 10-1 Fluoroscopic image-intensified system used for dynamic imaging of internal structures.

FIG. 10-2 Major components of an image intensifier.

throughout the fluoroscopic image. The electrons are focused by electrostatic focusing lenses and accelerated toward an anode. The **electrostatic focusing lenses** are not really lenses at all but are negatively charged plates along the length of the image-intensifier tube. These negatively charged plates repel the electron stream, focusing it toward the small output phosphor. To set the electron stream in motion at a constant velocity, an **accelerating anode** is located at the neck of the image intensifier near the output phosphor. This accelerating anode maintains a constant potential of approximately 25 kV.

These high-energy electrons result in hundreds of light photons being emitted from the output phosphor. The output phosphor is made of silver-activated zinc cadmium sulfide and is much smaller than the input phosphor. It is located at the opposite end of the image-intensifier tube, just beyond the accelerating anode. The **output phosphor** absorbs electrons and emits light in response. The result of this process is an increase in image brightness (Fig. 10-2).

The image light intensities from the output phosphor are converted to an electronic video signal and sent to a display monitor for viewing. Fig. 10-3 is an example of a typical radiographic and image-intensified fluoroscopic unit. Additional image recording devices, such as spot film or cine (movie film), can be attached to the fluoroscopic system to create permanent radiographic images of specific areas of interest.

 IMPORTANT RELATIONSHIP

Image-Intensified Fluoroscopy

Dynamic imaging of internal anatomic structures can be accomplished with the use of an image intensifier. The exit radiation is absorbed by the input phosphor, converted to electrons, sent to the output phosphor, released as visible light, and converted to an electronic video signal for transmission to the display monitor.

Brightness Gain

A brighter image is a result of high-energy electrons striking a small-output phosphor. Accelerating the electrons increases the light intensities at the output phosphor (**flux gain**). The reduction in the size of the output phosphor image compared with that of the input phosphor image also increases the light intensities (**minification gain**). **Brightness gain** is the product of both flux gain and minification gain and results in a brighter image on the output phosphor.

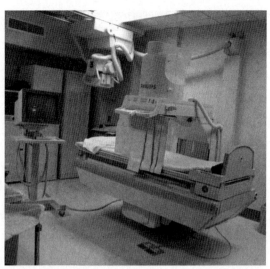

FIG. 10-3 A typical radiographic and image-intensified fluoroscopic unit. (From Ehrlich RA: *Patient Care in Radiography: With an Introduction to Medical Imaging,* ed 10, St. Louis, 2021, Elsevier Inc.)

 IMPORTANT RELATIONSHIP

Brightness Gain

A brighter image is created on the output phosphor when accelerated electrons strike a smaller output phosphor.

Although the term *brightness gain* continues to be used, it is now a common practice to express this increase in brightness with the term *conversion factor*. **Conversion factor** is an expression of the luminance at the output phosphor divided by the input exposure rate, and its unit of measure is the candela per square meter per milliroentgen per second ($cd/m^2/mR/s$). The numeric conversion factor value is roughly equal to 1% of the brightness gain value. For example, a brightness gain of 20,000 would have a conversion factor of 200. The higher the conversion factor or brightness gain value, the greater the efficiency of the image intensifier. See Box 10-1 for brightness gain and conversion factor formulas.

Automatic Brightness Control

The radiographer must also be familiar with **automatic brightness control (ABC)**, a function of the fluoroscopic unit that maintains the overall appearance of the fluoroscopic image (contrast and brightness) by automatically adjusting the kilovoltage peak (kVp), mA, or both. ABC (also known as automatic brightness stabilization [ABS]), generally operates by monitoring the current through the image intensifier or the output phosphor intensity and adjusting the exposure factor if the monitored value falls below preset levels. The fluoroscopic unit allows the operator to select a desired brightness level, and this level is subsequently maintained by ABC. ABC is slightly slow in its response to changes in patient tissue thickness and tissue density as the fluoroscopy tower is moved about over the patient; this is visible to the radiographer as a lag in the image brightness on the monitor as the tower is moved.

BOX 10-1   Brightness Gain and Conversion Factor Formulas

$$\text{Brightness gain} = \text{Minification gain} \times \text{Flux gain}$$

$$\text{Flux gain} = \frac{\text{Number of output light photons}}{\text{Number of input x} - \text{ray photons}}$$

$$\text{Minification gain} = \left(\frac{d_i}{d_0}\right)^2$$

$$\text{Conversion factor} = \frac{\text{Output phosphor illumination } (cd/m^2)}{\text{Input exposure rate } (mR/s)}$$

Example:
Input phosphor = 20 cm $\dfrac{20^2}{3^2} = \dfrac{400}{9} = 44.4 \times 400 = 13{,}320$ brightness gain
Output phosphor = 3 cm
Flux gain = 400

$$\text{Conversion factor} = 133.2 \left(13{,}320 \times 0.01 \left[1\% \text{ of brightness gain}\right]\right)$$

d_i, Input phosphor diameter; d_0, output phosphor diameter

FIG. 10-4 Magnification mode. When the image intensifier is operated in magnification mode, the voltage to the electrostatic focusing lenses is increased. This increase tightens the diameter of the electron stream, and the focal point is shifted farther from the output phosphor, resulting in a magnified image. (From Johnston JN, Fauber TL: *Essentials of Radiographic Physics and Imaging*, ed 2, St. Louis, 2016, Mosby.)

Magnification Mode

Another function of most image intensifiers is the multifield mode or magnification mode. When operated in **magnification mode**, the voltage to the electrostatic focusing lenses is increased. This increase tightens the diameter of the electron stream, and the focal point is shifted farther from the output phosphor (Fig. 10-4). The effect is that only the electrons from the central area of the input phosphor interact with the output phosphor and contribute to the image, giving the appearance of magnification. For example, a 30/23/15-cm (12/9/6-inch) trifocus image intensifier can be operated in any of these three modes. When operated in the 23-cm (9-inch) mode, only the electrons from the central 23 cm (9 inch) of the input phosphor interact with the output phosphor; the electrons about the periphery miss and do not contribute to the image. The same is true for the 15-cm (6-inch) mode. The degree of magnification (magnification factor [MF]) may be found by dividing the full-size input diameter by the selected input diameter. For example: MF = 30 ÷ 15 = 2× magnification.

This magnification improves the operator's ability to see small structures (spatial resolution, discussed shortly) but at the expense of increasing the patient dose. Remnant x-ray photons are converted to light and then to electrons and are focused on the output phosphor. If fewer electrons are incident on the output phosphor, the output intensity decreases. To compensate, more x-ray photons are needed at the beginning of the process to produce more light, resulting in more electrons at the input end of the image intensifier. ABC automatically increases x-ray exposure to achieve this. Again, with an increase in x-rays used comes an increase in patient dose.

IMPORTANT RELATIONSHIP

Magnification Mode and Patient Dose

> Operating the image intensifier in one of the magnification modes increases the operator's ability to see small structures but at the price of increasing the radiation dose to the patient.

Magnification modes improve **spatial resolution**, which refers to the smallest structure that may be detected in an image. Spatial resolution is measured in line pairs per millimeter (lp/mm), and typical fluoroscopic systems have spatial resolution capabilities of 4 to 6 lp/mm but greatly depend on the rest of the imaging chain (i.e., the viewing and recording systems).

Distortion is also an issue with image-intensified fluoroscopy. In radiography, distortion is a misrepresentation of the true size or shape of an object. In the case of fluoroscopy, shape distortion can be a problem. In fluoroscopy, distortion is a result of inaccurate control or focusing of the electrons released at the periphery of the photocathode and the curved shape of the photocathode. The combined result is an unequal magnification (distortion) of the image, creating what is called a "pincushion appearance" (Fig. 10-5). This problem also causes a loss of brightness around the periphery of the image, which is referred to as *vignetting*.

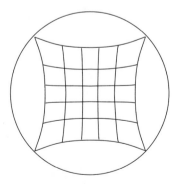

Image displaying
"pincushion" distortion

FIG. 10-5 Pincushion distortion. Appearance of the pincushion effect. The *circle* represents the television monitor display, and the grid represents the effect on the image. (From Johnston JN, Fauber TL: *Essentials of Radiographic Physics and Imaging*, ed 2, St. Louis, 2016, Mosby.)

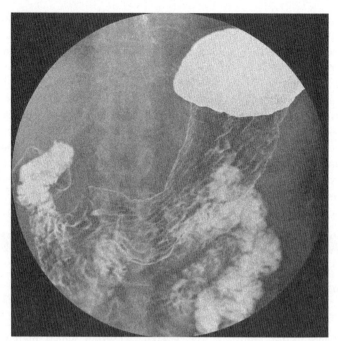

FIG. 10-6 Quantum noise. If too few x-rays exit the patient and expose the input phosphor, not enough light will be produced, decreasing the number of electrons released by the photocathode to interact with the output phosphor. A "grainy" or "noisy" image results. (From Bontrager K, Lampignano J: *Textbook of Radiographic Positioning and Related Anatomy*, ed 7, St. Louis, 2010, Mosby.)

One last factor to consider with image intensifiers is noise. Image noise results when insufficient information is present to create the image. In the case of fluoroscopy, this lack of image-forming information ultimately goes back to an insufficient quantity of x-rays. If too few x-rays exit the patient and expose the input phosphor, not enough light will be produced, decreasing the number of electrons released by the photocathode to interact with the output phosphor. This results in a "grainy" or "noisy" image (Fig. 10-6). Although other factors in the fluoroscopic chain may contribute to noise, the solution generally comes back to increasing the mA (quantity of radiation). For image-intensified fluoroscopy this is a small increase in mA because these systems operate at 2 to 5 mA. Because older image intensifier units are operated as **continuous fluoroscopy**, to minimize radiation dose, the operator should intermittently pulse the x-ray beam by activating the exposure switch on and off rapidly.

Viewing Systems

The original image intensifiers produced an image that was viewed using a mirror optics system—something akin to a sophisticated way of looking at the output phosphor with a "rearview mirror." With advancements in technology, the viewing system became a television monitor (older method) and now referred to as a display monitor. To view the image from the output phosphor on a display monitor, it must first be converted to an electrical signal (often referred to as *video signal*) by the television camera. Two devices are commonly used today to accomplish this: a camera tube and a **charge-coupled device (CCD)**. The camera tube and CCD differ in their size and readout process.

Television Cameras

Television cameras used to display the fluoroscopic image include the older camera tube (vidicon or Plumbicon) and the newer CCD. The **camera tube** has a vacuum tube approximately 15 cm (6 inch) in length that encloses an electron gun and a photoconductive target assembly. The diameter of the tube is the same size as that of the output phosphor. The camera tube most often used is the vidicon tube (Fig. 10-7). The vidicon tube is connected to the output phosphor of the image intensifier by either a fiberoptic bundle or an optical lens system (Fig. 10-8). The vidicon tube is a diode tube (cathode and anode) contained in a glass envelope to maintain a vacuum. The cathode consists of an electron gun that provides a continuous stream of electrons and a control grid that forms the electron stream into a "beam." The anode of the tube consists of a face plate, a signal plate, and a target. A steady stream of electrons from the

FIG. 10-7 A, Vidicon-type camera tube. **B,** The vidicon tube has a vacuum tube that encloses an electron gun and a photoconductive target assembly. The electrical signal leaving the camera tube varies in strength proportionally based on the varying brightness of the image being scanned. (Part A Modified from Copyright User: Sphl/Wikimedia Commons/CC-BY-SA 3.0; https://commons.wikimedia.org/wiki/File:Vidicon_tube-2.jpg. Part B from Curry T, Dowdey J, Murry R: *Christensen's Physics of Diagnostic Radiology*, ed 4, Philadelphia, 1990, Lippincott Williams & Wilkins.)

FIG. 10-8 Camera tube. The output phosphor is connected to the "photoelectric surface" end of the camera tube using a lens system or fiberoptics. (From Johnston JN, Fauber TL: *Essentials of Radiographic Physics and Imaging*, ed 3, St. Louis, 2020, Elsevier.)

electron gun scans the target assembly very quickly from left to right and top to bottom (raster pattern). As the stream of electrons bombards the target, anywhere there is light intensity from the output phosphor image, there will be an electrical signal leaving the tube. Scanning a brighter or higher light intensity results in the electrical signal leaving the camera tube with a higher strength. The darker or lower the light intensities scanned, the lower the strength of the electrical signal. The electrical signal leaving the camera tube varies in strength in proportion to the varying brightness of the image being scanned. This electrical (video) signal goes to the display monitor to complete the display process.

A CCD is a light-sensitive semiconducting device that generates an electrical charge when stimulated by light and stores this charge in a capacitor. The charge is proportional to the light intensity and is stored in rows of pixels. A CCD consists of a series of semiconductor capacitors, with each capacitor representing a pixel. Each pixel is composed of photosensitive material that dislodges electrons when stimulated by light photons. To digitize the charge from this device, the electrodes between each pixel, called *row gates*, are charged in sequence, moving the signal down the row, where it is transferred into the capacitors. From the capacitors, the charge is sent as an electronic signal to the display monitor. In this way, each pixel is individually "read" and sent to the display monitor (Fig. 10-9).

Compared with the vidicon-type camera tube, the CCD is read out by the charge in each pixel, whereas the vidicon is read out by an electronic beam. CCD TV cameras have some advantages over the camera tubes in that they are more sensitive to a wider range of light intensities and show no geometric distortion of the fluoroscopic display image. The CCD is smaller in size than the vidicon camera tube and works well in digital imaging.

FIG. 10-9 A, The charge-coupled device (CCD). **B,** The CCD is a light-sensitive semiconducting device that generates an electrical charge when stimulated by light and stores this charge in a capacitor until the charge is sent as an electronic signal to the display monitor. (From Johnston JN, Fauber TL: *Essentials of Radiographic Physics and Imaging*, ed 3, St. Louis, 2020, Elsevier.)

IMPORTANT RELATIONSHIP

Television Cameras and the Display Monitor

The camera tube and CCD are devices that convert the light image from the intensifier's output phosphor to an electronic signal that can be reconstructed on the display monitor.

Serving a similar purpose as the CCD is the **complementary metal oxide semiconductor (CMOS)**. CMOS devices are scintillators made up of a crystalline silicon matrix. Each detector element has its own amplifier, photodiode, and storage capacitor and is surrounded by transistors.

They do not have quite the light sensitivity or resolution of CCDs, but they use a fraction of the power to run, are very inexpensive to manufacture, and are improving.

Coupling of Devices

As mentioned earlier, the camera tube or CCD may be coupled to the output phosphor of the image intensifier by either a fiber-optic bundle or an optical lens system. The fiber-optic bundle is simply a bundle of very thin optical glass filaments. This system is very durable and simple in design but does not allow spot filming.

The optical lens system is a series of optical lenses that focus the image from the output phosphor on the television camera (camera tube or CCD). When spot filming is desired, a beam-splitting mirror (a partially silvered mirror that allows some light to pass through and reflects some in a new direction) is moved into the path of the output image and diverts some of the light to the desired spot-filming device (e.g., the photospot or cine camera) (Fig. 10-10). This system, although allowing spot filming of this type, is more susceptible to rough handling, which may cause maladjustment of the mirror and lenses and result in a blurred image.

Display Monitor

The purpose of the display monitor is to convert the electronic signal from the camera tube or CCD back into a visible image. In older image-intensified units, this monitor was a cathode ray tube (CRT) (Fig. 10-11), which includes an electron gun that scans the phosphor layer found on the inside of the glass front of the monitor, again in a raster pattern. As the video signal increases and decreases, so does the number of electrons emitted from the electron gun. The greater the number of electrons leaving the gun, the brighter the fluorescence of the phosphor, resulting in a bright spot on the display monitor. The lower the video signal, the fewer the electrons emitted from the gun and the lower the brightness of the displayed image.

In essence, the monitor reconstructs the image from the output phosphor as a visible image. The image is created on the fluorescent screen one line at a time starting in the upper left-hand

FIG. 10-10 Beam-splitting mirror. If the image intensifier is equipped with a spot-filming device, it diverts some of the light to the device for permanent images. (From Johnston JN, Fauber TL: *Essentials of Radiographic Physics and Imaging*, ed 3, St. Louis, 2020, Elsevier.)

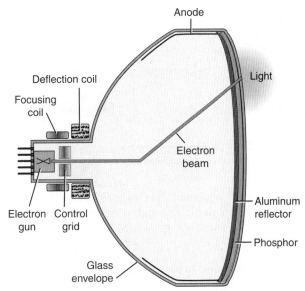

FIG. 10-11 Cathode ray tube (CRT) display monitor. The display monitor reconstructs the image from the output phosphor as a visible image. The CRT includes an electron gun that scans the phosphor layer found on the inside of the glass front of the monitor in a raster pattern. (From Johnston JN, Fauber TL: *Essentials of Radiographic Physics and Imaging*, ed 2, St. Louis, 2016, Mosby.)

corner and moving to the right (active trace). It then blanks (turns off) and returns to the left side (horizontal retrace). This process continues to the bottom of the screen. It then returns to the top (vertical retrace) and begins again by placing a line between each of the previously drawn lines. This action creates a line frame. Typical display monitors are called *525-line systems* because the traces create a 525-line frame. High-resolution monitors have 1024 lines per frame. However, the monitor continues to be the weak link in terms of the resolution of the fluoroscopic chain. The image intensifier is capable of resolving approximately 5 lp/mm, whereas the monitor can display only 1 to 2 lp/mm.

CRT monitors have been replaced with more advanced display monitors and are discussed later in this chapter.

Recording Systems

Cassette spot filming was a standard of image-intensified fluoroscopy for many years (Fig. 10-12). This was a static imaging process in which a standard radiographic cassette was used to obtain an image. With this system, the cassette is loaded into the lower part of the fluoroscopic tower and "parked" in a protective envelope in the back. When the spot-film exposure button is pressed, the cassette is moved into position between the patient and image intensifier, and the machine shifts from fluoroscopic to radiographic mode and exposes the film. In the shift to radiographic mode, the mA increases from one of the 0.5- to 5-mA fluoroscopic modes to one of the 50- to 1200-mA radiographic modes. Because this method of imaging uses the radiographic mode, it requires a much higher radiation dose to the patient than the other methods. As an alternative to exposing the entire film, the tower is generally equipped with a series of masking shutters that can "divide" the cassette and allow numerous exposures on one cassette, such as two exposures on one cassette,

FIG. 10-12 A typical image-intensified fluoroscopic unit showing two types of recording systems, cassette spot filming and a photo-spot camera. (From Johnston JN, Fauber TL: *Essentials of Radiographic Physics and Imaging*, ed 2, St. Louis, 2016, Mosby.)

four on one, and six on one. In each setting, the image is smaller and organized as one of multiple images on one film.

IMPORTANT RELATIONSHIP

Cassette Spot Filming

Cassette spot-film devices were a means of recording static images during an image-intensified fluoroscopic examination. The unit shifts to radiographic mode (using a higher mA), and the radiation dose to the patient is much higher than in the fluoroscopic mode.

Film cameras (sometimes called *photo-spot cameras*) were also a mainstay of image-intensified fluoroscopy (see Fig. 10-10). They most commonly used 105-mm "chip" film or 70-mm roll film. The photo-spot camera was also a static imaging system that was used with an optical lens system incorporating a beam-splitting mirror. When the spot-film exposure switch is pressed, the beam-splitting mirror is moved into place, diverting some of the beam toward the photo camera and exposing the film. This device uses the visible light image from the output phosphor of the image intensifier and photographically exposes the 105-mm (or 70-mm) film, similar to a 35-mm film camera used in photography. This system allows very fast imaging of up to 12 frames per second, and because it is "photographing" the image off the output phosphor of the image intensifier, it requires approximately half the radiation dose of the cassette spot-filming system.

With image-intensified fluoroscopy, videotape or DVD recording was an option when dynamic imaging is desired. This process used a VHS videotape or DVD recorder connected to the display monitor. From this point, it operates quite like a home recording system. During fluoroscopic examinations, the "record" button is pressed on the system, and it records the image from the monitor. Although not typically used in today's fluoroscopic systems, such imaging is useful in functional studies of the esophagus or for placement of catheters or medical devices.

As more departments transition to fully digital environments and eliminate film and chemical processing, a greater dependence is being placed on digital imaging and storage means. Without chemical processing and film, cassette spot filming and photo-spot imaging go away. If the fluoroscopic signal is in digital form, the size of the data files makes it impossible to record any length of dynamic images on a VHS tape.

DIGITAL FLUOROSCOPY

Similar to image-intensified fluoroscopy, digital fluoroscopy has evolved over time. Early versions of digital fluoroscopy used an image-intensified fluoroscopic chain but added an **analog-to-digital converter (ADC)** and a computer between the TV camera and the monitor (Fig. 10-13). An ADC is a device that takes the video (analog) signal and divides it into a series of bits (1s and 0s) that the computer "understands." The number of bits into which the signal is divided determines the contrast resolution (number of shades of gray) of the system. The ADC is necessary for the computer to process and display the image. When in digital form, the image can be postprocessed and stored in that format or printed onto film using a dry laser printer.

The incorporation of a CCD into this setup further improved digital fluoroscopy. The CCD eliminated some of the problems associated with the camera tube. The CCD is more light sensitive (higher detective quantum efficiency [DQE]) and exhibits less noise and no spatial distortion. It also has a higher spatial resolution and requires less radiation in the system, reducing patient dose.

Flat-Panel Detector Fluoroscopy

A more recent advance in digital fluoroscopy is the introduction of a flat-panel detector in place of an image intensifier (Fig. 10-14). Two forms of flat-panel detectors may be used for fluoroscopic applications: the cesium iodide amorphous silicon indirect-capture detector and the amorphous selenium direct-capture detector. A commonly used flat-panel detector for fluoroscopic applications is the cesium iodide amorphous silicon indirect-capture detector. The scintillator of this system uses cesium iodide or gadolinium oxysulfide as the phosphor. The photodetector is amorphous silicon, which is a liquid that can be painted onto a substrate (foundation or underlying layer) and is the material that makes flat-panel detectors possible. The other component is

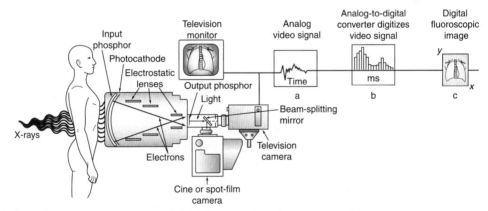

FIG. 10-13 Analog and digital signals in fluoroscopy. The video signal from the television camera is analog, whereas the voltage signal continuously varies. This analog signal is sampled *(a)*, producing a stepped representation of the analog video signal *(b)*. The numerical values of each step are stored *(c)*, producing a matrix of digital image data. The binary representation of each pixel value in the matrix is stored and can be manipulated by a computer. The value of each pixel can be mapped to a brightness level for viewing on a display monitor or to an optical density for hard copy on film. (From Eastman Kodak Company, Dayton, OH.)

FIG. 10-14 Digital fluoroscopy using flat-panel-detector technology. (Courtesy of Siemens Healthcare, Malvern, PA.)

a thin-film-transistor (TFT) array. TFTs are electronic components layered onto a glass substrate that includes a readout, charge collector, and light-sensitive elements. The panel is configured into a network of pixels (or detector elements [DELs]) covered by the scintillator plate with each pixel containing a photodetector and a TFT. With this system, x-ray energy is absorbed by the scintillator and converted to light energy. This light is then absorbed by the photodetectors and converted to electrical charges, which are in turn captured and transmitted by the TFT array to the monitor for display.

Flat-panel detectors are very popular in full-field digital mammography, interventional, and cardiology applications and are gaining ground in general fluoroscopy. They are much lighter and more compact, they produce a digital signal directly (no need for a camera tube or CCD), and because it is a digital system producing a digital signal (without the electronic components of the old image-intensified system), there is less electronic noise. Detector arrays are currently available in field-of-view (FOV) sizes of 25 × 25 cm to 43 × 43 cm (10 × 10 inches to 17 × 17 inches).

Although the cesium iodide amorphous silicon indirect-capture detector is essentially the same as that for DR (digital radiography), there are a few differences for use as a dynamic digital detector in digital fluoroscopy applications. In general, dynamic versions of these detectors must respond in rapid sequences to create a dynamic image. Current dynamic versions are capable of up to 60 frames per second. To accomplish this, rapid readout speeds (how the active matrix processes the image data) are necessary. The design is a two-dimensional rectilinear array of pixels that can be electronically processed line by line in a fraction of a second. Furthermore, for fluoroscopic applications, very-low-noise flat-panel-detector systems are needed. Fluoroscopy generally operates at a low-dose output; hence, any operational noise degrades the fluoroscopic image, making noise a greater factor in detectors used for this application. Application-specific integrated circuits (ASICs) are used to minimize noise and amplify signal from the active matrix. These circuits are particularly important in fluoroscopic applications because they minimize noise, maximize readout speed, and allow for switching from low-dose to high-dose inputs (for static imaging). Another consideration with the low-dose fluoroscopic applications is the need to maintain a large fill factor (the area of each pixel that is sensitive to x-ray detection materials). With general radiography that uses a larger dose output, this is generally not a problem, but it becomes a problem with fluoroscopic applications because of the lower radiation doses used in fluoroscopic imaging, particularly with indirect-capture detectors. Other features such as a light-emitting diode array "backlighting system" have also been incorporated to erase the detector between frames to prevent "ghosting" caused by any residual exposure charge from the previous frame.

 IMPORTANT RELATIONSHIP

Flat-Panel Detectors for Dynamic Imaging

> Fluoroscopic versions of flat-panel detectors must respond in rapid sequences to create dynamic images, are needed to maintain a large fill factor to reduce image noise caused by low-dose fluoroscopic applications, and must erase the detector between frames to prevent "ghosting" caused by any residual exposure charge from the previous frame.

The use of flat-panel detectors in place of an image intensifier offers several advantages. The first is a reduction in the size, bulk, and weight of the fluoroscopic tower. A flat-panel detector greatly reduces all three, allowing easier manipulation of the tower, greater flexibility of movement, and greater access to the patient during the examination. A flat-panel detector with a 30- × 43-cm (12- × 17-inch) active area occupies less than 25% of the volume of a 30-cm (12-inch) image-intensifier tube and less than 15% of the volume of a 43-cm (17-inch) image-intensifier tube. The flat-panel detectors also replace the spot filming and other recording devices. Some flat-panel detector units operate in the radiographic mode (50–1200 mA) so that in many cases additional radiographic images are not needed. The images, both dynamic and static, are recorded by the system and can be readily archived with the patient record in a picture archiving and communication system (PACS). It should be noted that the images produced are very large data files because spot images can be 8 MB or larger and dynamic images as large as 240 MB per second.

Furthermore, flat-panel detectors are less likely to degrade with age; are more durable; present a rectangular field providing more information; and have better contrast resolution, higher DQE, wider dynamic range, and all the postprocessing options common to digital images. The spatial resolution of flat-panel detectors is the same for all FOV options provided binning (the process of grouping and averaging adjacent DELS) is not used and is higher than that of an image-intensified system (2.5–3.2 lp/mm versus 1–2 lp/mm). Finally, flat-panel detectors do not exhibit most image artifacts seen with image intensifiers. Flat-panel detectors have a 60 times larger operational dynamic range than image-intensifier systems and, because of this, do not exhibit veiling glare. Because the DELs of a flat-panel detector are arranged in a grid pattern (uniform columns and rows), they do not exhibit the pincushion and S distortion artifacts. Vignetting (unequal brightness) and defocusing artifacts are also eliminated with flat-panel detectors. Like image-intensified fluoroscopic units, the use of a "dead-man" exposure switch (one that turns the exposure off when the switch is released) has long been a part of all fluoroscopy systems.

 IMPORTANT RELATIONSHIP

Digital Fluoroscopic Systems

> The use of flat-panel detectors in place of an image intensifier offers several advantages, such as a reduction in the size, bulk, and weight of the fluoroscopic tower; allowing for easier manipulation of the tower; and greater access to the patient during the examination. The flat-panel detectors also replace the spot filming and other recording devices, and, because they operate in radiographic mode, in many cases, additional radiographic images are not needed. The images, both dynamic and static, can also be readily archived with the patient record in a PACS.

FLUOROSCOPIC FEATURES

Modern fluoroscopic equipment offers several features that impact the quality of the fluoroscopic image and radiation dose to the patient. There are several controls and settings, both on the control console and tower, that allow adjustment of the radiation output and image quality. The consideration for selecting kVp is the same as for general radiography. Using higher kVp settings (appropriate for the examination) results in a higher energy beam and lower patient dose.

Collimation of the fluoroscopic beam reduces the field size exposing the patient. Fully open, the unit exposes the patient to a beam adequate to cover the full size of the image intensifier or detector. With the newest units, lines appear on the **last image hold (LIH)** displayed on the monitor, indicating the position of the collimator plates. This allows the collimator to be further adjusted without exposing the patient to additional radiation (**virtual collimation**). The collimator should be adjusted to eliminate all anatomic structures not necessary to the exam being performed. Collimation changes the FOV displayed, but it does not magnify the image (Fig. 10-15). By reducing the area of tissue being exposed, overall patient dose is reduced.

Frame averaging is an operation that reduces overall patient dose and image noise by averaging multiple image frames together. Because the combining of frames reduces noise, less radiation is needed to maintain image quality; however, spatial resolution is decreased.

The option to include the grid is also a control feature. The grid reduces the amount of scatter reaching the image intensifier or detector and improves image quality. But because it also removes some useful radiation from the remnant beam, mA (quantity of radiation) must be increased to maintain overall exposure to the image intensifier or detector. In general, its use increases radiation dose to the patient. The decision to use it should be based on the exam and the anatomic area's capacity to produce scatter radiation. The abdomen, for example, produces more scatter radiation, and the grid should be selected; however, the extremities or pediatric patients may not require its use.

Modern fluoroscopic units also allow for the selection and interchangeability of added filtration thickness or material. The operation of this control may entail the substitution of filters of different thicknesses or switching of filtration material. The typical material used for beam filtration is aluminum, which has an atomic number ideally suited to removing low-energy x-ray photons. It is important to remove these low-energy photons from the beam before they can expose the

FIG. 10-15 Collimation and field of view (FOV). **A,** Full FOV image without collimation. **B,** Smaller FOV with increased collimation. Note the anatomy visualized is not magnified. (From Johnston JN, Fauber TL: *Essentials of Radiographic Physics and Imaging*, ed 3, St. Louis, 2020, Elsevier.)

patient and contribute only to patient dose. This filtration acts to increase the average energy of the beam by removing low-energy photons. Higher atomic materials such as copper are used in some units and may be selected when additional filtration and beam hardening are desired. Advancements in the type and combination of materials used in *spectral filtration* are incorporated into the design of modern fluoroscopic equipment and assists in reducing patient skin dose while maintaining quality fluoroscopic images.

Anatomic programs are also available on modern fluoroscopic units. These programs are pre-set fluoroscopic exam settings established and programmed into the unit at the time of manufacture or at the time of installation as dictated by the facility. Each preset brings up a predetermined set of exposure factors, filter thickness and type, and so on, just as they do on radiographic units. Along this same line are the default settings on the unit. These defaults are intended to be "ideal" or "standard" values for minimizing dose and maximizing image quality. They are not hard and fast rules of operation and should be changed depending on circumstances and the exam to be performed. The operator should evaluate the default settings when they appear on the control panel or tower to be sure they match the exam and patient (e.g., size, pediatric versus adult, pathology, anatomy of interest).

 IMPORTANT RELATIONSHIP

Fluoroscopic Features

> Use of virtual collimation during LIH, frame averaging, and added filtration reduces the patient dose. Conversely, use of a grid increases the patient dose.

Automatic Exposure Rate Control

Like ABC used in older image-intensified units, **automatic exposure rate control (AERC)** serves a similar function in modern fluoroscopy. AERC automatically adjusts the tube current (mA), voltage (kVp), filtration, and pulse width to maintain radiation exposure to the flat-panel detector. A variety of variables during a fluoroscopic exam can result in changes in the radiation exposure reaching the flat-panel detector. Changes in patient thickness, tissue attenuation, object-to-image-receptor distance (OID), collimation, and FOV may require an increase or decrease in the radiation reaching the detector.

Magnification

Electronic magnification is the selection of a smaller FOV. When a smaller FOV is selected, an area smaller than the size of the detector is exposed by the x-ray beam, but the area is enlarged to fill the display monitor area magnifying the anatomic structures (Fig. 10-16). Like intensified fluoroscopy, flat-panel detectors provide several different magnification modes. However, the spatial resolution of flat-panel detectors is the same for some FOV options, and the patient radiation dose is not significantly increased provided binning (the process of grouping and averaging adjacent DELS to reduce noise) is not used. For some FOVs, binning reduces the spatial resolution; however, for a smaller FOV, spatial resolution is increased, and noise is increased, resulting in increased radiation exposure to reduce the noise. However, the increase in radiation dose is less compared with magnification during image-intensified fluoroscopy. Selecting the magnification mode automatically adjusts the x-ray beam collimation to match the displayed tissue image and avoids irradiating tissue that does not appear in the image. The largest FOV should be used whenever possible to reduce patient radiation dose along with increased collimation to reduce irradiation of unnecessary patient tissues.

FIG. 10-16 Electronic magnification. **A,** Full FOV image. **B,** Electronic magnification mode results in a magnified image displayed. (From Johnston JN, Fauber TL: *Essentials of Radiographic Physics and Imaging*, ed 3, St. Louis, 2020, Elsevier.)

Pulsed Fluoroscopy

An operational feature of modern fluoroscopy units is **pulsed fluoroscopy**, using a pulsed beam technology to reduce radiation output necessary for the fluoroscopic image and patient radiation dose. This is simply a design of the unit that rapidly turns the x-ray beam on and off during operation. This operation introduces two concepts necessary to understanding its value, pulse rate and pulse width. **Pulse rate** refers to how many pulses occur per second of operation. Think of this as how many exposures occur per second. **Pulse width** refers to the length of each pulse. Think of this as how long each exposure lasts. The operator can select pulse rates generally from 1 pulse per second to 30 pulses per second. Pulse widths are generally less than 6 milliseconds for pediatrics and less than 10 milliseconds for adults. Because the pulse widths are much lower than 33 ms when compared with image-intensified fluoroscopy, the mA used is higher (50–1200) to maintain enough exposure to the detector for image quality (maintaining the needed signal-to-noise ratio [SNR] or contrast-to-noise ratio [CNR]). If the unit is operated at 30 pulses per second, the radiation dose is no different than continuous fluoroscopy, yet image quality is improved due to reduced motion artifacts. However, if operated at pulse rates below 30, a radiation dose reduction is realized (Fig. 10-17).

◤ IMPORTANT RELATIONSHIP

Pulsed Fluoroscopy

Operating the fluoroscope in a pulsed mode reduces the number of images each second, decreases the patient dose, and reduces the visibility of patient motion.

FIG. 10-17 Continuous versus pulsed fluoroscopy. **A,** Continuous fluoroscopy produces 30 images (frames) during a period of 1 second. **B,** Pulsed fluoroscopy can vary the number of images (frames) per second. This example has 7 frames per second.

Dose Rates

Most fluoroscopic units today allow for the selection of dose rates. The dose rate setting may be labeled as low, medium, or high (or icons may be used to imply the same). These settings change the dose generally by a percentage such as 50% (medium is 50% of high, and low is 50% of medium). These selections control the radiation dose rate at the detector, and automatic changes in the filter may occur along with changes in the pulse rate.

As with radiography, the operator should select the dose rate depending on the exam to be performed. For example, differentiation of soft tissue structures with lower subject contrast requires a higher dose rate, and barium studies (higher subject contrast) require a comparatively lower dose rate.

 IMPORTANT RELATIONSHIP

Pulsed Fluoroscopy and Dose Rates

Using pulsed fluoroscopy along with lower dose rates appropriate to the procedure reduces the patient radiation dose.

Image Recording

A sequence of digital radiographic images can be recorded per second with flat-panel detector fluoroscopy, which reduces the need for follow-up radiographic images. These radiographic images have improved quality (less noise) than fluoroscopic images; however, patient radiation exposure is significantly increased. Use of features such as LIH or last frame hold along with **fluoro loop save** saves single images or a fluoro sequence loop to memory (based on the equipment's memory capacity). Saved fluoro images have increased noise but significantly less exposure to the patient. These fluoroscopic images can be postprocessed and maintained in the patient's permanent record.

Dose Monitoring

Air kerma (**k**inetic **e**nergy **r**eleased in **m**atter) specifies the intensity of x-rays at a given point in air at a known distance from the focal spot or source of x-rays, and the cumulative or total air kerma is monitored during the fluoroscopic procedure. Other dose displays such as **dose-area product (DAP)** and **kerma area product (KAP)** provide indicators of patient radiation risk and should be documented in the patient's record. DAP meters (measure exposure in air followed by a computation to estimate absorbed dose to the patient) are required on all new fluoroscopes in the United States and internationally. KAP is the same as DAP and is the product of the total air kerma and the area of the x-ray beam at the entrance of the patient. Units of DAP and KAP are expressed in micro or milli gray (Gy) per area squared but can vary by manufacturer (Box 10-2). A cumulative dose (more recently referred to as *reference dose*) may also be displayed in Gy that estimates the patient's skin dose for the fluoroscopic procedure. These radiation dose units (DAP or KAP and reference dose) should be monitored during the procedure and the operator notified if an agreed upon *radiation or dose threshold* has been reached. The radiographer may be responsible for monitoring and documenting these radiation dose units in the patient's medical record. In addition to dose displays, the total amount of fluoro time for the procedure should be documented in the patient's record. An important quality control check on the fluoro unit is the fluoroscopic

---

BOX 10-2   Dose Monitoring

Air kerma: kinetic energy released in mass and specifies the intensity of x-rays at a given point in air at a known distance from the source of x-rays.

Kerma area product (KAP), also known as dose area product (DAP), is the product of cumulative air kerma and the area of the x-ray beam at the entrance of the patient.

Dose monitoring units may vary by manufacturer:

$$1\,\mu Gy\text{-}m^2 \;\; = \;\; 1\,cGy\text{-}cm^2 \;\; = \;\; 10\,mGy\text{-}cm$$

$$1\,centi = 10\,milli = 10{,}000\,micro \quad 1\,centimeter\ squared\left(cm^2\right) = 0.0001 m^2$$

Cumulative air kerma (reference dose) is measured in Gy and provides an estimate about the total patient skin dose for the fluoroscopic procedure.

---

exposure rate that measures the intensity of the x-ray beam and should not exceed 10 R/min or approximately 88 mGy/min in the United States.

Technological advancements continue in software that will provide for improvements in fluoroscopic image quality, noise reduction, and minimizing patient radiation dose.

Viewing Systems

Advancements in monitors have improved the quality of the displayed fluoroscopic image. These improved display monitors are currently used with both image-intensified units and digital fluoroscopic units (Fig. 10-18).

Liquid crystal display (LCD) monitors are one of the modern display options. LCD monitors offer superior resolution and brightness over CRT monitors. They work in a completely different way than CRT monitors. LCD monitors are made up of several layers (Fig. 10-19). The heart of the LCD is the liquid crystal layer sandwiched between polarizing layers that contain nematic liquid crystals. These crystals are typically rod shaped, are semi-liquid, and can change the direction of light (unpolarized EMR waves traveling in two planes) that passes through them. The crystals exist in an unorganized "twisted" state. When an electric current is applied, they organize or "untwist." In the untwisted state, they organize into configurations that block or allow light to pass through depending on the polarizing filters. The polarized layers on each side are oriented perpendicular to one other, meaning that light that may be able to pass through one would be at the wrong orientation to pass through the other. When electric current is applied to the liquid crystal layer, the "untwisting" changes the orientation of light passing through (polarizing the EMR waves to travel in one plane) the back layer and allows it to pass through the front. A TFT panel is located behind the liquid crystal layer. The number of TFTs is equal to the number of pixels displayed. The TFTs control the current to each pixel and switch it on or off by causing the liquid crystals to twist or untwist. A monochromatic LCD monitor displays the light as shades of gray. A color LCD monitor has a color filter layer added to display shades of color. The intensity of light is controlled by the current to the crystals, which is controlled by the TFTs. This in turn determines the shade of gray if monochromatic or the shade of color if using a color monitor.

Plasma monitors may also be an option for display monitors. Plasma monitors are very similar in construction to LCD monitors, but instead of a liquid crystal layer, they have a thin layer of pixels (Fig. 10-20). Each pixel contains three neon- and xenon-gas-filled cells (subpixels). Each of these cells is coated with a different phosphor layer formula that produces red, green, or blue light when stimulated. On each side of this layer of pixels are dielectric layers. When electricity is

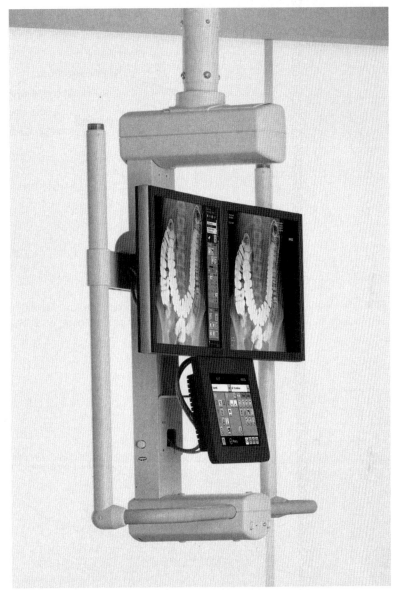

FIG. 10-18 Display monitor. Modern high-resolution liquid crystal display (LCD) monitor with a touch screen display. (Courtesy of Siemens Healthcare, Malvern, PA.)

passed between these dielectric layers through the pixels, the gas within is ionized. The liberated electrons release ultraviolet radiation to return to the shell of an atom. The ultraviolet radiation in turn stimulates the phosphor coating in the cell, producing visible light of a color corresponding to the phosphor formula. The current through the pixels (and subpixels) is modulated by the electrodes several thousand times per second, thereby controlling the intensity of light produced. This control and modulation process make it possible for plasma monitors to produce billions of different shades of color.

FIG. 10-19 LCD monitor. LCD monitors are composed of several layers. (From Johnston JN, Fauber TL: *Essentials of Radiographic Physics and Imaging*, ed 2, St. Louis, 2016, Mosby.)

FIG. 10-20 Plasma monitor. Plasma monitors are very similar in construction to LCD monitors, but instead of a liquid crystal layer, they have a thin layer of pixels. (From Johnston JN, Fauber TL: *Essentials of Radiographic Physics and Imaging*, ed 2, St. Louis, 2016, Mosby.)

SPECIALIZED FLUOROSCOPIC UNITS

Mobile C-arm units have fluoroscopic capabilities that are typically used in the operating room when imaging is necessary during surgical procedures. Display monitors are also included, offering both static and dynamic imaging during the procedure. Because it is a fluoroscopic system, many of the features of a fixed fluoroscopic unit are also made available with a C-arm. A C-arm unit is designed with an x-ray tube and image intensifier or digital detector attached in a C configuration (Figs. 10-21 and 10-22). As a result, the unit can be positioned in a variety of planes, enabling viewing from different perspectives. Generally, three sets of locks are provided to move and hold the C-arm in place. One set moves the entire "C" toward or away from the base (the equivalent of moving a table side to side). Another set allows the "C" to pivot about its axis (the equivalent of angling a general radiographic tube head assembly). The last set allows the "C" to slide along its arc (the equivalent of moving the patient from anteroposterior or posteroanterior positions to oblique to lateral positions without having to move the patient).

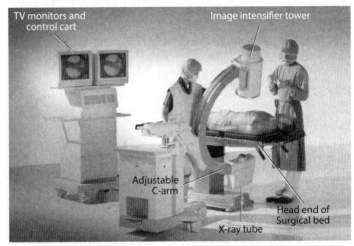

FIG. 10-21 A mobile C-arm unit. (Courtesy of Philips Healthcare, Andover, MA.)

FIG. 10-22 OEC Elite CFD C-arm Unit. (Courtesy of GE Healthcare © General Electric Company.)

FIG. 10-23 Mini C-arm unit. (Courtesy of Hologic, Inc.)

Generally, the x-ray tube should be positioned under the patient and the image intensifier or digital detector above the patient. Positioning the C-arm in this manner during the imaging procedure reduces the radiation exposure to the operator. Because the C-arm uses fluoroscopy, standard radiation exposure techniques and safety practices used during fluoroscopy in the radiology department must also be adhered to during operation of a C-arm unit. The radiographer should also pay attention to the distance between the patient and the x-ray tube as well as to total fluoroscopy time. In this situation, fluoroscopy is being used in an "uncontrolled" environment, and it is the radiographer's responsibility to monitor and apply radiation safety measures.

Significant advancements have been made with C-arm type fluoroscopic units used for a variety of anatomic areas. For example, the **mini C-arm** (Fig. 10-23) provides a lower dose rate and greater equipment flexibility while providing quality images of extremities. The mini C-arm is available with flat-panel detector fluoroscopy, rotating detectors, both full FOV and magnification modes, and a touch-screen display.

Surgical procedures have multiple imaging needs and the **O-arm** system (Fig. 10-24) can provide both static and dynamic images along with two- and three-dimensional images. Equipment movement is motor controlled, the gantry opens for easy patient access laterally, and specialized draping is used to maintain sterility when the gantry is closed. Fluoroscopic and radiographic images are obtained with flat-panel detector technology, which allows the surgeon to assess the outcome of the procedure before closing the patient.

RADIATION SAFETY

Radiation safety is just as important during fluoroscopic imaging as it is with radiographic imaging. It is the fluoroscopic operator's responsibility to be knowledgeable about the equipment and methods to reduce patient radiation dose. A few methods of minimizing radiation dose to the patient during fluoroscopic procedures include omission of the grid during fluoroscopy (when appropriate), minimal use of the magnification feature, and use of LIH when the x-ray exposure

FIG. 10-24 O-arm unit. (From Lampignano: *Bontrager's Textbook of Radiographic Positioning and Related Anatomy*, ed 9, St. Louis, 2018, Elsevier.)

is not activated while the operator reviews the image. In addition, maneuvering the equipment or patient to distribute the radiation exposure over a wider area of skin, minimizes the dose.

Because older image-intensified fluoroscopic units use a continuous stream of x-rays, the exposure should be intermittently pulsed by the operator. Applying pressure to the exposure switch or pedal intermittently significantly reduces the exposure of both patients and personnel and reduces the heat load on the x-ray tube. Modern image-intensified and digital fluoroscopy use a controlled pulsed x-ray exposure, and the operator is not required to intermittently release the pressure. Operating the fluoroscope in the lowest pulsed mode along with a lower dose rate will minimize patient radiation dose.

Time, distance, and shielding are the standard radiation safety practices used during fluoroscopic imaging. Reducing the x-ray exposure time reduces the exposure to the patient and any personnel remaining in the room. The control panel timer produces an audible noise when 5 minutes of x-ray fluoroscopic time has been used. It is the operator's responsibility to minimize the x-ray fluoroscopy, and the radiographer should document the total amount of x-ray fluoroscopic time used during the procedure. Modern fluoroscopic units provide dose monitoring in addition to the cumulative fluorotimer. The DAP or KAP and cumulative air kerma (reference dose) provide radiation exposure data and need to be recorded in the patient's medical record. If these dose-monitoring systems are not available, then the cumulative exposure time and number of acquired static images need to be documented. In addition, the intensity of the x-ray exposure at the tabletop should not exceed 10 R/min (~88 mGy/min) for routine fluoroscopic units equipped with ABC. Whenever the patient's exposure is reduced, personnel exposure also is reduced.

The source-to-skin distance (SSD) should be no less than 38 cm (15 inches) for stationary fluoroscopic units and no less than 30 cm (12 inches) on a mobile C-arm fluoroscopic unit. Increasing the SSD and decreasing the distance between the patient and the radiation detector (OID) will decrease patient exposure. Increasing collimation and decreasing the number of static (radiographic) images will reduce patient exposure. If the fluoroscopic unit has features such as virtual collimation (x-ray field size can be adjusted without irradiating the patient) and the ability to save a sequence of fluoroscopic images without acquiring radiographic images, patient exposure will be further decreased. In addition, personnel other than the operator should increase their distance from the patient to reduce exposure to scatter radiation from the patient.

TABLE 10-1   **Methods of Reducing Patient and Personnel Exposure During Fluoroscopy**
• Operating the fluoroscopic exposure intermittingly or in the lowest pulsed mode along with a lower dose rate and the use of last image hold minimizes the patient radiation dose.
• Evaluate and use preset or default settings available to minimize the patient dose.
• Reducing the amount of x-ray fluoroscopic time reduces patient and personnel exposure.
• Increase collimation with virtual collimation, remove the grid, and minimize the use of magnification.
• Monitor and document the amount of total x-ray fluoroscopic time displayed in 5-minute increments on the control panel in addition to the number of acquired radiographic images. If provided, cumulative radiation dose data should be recorded.
• The intensity of x-ray exposure at the tabletop should not exceed 10 R/min (88 mGy/min) for units equipped with ABC or AERC.
• The SSD should be not less than 38 cm (15 inches) for stationary fluoroscopic units and not less than 30 cm (12 inches) on mobile C-arm fluoroscopic units.
• Personnel in the fluoroscopic room during procedures should increase their distance from the patient to reduce exposure to scatter radiation.
• Personnel should wear appropriate lead shielding during fluoroscopic procedures.
• The Bucky slot cover must contain at least 0.25 mm of lead-equivalent shielding and cover the opened space on the side of the table.
• A protective curtain placed between the patient and operator must have at least 0.25 mm of lead equivalent.

ABC, Automatic brightness control; *AERC,* automatic exposure rate control; *SSD,* source-to-skin distance.

In addition to all personnel in the room wearing lead aprons (recommended 0.5 mm of lead equivalent), two additional types of shielding are required during fluoroscopy. Because the Bucky tray is positioned at the end of the table for operation of the under-table x-ray tube in a fixed fluoroscopic unit, a Bucky slot cover with at least 0.25 mm of lead equivalent should automatically cover the opened space at the side of the table. In addition, a protective lead curtain with at least 0.25 mm of lead equivalent must be placed between the patient and the operator to reduce exposure to the operator. Table 10-1 lists methods of reducing patient and personnel exposure during fluoroscopy.

QUALITY CONTROL

Quality control programs are vitally important for all ionizing radiation–producing equipment to monitor equipment performance and minimize patient dose. Fluoroscopic equipment is used extensively in health care and contributes significantly to the radiation dose received by the general population. Quality control is a team effort among the radiographer, radiologist, and medical physicist. Although some equipment monitoring and data may be collected by a radiographer, performance tests and their interpretation are typically performed by a medical physicist. However, the radiographer should be familiar with the monitoring and testing necessary to ensure that the fluoroscopic unit is operating correctly.

The radiographer, in particular, a quality control radiographer, may be responsible for the operational inspection of the equipment. This inspection should be conducted using a checklist of the items found in Box 10-3 at least every 6 months. The radiographer may also be responsible for an inspection of the imaging suite itself to examine the general physical condition of the room, unit, supporting electrical cables, and control booth, noting any wear or deterioration. This inspection of the physical condition should be placed on the same schedule and conducted along with the operational inspection.

BOX 10-3   Fluoroscopic Equipment Inspection Checklist

Inspect	Ensure that
Bucky slot cover	When the Bucky is parked at the foot of the table, the metal cover should expand and cover the entire opening.
Protective curtain	The curtain should be in good condition and move freely into place when the tower is moved to the operating position.
Tower: locks, power assist, control panel	The electromagnetic locks are in good working order, the power assist moves the tower about easily in all directions, and all control panel indicator lights are operational.
Exposure switch (dead-man switch)	The switch is not sticking and operates the x-ray tube only while in the depressed position. (Also test the switch with the tower in the park position; it should not activate the x-ray tube while parked.)
Collimator shutters	In the fully open position, the shutters should restrict the beam to the size of the input phosphor and be accurate to within ±3%.
Fluoroscopic timer	The timer should buzz audibly after 5 minutes of fluoroscopic "beam-on" time.
Monitor brightness	While exposing a penetrometer through a fluoroscopic phantom, the monitor image is adjusted to display as many of the penetrometer steps as possible.
Table tilt motion	The table tilts smoothly to its limit in both directions, and the angulation indicator is operational.

BOX 10-4   Quality Control (QC) Specific to Fluoroscopic Equipment

QC Test	Description
Fluoroscopic system resolution	Tests the system's ability to display details of small objects (high-contrast resolution) and larger objects (low-contrast resolution)
Fluoroscopic ABC/AERC performance	Evaluates image quality for changes in exposure parameters such as high dose rate, pulsed modes, and FOV
Fluoroscopic phantom image quality	Evaluates the quality of the displayed fluoroscopic image, including image distortion or lag
Fluoroscopic exposure rates	Measures the intensity of the x-ray beam; fluoroscopic exposure rate should not exceed 10 R/min (~88 mGy/min)
Fluoroscopic alignment test	Ensures the radiation beam aligns with the center of the image intensifier or flat-panel detector within 2% of the SID
Patient dose monitoring system calibration, if present	Evaluates proper function of patient dose monitoring systems such as DAP meters
Display monitor performance	Evaluates the display characteristics of the monitor (described in Chapter 5)

The other important part of the quality control program is the performance inspection and equipment testing. Box 10-4 lists a few common fluoroscopic quality control tests. Although a quality control radiographer may perform some of these tests, an appropriately trained and licensed medical physicist should conduct and interpret this portion of the program and oversee the entire quality control monitoring program.

CHAPTER SUMMARY

- Fluoroscopy allows imaging of the movement of internal structures by its use of a continuous beam of x-rays.
- Image intensification provides a brighter image for viewing. The exit radiation is absorbed by the input phosphor, converted to electrons, sent to the output phosphor, released as visible light, and converted to an electronic video signal for transmission to the television or computer monitor.
- Brightness gain is the product of flux gain and minification gain and results in a brighter image on the output phosphor.
- ABC maintains the overall appearance of the image by monitoring the current through the image intensifier or the output phosphor intensity and adjusting exposure factors if the monitored values fall below preset levels.
- Image intensifiers provide a multifield mode that magnifies the image. When operating the unit in the magnification mode, spatial resolution improves but patient exposure increases.
- To view the image-intensified fluoroscopic image on a display monitor, it must be converted to an electrical signal by a camera tube or CCD.
- Cassette spot film, photo-spot cameras, cine film, and videotape or DVD are all methods of recording static or dynamic images during image-intensified fluoroscopy.
- Cassette spot filming shifts to the radiographic mode using a higher mA and increases patient exposure.
- Digital fluoroscopy can be accomplished by attaching an ADC between the camera tube or CCD and the television or computer monitor.
- The use of flat-panel detectors in place of an image intensifier offers several advantages, such as reductions in the size, bulk, and weight of the fluoroscopic tower; allowing easier manipulation of the tower; and greater access to the patient during the examination.
- Flat-panel detectors also replace spot filming and other recording devices, and because they are capable of operating in radiographic mode, additional radiographic images are not needed in many cases. The images, both dynamic and static, can also be readily archived with the patient record in a PACS.
- Image-intensified fluoroscopy uses a lower mA (0.5–5 mA), whereas digital fluoroscopy uses a higher mA (50–1200 mA). A higher mA is needed for the lower pulse width to maintain sufficient exposure to the IR for a diagnostic image (maintaining the needed SNR).
- Modern fluoroscopic units use a pulsed x-ray beam, whereas older image intensifiers operate as a continuous x-ray beam exposure unless the operator produces intermittent x-ray exposures.
- Modern fluoroscopic units have features such as AERC, the ability to select dose rates, virtual collimation, change filtration, and select predetermined set of exposure factors, in addition to pulsed fluoroscopy, frame averaging, electronic magnification, fluoro loop save, and dose monitoring.
- LCD and plasma monitors are modern display options. They offer superior resolution, brightness, and work in a different way than CRT monitors.
- Several specialized fluoroscopic units are available for use outside the radiology department such as mobile C-arm, mini C-arm, and O-arm.
- Radiation safety practices include reducing the amount of fluoroscopic time and shielding the operator with the Bucky slot cover and a protective curtain placed between the patient and the operator. The SSD should be not less than 38 cm (15 inches) for stationary fluoroscopic units and not less than 30 cm (12 inches) on a mobile fluoroscopic unit, and the intensity of the x-ray exposure at the tabletop should not exceed 10 R/min (~88 mGy/min).
- Quality control procedures are important for monitoring the performance of the fluoroscopic unit.

REVIEW QUESTIONS

1. In image-intensified fluoroscopy, the mA range is typically _____.
   A. 0.5 to 5 mA
   B. 20 to 50 mA
   C. 100 to 300 mA
   D. 400 to 600 mA

2. During fluoroscopy, releasing the pressure applied to the pedal or switch terminates the radiation exposure and is known as the _____.
   A. fluoroscopic timer
   B. intensification switch
   C. activation switch
   D. dead-man switch

3. What component of the image intensifier converts the exit or remnant radiation into visible light?
   A. Output phosphor
   B. Photocathode
   C. Input phosphor
   D. Electrostatic focusing lenses

4. What component of the image intensifier converts the visible light into electrons?
   A. Output phosphor
   B. Photocathode
   C. Input phosphor
   D. Electrostatic focusing lenses

5. In image-intensified fluoroscopy, to view the images on a display monitor, the light intensities are converted by a _____.
   A. camera tube
   B. electrostatic lens
   C. CCD
   D. A or C

6. Brightness gain is a product of _____.
   A. minification gain and ABC
   B. flux gain and ABC
   C. minification gain and flux gain
   D. ABC and mA

7. The numeric conversion factor value is equal to _____ of the brightness gain value.
   A. 0.001
   B. 0.01
   C. 0.1
   D. 1.0

8. A brightness gain of 40,000 would have a conversion factor of _____.
   A. 40
   B. 400
   C. 4000
   D. 40,000

9. A disadvantage of using the magnification mode during image-intensified fluoroscopy is _____.
   A. decreased spatial resolution
   B. increased patient exposure
   C. decreased brightness
   D. decreased contrast

10. When spot filming during image-intensified fluoroscopy, the radiation dose to the patient is decreased.
    A. True
    B. False

11. Which of the following fluoroscopic features will decrease patient radiation dose?
    1. Virtual collimation
    2. Pulsed fluoroscopy
    3. Frame averaging
       A. 1 and 2 only
       B. 1 and 3 only
       C. 2 and 3 only
       D. 1, 2, and 3

12. When operating a stationary fluoroscopic unit, the SSD should not be less than _____.
    A. 25 cm (10 inches)
    B. 30 cm (12 inches)
    C. 38 cm (15 inches)
    D. 45 cm (18 inches)

13. During fluoroscopy, the x-ray exposure at the tabletop should not exceed _____.
    A. 0.01 R/min
    B. 0.1 R/min
    C. 1.0 R/min
    D. 10 R/min

14. The Bucky slot cover must have a lead equivalent thickness of _____.
    A. 0.10 mm
    B. 0.25 mm
    C. 0.50 mm
    D. 2.5 mm

15. Which of the following combinations reduces patient radiation exposure during fluoroscopy?
    A. Highest pulse mode and highest dose rate
    B. Highest pulse mode and lowest pulse rate
    C. Lowest pulse mode and highest dose rate
    D. Lowest pulse mode and lowest dose rate

16. In comparing flat-panel detector fluoroscopy with image-intensified fluoroscopy, which is NOT correct about flat-panel detector fluoroscopy?
    A. Spatial resolution is less than image intensified
    B. The size of the fluoroscopic tower is less
    C. Higher detective quantum efficiency
    D. Less image distortion artifacts

Summary of Important Relationships

CHAPTER 1: RADIATION AND ITS DISCOVERY

The Dual Nature of X-ray Energy

X-rays act like both waves and particles.

Wavelength and Frequency

Wavelength and frequency are inversely related. Higher-energy x-rays have decreased wavelength and increased frequency. Lower-energy x-rays have increased wavelength and decreased frequency.

CHAPTER 2: THE X-RAY BEAM

Filament

The filament is the source of electrons during x-ray production.

Target

The target is the part of the anode that is struck by the focused stream of electrons coming from the cathode. The target stops the electrons and creates the opportunity for the production of x-rays.

Tungsten

Because tungsten has a high atomic number (74) and a high melting point (3400°C [6152°F]), it efficiently produces x-rays.

Dissipating Heat

The heat produced when the x-ray exposure is activated is transferred to the insulating oil that surrounds the x-ray tube.

Rotating Anodes

Rotating anodes can withstand higher heat loads than stationary anodes because the rotation causes a greater physical area, or focal track, to be exposed to electrons.

Production of X-rays

As electrons strike the target, their kinetic energy is transferred to the tungsten atoms in the anode to produce x-rays.

Interactions that Produce X-ray Photons

Bremsstrahlung interactions and characteristic interactions both produce x-ray photons.

Bremsstrahlung Interactions

Bremsstrahlung interactions occur when a projectile (incident) electron completely avoids the orbital electrons of a tungsten atom and travels very close to its nucleus. The closer the projectile electron travels to the nucleus, the stronger the attraction. The stronger this attraction, the more energy the projectile electron loses and the stronger the resultant x-ray photon (higher energy). Projectile electrons that travel farther from the nucleus create x-ray photons with less energy. Most x-ray interactions in the diagnostic energy range are bremsstrahlung.

Characteristic Interactions

Characteristic interactions are produced when a projectile (incident) electron interacts with an electron from the inner shell (K-shell) of a tungsten atom. Characteristic x-rays can be produced in a tungsten target only when the kilovoltage peak (kVp) is set at 70 or greater because the binding energy of the K-shell electron is 69.5 keV.

Thermionic Emission

When the tungsten filament gains enough heat (therm), the outer-shell electrons (ions) of the filament atoms are boiled off, or emitted, from the filament.

Tube Current

Electrons flow only in one direction in the x-ray tube—from cathode to anode. This flow of electrons is called the *tube current* and is measured in milli-amperage (mA).

Energy Conversion in the X-ray Tube

As electrons strike the anode target, more than 99% of their kinetic energy is converted to heat, whereas less than 1% of their energy is converted to x-rays.

Kilovoltage and the Speed of Electrons

The speed of the electrons traveling from the cathode to the anode increases as the kilovoltage applied across the x-ray tube increases.

Speed of Electrons and Quality of X-rays

The speed of the electrons in the tube current determines the quality or energy of the x-rays that are produced. The quality or energy of the x-rays in turn determines the penetrability of the primary beam (ease with which it moves through tissue).

kVp and Beam Penetrability

As kVp increases, beam penetrability increases; as kVp decreases, beam penetrability decreases.

Milliamperage, Tube Current, and X-ray Quantity

The quantity of electrons in the tube current and quantity of x-rays produced are directly proportional to the milliamperage.

Exposure Time, Tube Current, and X-ray Quantity

The quantity of electrons flowing from the cathode to the anode and the quantity of x-rays produced are directly proportional to the exposure time.

Quantity of Electrons, X-rays, and mAs

The quantity of electrons flowing from the cathode to the anode and the quantity of x-rays produced are directly proportional to milliamperage-seconds (mAs).

Line-focus Principle

The line-focus principle describes the relationship between the actual focal spot, where the electrons in the tube current bombard the target, and the effective focal spot, which is the same area as seen from directly below the tube.

Anode Angle and Effective Focal Spot Size

Based on the line-focus principle, the smaller the anode target angle, the smaller the effective focal spot size.

Anode Heel Effect

X-rays are more intense on the cathode side of the tube; their intensity decreases toward the anode side.

Low-Energy Photons, Patient Dose, and Image Formation

Low-energy photons serve only to increase patient dose and do not contribute to image formation.

CHAPTER 3: IMAGE FORMATION AND RADIOGRAPHIC QUALITY

Differential Absorption and Image Formation

A radiographic image is created when an x-ray beam passes through a patient and then interacts with an image receptor (IR), such as a digital imaging system. The variations in the absorption and transmission of the exiting x-ray beam structurally represent the anatomic area of interest.

X-ray Photon Absorption

During attenuation of the x-ray beam, the photoelectric effect is responsible for total absorption of the incoming x-ray photon.

X-ray Beam Scattering

During attenuation of the x-ray beam, the incoming x-ray photon may lose energy and change direction as a result of the Compton effect.

Factors Affecting Beam Attenuation

Increasing tissue thickness, atomic number, and tissue density increases x-ray beam attenuation because more x-rays are absorbed by the tissue. Increasing the quality of the x-ray beam decreases beam attenuation because the higher-energy x-rays penetrate the tissue.

X-ray Interaction with Matter

When the diagnostic primary x-ray beam interacts with anatomic tissues, three processes occur: absorption, scattering, and transmission.

Image Brightness

The range of image brightness levels visible after processing is a result of the variation in x-ray absorption and transmission as the x-ray beam passes through anatomic tissues.

Brightness and Radiographic Quality

A radiographic image must have sufficient brightness to visualize the anatomic structures of interest.

Differentiating Among Anatomic Tissues

The ability to distinguish among types of tissues is determined by the differences in brightness levels in the image or contrast. Anatomic tissues that attenuate the beam similarly have low subject contrast. Anatomic tissues that attenuate the beam very differently have high subject contrast.

Sharpness of Anatomic Detail

The accuracy of the anatomic structural lines displayed in the radiographic image is determined by its spatial resolution.

Size Distortion

Radiographic images of objects are always magnified in terms of the true object size. The source-to-image receptor distance (SID) and object-to-image receptor distance (OID) have a geometric relationship and play an important role in minimizing the amount of size distortion of the radiographic image.

Shape Distortion

Shape distortion can occur from inaccurate central ray (CR) alignment of the tube, the part being radiographed, or the IR. Elongation refers to images of objects that appear longer than the true objects. Foreshortening refers to images that appear shorter than the true objects.

Number of Photons and Quantum Noise

Decreasing the number of photons reaching the IR may increase the amount of quantum noise within the radiographic image; increasing the number of photons reaching the IR may decrease the amount of quantum noise within the radiographic image.

Dynamic Range and Film-Screen Imaging

The range of exposure intensities that film can accurately detect is limited (limited dynamic range). This renders film more susceptible to overexposure and underexposure and restricts its ability to display tissues that vary greatly in x-ray attenuation.

Fluoroscopy

Dynamic imaging of internal anatomic structures can be visualized with the use of a flat-panel detector or image intensifier. The exit radiation interacts with the acquisition device, is processed or converted, and then transmitted to the display monitor for viewing.

Image Formation

The process of differential absorption for image formation remains the same regardless of the type of imaging system, digital, film, or fluoroscopic. The varying x-ray intensities exiting the anatomic area of interest form the image that is displayed on a monitor or film.

CHAPTER 4: DIGITAL IMAGE CHARACTERISTICS, RECEPTORS, AND IMAGE ACQUISITION

Pixel Size, Field of View (FOV), and Matrix Size

The pixel size is directly related to the FOV displayed and inversely related to the matrix size. Increasing the FOV for the same matrix size will increase the size of the pixel and decrease spatial resolution, whereas increasing the matrix size for the same FOV will decrease the pixel size and increase spatial resolution.

Pixel Bit Depth and Contrast Resolution

The greater the pixel bit depth (i.e., 16 bit), the more precise the digitization of the analog signal and the greater the number of shades of gray available for image display. Increasing the number of shades of gray available to display in a digital image improves its contrast resolution.

Pixel Density and Pitch and Spatial Resolution

Increasing pixel density and decreasing pixel pitch increases spatial resolution. Decreasing pixel density and increasing pixel pitch decreases spatial resolution.

Spatial Frequency and Spatial Resolution

The unit of measure for spatial frequency is line pairs per millimeter (lp/mm). Increasing the number of lp/mm resolved in the imaging system (higher spatial frequency) results in improved spatial resolution.

Digital Detectors, Dynamic Range, and Exposure Latitude

Digital IRs have a wide dynamic range; that is, they can accurately capture a wide range of x-ray intensities exiting the patient. The computer then processes the raw pixel data to compensate for an exposure error and create a diagnostic radiographic image. However, lower- or higher-than-necessary exposure techniques do not guarantee a quality digital image. Exposure latitude is the range of exposures that should be used to produce a diagnostic image.

Modulation Transfer Function (MTF) and Anatomic Detail

MTF is a measure of the imaging system's ability to accurately display small anatomic objects having high spatial frequency. An imaging system that has a high MTF can display anatomic detail with improved visibility.

Detective Quantum Efficiency (DQE) and X-ray Exposure

An IR with a higher DQE requires less x-ray exposure to produce a quality radiographic image when compared with an IR with a lower DQE value.

Signal-to-Noise Ratio (SNR) and Image Quality

Increasing the SNR increases the visibility of anatomic details, whereas decreasing the SNR decreases the visibility.

Contrast-to-Noise Ratio (CNR) and Image Quality

Increasing the CNR increases the visibility of anatomic details, whereas decreasing the CNR decreases the visibility.

Computed Radiography Digital IRs

The CR latent image is acquired in the photostimulable phosphor (PSP) layer of the imaging plate (IP). Most energy from the exit radiation intensities is stored in the PSP for extraction in the reader unit.

Sampling Frequency and Spatial Resolution

Increasing the sampling frequency results in more sampling points and decreased pixel pitch, which improves the spatial resolution of the digital image. Decreasing the sampling frequency results in fewer sampling points and increased pixel pitch and decreased spatial resolution.

IR Size and Matrix Size

For a fixed matrix size CR system, using a smaller IR for a given FOV results in improved spatial resolution of the digital image. Increasing the size of the IR for a given FOV results in decreased spatial resolution.

Indirect Conversion Detectors in Direct Radiography

Indirect conversion detectors involve a two-stage process of converting x-ray intensities first to visible light and then to electrical charges. A scintillator type material is used to absorb the x-ray energy, emits light in response, and then the light is converted to electrical signals. The electrical signals are then directed to amplifiers and the analog-to-digital converter (ADC) to produce a raw digital image. Flat-panel thin-film transistor (TFT) detectors are common in direct radiography, but charge-coupled device (CCD) and complementary metal oxide semiconductor (CMOS) indirect conversion detectors are also used in digital radiography (DR).

Direct Conversion Detectors in DR

Direct conversion uses amorphous selenium-coated (a-Se) detectors to directly convert the exit radiation to electrical charges. Similar to indirect conversion detectors, the electronic charge is stored in a TFT array before it is amplified, digitized, and processed in the computer.

CHAPTER 5: DIGITAL IMAGE PROCESSING, DISPLAY, AND DATA MANAGEMENT

Preprocessing: Corrections and Histogram

Several operations occur on the raw image data to prepare for further processing to display a quality image. Software corrections can be applied to account for imperfections (bad or dead pixels) that only occur with DR type IRs, and flat fielding is a process of correcting the non-uniformity of pixel values throughout the entire image. A histogram is created that represents the range of digital pixel values versus the relative prevalence of the pixel values in the latent image. Scanning the entire IR to identify the exposure field brightness levels and the edges of the collimated image (exposure field recognition and segmentation) is necessary to identify only the image data representing the anatomic area.

Histogram Analysis

During histogram analysis, the exposure histogram is compared with a stored (reference) histogram for that anatomic part; values of interest (VOIs) are identified in preparation for image processing and display.

Exposure Indicator

The exposure indicator provides a numeric value indicating the level of radiation exposure to the digital IR. These values may be vendor specific and have a direct, logarithmic, or inverse relationship to the IR exposure. A universal standard exposure indicator (deviation index) has been developed and provides the radiographer with important information about the IR exposure. The radiographer should assess the exposure indicator along with image quality before considering a repeat image.

Lookup Tables (LUTs)

LUTs provide the means to alter the original pixel values to improve the brightness and contrast of the displayed image.

Window Level and Image Brightness

A relationship exists between window level and image brightness on the display monitor. Changing the window level on the display monitor allows the image brightness to be increased or decreased throughout the entire range.

Window Width and Image Contrast

A narrow (decreased) window width displays higher radiographic contrast, whereas a wider (increased) window width displays lower radiographic contrast.

Display Monitor

A high-resolution 5-megapixel (2048 × 2560 pixels) display monitor is recommended for diagnostic interpretation. In addition, a display monitor having diagonal dimensions of 54 cm (21 inches) is adequate for viewing images sized 35 × 43 cm (14 × 17 inches) with a recommended pixel pitch of 0.200 mm at a standard viewing distance of about 60 cm (24 inches).

Display Monitor Luminance

Luminance is a measurement of the light intensity (brightness) emitted from the surface of the monitor and is expressed in units of candela per square meter (cd/m^2). Primary display monitors should exhibit a minimum luminance of 1.0 cd/m^2 and a maximum luminance of 350 cd/m^2. A ratio of the maximum to minimum luminance, luminance ratio (LR), is recommended to be greater than 250 and a display monitor with an LR of 350 has improved image contrast.

Data Management

Data management is a complex system-wide effort to ensure that people, equipment, and processes are in place to expand health care communication and improve patient outcomes. Imaging informatics requires efficient and effective methods for acquisition, storage, retrieval, transmission, and display of digital image data from multiple imaging modalities and throughout healthcare systems. Health Insurance Portability and Accountability Act (HIPAA) established national standards to protect the privacy and confidentiality of patients' protected health information (PHI).

Patient Health Information

PHI is collected and stored in the hospital information system (HIS) and shared with the radiology information system (RIS). The electronic health record (EHR) is the system for patient PHI that can be shared outside the facility and among many healthcare systems.

Picture Archival and Communication System (PACS)

A PACS is a computer system designed for digital imaging that can receive, store, archive, distribute, and display digital images. The major components of PACS include the imaging modalities, digital communication networks, display workstations, and archival capabilities for storage and retrieval.

Digital Communication Networks

Digital Imaging and Communications in Medicine (DICOM) is an international communication standard for information sharing between PACS and imaging modalities to transmit, store, retrieve, print, process, and display medical imaging information.

The Health Level Seven standard (HL7) is a communication standard for medical information. Connectivity and communication among these systems are necessary for radiology to realize the full potential of imaging informatics. Integrating the Healthcare Enterprise (IHE) promotes the coordinated use of established standards such as DICOM and HL7 to address specific clinical needs in support of optimal patient care.

Display Workstation

A display workstation is simply a desktop computer that allows for the retrieval and viewing of medical images from one of the modalities or storage components of the PACS. Quality-control (QC) display stations and interpreting stations have greater function and capability, such as more advanced image manipulation (windowing: level and width), annotation, patient demographic information, cropping, panning, and magnification (zoom). In addition to other standards of communication, DICOM specifies information included as a header on digital images (DICOM header) and the Grayscale Standard Display Function (GSDF) is the DICOM recommended standard for consistent display characteristics such as, grayscale appearance and image quality.

Transmission, Storage, and Archive

Transmission devices need to have the capacity to handle the volume of images, delivered within a reasonable time frame and, can check for errors. To improve transmission of the data to the various end users of the imaging data, compression (reversible or irreversible) may be used. Policies and procedures are also needed to effectively and appropriately archive (current and previous exams) and store digital image data for years.

Teleradiology

Teleradiology is the practice of diagnostic image interpretation outside the facility (offsite) from where the imaging data are acquired. Communication needs between teleradiologists and the imaging professionals include providing timely and relevant patient information, ability to answer questions regarding the procedure, and maintaining standard QC practices. The practice of teleradiology should maintain the same high standards, safety, and quality as onsite radiology services.

Quality Control

QC is an important activity to ensure that radiographic equipment is functioning properly and should occur routinely and consistently. QC activities are equally important for digital image data management and are most likely performed by an imaging informatics professional.

Security of PHI

Radiographers have routine access to PHI in performance of their duties and must take responsibility for adhering to the department's policies and procedures. Patients must be confident that radiographers have the skills to perform their imaging procedures and believe that their PHI will be secure.

CHAPTER 6: EXPOSURE TECHNIQUE FACTORS

mAs and Quantity of Radiation

As mAs increases, the quantity of radiation reaching the IR increases. As mAs decreases, the amount of radiation reaching the IR decreases.

mA and Exposure Time

mA and exposure time have an inverse proportional relationship when maintaining the same mAs.

mAs and Digital Image Brightness

The level of mAs does not control image brightness when using digital IRs. During computer processing, image brightness is maintained when the mAs is too low or too high. A lower-than-needed mAs produces an image with increased quantum noise, and a higher-than-needed mAs exposes a patient to unnecessary radiation.

Exposure Indicator Value

A numerical value or exposure indicator is displayed on the processed digital image to indicate the level of x-ray exposure received (incident exposure) on the IR. If the exposure indicator value falls outside the manufacturer's suggested range, exposure to the digital IR, image quality, and patient exposure could be affected.

kVp and the Radiographic Image

Increasing or decreasing the kVp changes the amount of radiation exposure to the IR and the subject contrast produced within the image.

Exposure Errors in Digital Imaging

kVp and mAs exposure errors should be reflected in the exposure indicator value; however, image brightness can be maintained during computer processing.

kVp and the 15% Rule

A 15% increase in kVp has the same effect on exposure to the IR as doubling the mAs. A 15% decrease in kVp has the same effect on exposure to the IR as halving the mAs.

kVp and Subject Contrast

A high kVp results in less absorption and more transmission in anatomic tissues, which results in less variation in the x-ray intensities exiting (remnant) the patient producing lower subject contrast. A low kVp results in more absorption and less x-ray transmission in the anatomic tissues but with more variation in the x-ray intensities exiting the patient resulting in higher subject contrast

Kilovoltage, Scatter Radiation, and Radiographic Contrast

At higher kVp, more x-rays are transmitted with fewer overall interactions; however, a greater proportion of the interactions are from Compton scattering (fog) than photoelectric absorption, which decreases the radiographic contrast. Decreasing the kVp will increase photoelectric absorption and increase the number of interactions, but the proportion of Compton scattering (fog) will decrease compared with photoelectric absorption, increasing radiographic contrast.

Focal Spot Size and Spatial Resolution

As focal spot size increases, unsharpness increases and spatial resolution decreases; as focal spot size decreases, unsharpness decreases and spatial resolution increases.

SID and X-ray Beam Intensity

As SID increases, the x-ray beam intensity becomes spread over a larger area. This decreases the overall intensity of the x-ray beam reaching the IR.

SID and mAs

Increasing the SID requires the mAs to be increased to maintain exposure to the IR, and decreasing the SID requires a decrease in the mAs to maintain exposure to the IR.

SID, Size Distortion, and Spatial Resolution

As SID increases, size distortion (magnification) decreases, and spatial resolution increases; as SID decreases, size distortion (magnification) increases, and spatial resolution decreases.

OID, Size Distortion, and Spatial Resolution

Increasing the OID increases magnification and decreases the spatial resolution, whereas decreasing the OID decreases magnification and increases the spatial resolution.

Grids, Scatter, and Contrast

Placing a grid between the anatomic part and the IR absorbs scatter radiation exiting the patient and increases radiographic contrast.

Grids and IR Exposure

Adding, removing, or changing a grid requires an adjustment in mAs to maintain radiation exposure to the IR.

Beam Restriction and IR Exposure

Changes in beam restriction alter the amount of tissue irradiated and therefore affect the amount of exposure to the IR. The effect of collimation is greater when imaging large anatomic areas, performing examinations without a grid, and using a high kVp.

Tube Filtration, Radiation Quantity, and Average Energy

Increasing tube filtration decreases radiation quantity and increases the average energy of the x-ray beam. Decreasing tube filtration increases radiation quantity and decreases the average energy of the x-ray beam.

CHAPTER 7: SCATTER CONTROL

kVp and Scatter

The amount and energy of scatter radiation exiting the patient depends, in part, on the kVp selected. Examinations using higher kVp produce a greater proportion of higher-energy scattered x-rays compared with examinations using low kVp.

X-ray-Beam Field Size, Thickness of the Part, and Scatter

The larger the x-ray-beam field size, the greater the amount of scatter radiation produced. The thicker the part being imaged, the greater the amount of scatter radiation produced.

Volume of Tissue Irradiated and Scatter

The volume of tissue irradiated is affected by both the part thickness and the x-ray-beam field size. Therefore, the greater the volume of tissue irradiated, because of either or both factors, the greater the amount of scatter radiation produced.

Beam Restriction and Patient Dose

As beam restriction or collimation increases, the field size and patient dose decrease. As beam restriction or collimation decreases, the field size and patient dose increase.

Collimation and Scatter Radiation

As collimation increases, the field size and quantity of scatter radiation decrease; as collimation decreases, the field size and quantity of scatter radiation increase.

Collimation and Radiographic Contrast

As collimation increases, the quantity of scatter radiation decreases and radiographic contrast increases; as collimation decreases, the quantity of scatter radiation increases and radiographic contrast decreases.

Collimation and Exposure to the IR

As collimation increases, exposure to the IR decreases; as collimation decreases, exposure to the IR increases.

Scatter Radiation and Image Quality

Scatter radiation adds unwanted exposure to the IR and decreases image quality.

Grid Ratio and Radiographic Contrast

As the grid ratio increases for the same grid frequency, scatter cleanup improves and radiographic contrast increases; as grid ratio decreases for the same grid frequency, scatter cleanup becomes less effective and radiographic contrast decreases.

Focused versus Parallel Grids

Focused grids have lead lines that are angled to approximately match the divergence of the primary beam. Thus, focused grids allow more transmitted photons to reach the IR than parallel grids.

Grid Ratio and Exposure to IR

As the grid ratio increases, exposure to the IR decreases; as the grid ratio decreases, exposure to the IR increases.

Grid Ratio and Patient Dose

As the grid ratio increases, patient dose increases because of the increase in mAs; as the grid ratio decreases, patient dose decreases because of the decrease in mAs.

Upside-Down Focused Grids and Grid Cutoff

Placing a focused grid upside down on the IR causes the edges of the IR to be significantly underexposed.

Off-Level Error and Grid Cutoff

Angling the x-ray tube across the grid lines or angling the grid itself during exposure produces an overall decrease in exposure across the entire IR.

Off-Center Error and Grid Cutoff

If the center of the x-ray beam is not aligned from side to side with the center of a focused grid, grid cutoff can occur as a loss of exposure across the entire IR.

Off-Focus Error and Grid Cutoff

Using an SID outside the focal range creates a loss of exposure at the periphery of the IR.

Air Gap Technique and Scatter Control

The air gap technique is an alternative to using a grid to control the scatter reaching the IR. By moving the IR away from the patient, more scatter radiation will miss the IR. The greater the gap, the lesser the scatter reaches the IR.

CHAPTER 8: EXPOSURE TECHNIQUE SELECTION

Principle of Automatic Exposure Control (AEC) Operation

Once a predetermined amount of radiation is transmitted through a patient, the x-ray exposure is terminated. This determines the exposure time and therefore the total amount of radiation exposure to the IR.

Radiation-Measuring Devices

Detectors are the AEC devices that measure the amount of radiation transmitted. The radiographer selects the combination of the detectors to use.

Function of the Ionization Chamber

The ionization chamber interacts with exit radiation before it reaches the IR. Air in the chamber is ionized, an electrical charge proportional to the amount of radiation is created, and this charge travels to the timer circuit where the exposure is terminated.

AEC and mAs Readout

If the radiographic unit has an mAs readout display, the radiographer should take note of the reading after an exposure is made. This information can be invaluable.

kVp and AEC Response

The radiographer must set the kVp as needed to ensure adequate penetration while producing the appropriate level of subject contrast. The kVp selected determines the length of exposure time when using AEC. A low kVp requires more exposure time to reach the predetermined amount of exposure. A high kVp decreases the exposure time to reach the predetermined amount of exposure and reduces the overall radiation exposure to the patient.

mA and AEC Response

If the radiographer can set the mA when using AEC, it will inversely affect the time of exposure for a given procedure. Increasing the mA decreases the exposure time to reach the predetermined amount of exposure. Decreasing the mA increases the exposure time to reach the predetermined amount of exposure.

Function of Backup Time

Backup time, the maximum exposure time allowed during an AEC examination, serves as a safety mechanism when AEC is not used properly or is not functioning properly.

Setting Backup Time

Backup time should be set to 150% to 200% of the expected exposure time. This allows the properly used AEC system to appropriately terminate the exposure but protects the patient and tube from excessive exposure if a problem occurs.

Detector Selection

The combination of detectors affects the amount of exposure reaching the IR. If the area of radiographic interest is not directly over the selected detectors, that area will likely be overexposed or underexposed. When performing a radiographic study where the IR is located outside the Bucky, the AEC system should be deactivated, and a manual technique should be used.

Patient Centering

Accurate centering of the area of interest over the detectors is critical to ensure proper exposure to the IR. If the area of interest is not properly centered to the detectors, overexposure or underexposure may occur.

Collimation and AEC Response

Excessive or insufficient collimation may affect the amount of exposure reaching the IR. Insufficient collimation may result in excessive scatter reaching the detectors, causing the exposure time to terminate too quickly. Excessive collimation may result in an extremely long exposure time.

Type of IR and AEC Response

The AEC system is calibrated based on the type of IR used. If an IR of a different type is used, the detectors will not sense the difference, and the exposure time will terminate at the preset value, which may jeopardize image quality.

Exposure Technique Charts and Radiographic Quality

Exposure technique charts are important for digital imaging because digital systems have a wide dynamic range and can compensate for exposure technique errors. Technique charts should be developed and used with all types of radiographic imaging systems to maintain patient radiation exposure *as low as reasonably achievable* (ALARA).

Variable kVp/Fixed mAs Technique Chart

The variable kVp chart adjusts the kVp for changes in part thickness while maintaining a fixed mAs (2 kVp change for every 1-cm [~0.5-inch] change in part thickness).

Fixed kVp/Variable mAs Technique Chart

The fixed kVp/variable mAs technique chart identifies optimal kVp values and alters the mAs for variations in part thickness (every 4- to 5-cm [1.6- to 2-inch] change in part thickness, the mAs should be adjusted by a factor of 2).

CHAPTER 9: FILM-SCREEN IMAGING

Sensitivity Specks and Latent Image Centers

Sensitivity specks serve as the focal points for the development of latent image centers. After exposure, these specks trap the free electrons and then attract and neutralize the positive silver ions. After enough silver is neutralized, the specks become a latent image center and are converted into metallic silver after chemical processing.

Silver Halide and Film Sensitivity

As the number and/or size of silver halide crystals increase, film sensitivity or speed increases. A faster film speed requires less radiation exposure to produce a specific density.

Screen Speed and Recorded Detail

As screen speed increases, recorded detail decreases; as screen speed decreases, recorded detail increases.

Screen Speed, Light Emission, and Patient Dose

The faster an intensifying screen, the more light is emitted for the same intensity of x-ray exposure. As the screen speed increases, less radiation is necessary, and the radiation dose to the patient is decreased; as screen speed decreases, more radiation is necessary, and the radiation dose to the patient is increased.

Film-Screen System Speed and mAs

Increasing the film-screen speed requires a decrease in the mAs to maintain density. Decreasing the film-screen speed requires an increase in the mAs to maintain density.

Developing or Reducing Agents

The developing agents are responsible for reducing the exposed silver halide crystals to metallic silver, visualized as radiographic densities. Phenidone is responsible for creating the lower densities, and hydroquinone is responsible for creating the higher densities. Their combined effect results in a range of visible densities on the radiograph.

Clearing the Unexposed Crystals

The fixing agent, ammonium thiosulfate, is responsible for removing the unexposed crystals from the emulsion.

Archival Quality of Radiographs

Maintaining the archival (long-term) quality of radiographs requires most of the fixing agent to be removed (washed) from the film. Staining or fading of the permanent image results when too much thiosulfate remains on the film.

Archival Quality of Radiographs

Permanent radiographs must retain a moisture content of 10% to 15% to maintain archival quality. Excessive drying can cause the emulsion layers to crack.

Replenishment and Solution Performance

The replenishment system provides fresh chemicals for the developing and fixing solutions to maintain their chemical activity and volume when they become depleted during processing.

Developer Temperature and Radiographic Quality

Variations in developer temperature can adversely affect the quality of the radiographic image. Increasing the developer temperature increases the density, and decreasing it decreases the density. Further, radiographic contrast may be adversely affected by changes in the developer temperature.

Silver Recovery

Silver is a natural resource and is a heavy metal that can be toxic to the environment, and it must be removed from the used fixer.

Dynamic Range

The range of exposure intensities an IR can accurately detect determines its dynamic range. Film-screen IRs have a narrow dynamic range when compared with digital IRs.

Light Transmittance and Optical Density (OD)

As the percentage of light transmitted decreases, the OD increases; as the percentage of light transmitted increases, the OD decreases.

OD and Light Transmittance

For every 0.3 change in OD, the percentage of light transmitted has changed by a factor of 2. A 0.3 increase in OD results from a decrease in the percentage of light transmitted by half, whereas a 0.3 decrease in OD results from an increase in the percentage of light transmitted by a factor of 2.

Exposure Intensity and OD

Increasing the exposure intensity to the film-screen IR increases the OD, whereas decreasing the exposure intensity to the film-screen IR decreases the OD.

CHAPTER 10: DYNAMIC IMAGING: FLUOROSCOPY

Image-Intensified Fluoroscopy

Dynamic imaging of internal anatomic structures can be accomplished with the use of an image intensifier. The exit radiation is absorbed by the input phosphor, converted to electrons, sent to the output phosphor, released as visible light, and converted to an electronic video signal for transmission to the display monitor.

Brightness Gain

A brighter image is created on the output phosphor when accelerated electrons strike a smaller output phosphor.

Magnification Mode and Patient Dose

Operating the image intensifier in one of the magnification modes increases the operator's ability to see small structures but at the price of increasing the radiation dose to the patient.

Television Cameras and the Display Monitor

The camera tube and CCD are devices that convert the light image from the intensifier's output phosphor to an electronic signal that can be reconstructed on the display monitor.

Cassette Spot Filming

Cassette spot-film devices were a means of recording static images during an image-intensified fluoroscopic examination. The unit shifts to radiographic mode (using a higher mA), and the radiation dose to the patient is much higher than in the fluoroscopic mode.

Flat-Panel Detectors for Dynamic Imaging

Fluoroscopic versions of flat-panel detectors must respond in rapid sequences to create dynamic images, are needed to maintain a large fill factor to reduce image noise due to low-dose fluoroscopic applications and must erase the detector between frames to prevent "ghosting" caused by any residual exposure charge from the previous frame.

Digital Fluoroscopic Systems

The use of flat-panel detectors in place of an image intensifier offers several advantages, such as a reduction in the size, bulk, and weight of the fluoroscopic tower; allowing for easier manipulation of the tower; and greater access to the patient during the examination. The flat-panel detectors also replace the spot filming and other recording devices, and, because they operate in radiographic mode, in many cases, additional radiographic images are not needed. The images, both dynamic and static, can also be readily archived with the patient record in a PACS.

Fluoroscopic Features

Use of virtual collimation during last image hold (LIH), frame averaging, and added filtration reduces the patient dose. Conversely, use of a grid increases the patient dose.

Pulsed Fluoroscopy

Operating the fluoroscope in a pulsed mode reduces the number of images each second, decreases the patient dose, and reduces the visibility of patient motion.

Pulsed Fluoroscopy and Dose Rates

Using pulsed fluoroscopy along with lower dose rates appropriate to the procedure reduces the patient radiation dose.

Summary of Mathematical Applications

CHAPTER 2: THE X-RAY BEAM

Characteristic X-ray Photons

To find the energy of a characteristic x-ray photon, one must know the shell-binding energies of the element and the shells involved. The projectile electron must possess kinetic energy equal to or greater than the shell-binding energy to remove it from orbit. The photon energy is then equal to the difference in the binding energy of the shells involved.

Example:
A projectile electron removes a K-shell electron, and an L-shell electron fills the vacancy:

$$\text{K-shell binding energy} = 69.5 \text{ keV}$$

$$\text{L-shell binding energy} = 12.1 \text{ keV}$$

$69.5 - 12.1 = 57.4 \text{ keV}$

The energy of the K-shell characteristic x-ray photon produced is 57.4 keV.

Calculating Milliamperage-Seconds (mAs)

$$\text{mAs} = \text{mA} \times \text{seconds}$$

Examples:

$$200 \text{ mA} \times 0.25 \text{ s} = 50 \text{ mAs}$$

$$500 \text{ mA} \times 2 / 5 \text{ s} = 200 \text{ mAs}$$

$$800 \text{ mA} \times 100 \text{ ms (milliseconds or } 0.1 \text{ s)} = 80 \text{ mAs}$$

Calculating Heat Units

An exposure is made with a three-phase x-ray unit at 600 mA and 75 kilovoltage peak (kVp) over 0.05 s. How many heat units are produced from this exposure?

$$\text{HU} = \text{mA} \times \text{time} \times \text{kVp} \times \text{generator factor}$$
$$\text{HU} = 600 \times 0.05 \times 75 \times 1.35$$
$$3037.5 \text{ HU}$$

CHAPTER 4: DIGITAL IMAGE CHARACTERISTICS, RECEPTORS, AND IMAGE ACQUISITION

Pixel Size and Field of View (FOV)

FOV = 17 in (431.8 mm) and matrix size = 1024:

$$\frac{431.8}{1024} = 0.42 \text{ mm pixel size}$$

If the FOV was decreased to 12 inches (304.8 mm) for the same matrix size of 1024:

$$\frac{304.8}{1024} = 0.30 \text{ mm pixel size}$$

Decreasing the displayed FOV for a given matrix size will decrease the size of the pixels and increase spatial resolution.

Pixel Size and Matrix Size

FOV = 17 inches (431.8 mm) and matrix size = 1024:

$$\frac{431.8}{1024} = 0.42 \text{ mm pixel size}$$

If the matrix size was increased to 2048 for the same FOV:

$$\frac{431.8}{2048} = 0.21 \text{ mm pixel size}$$

Increasing the matrix size for a given FOV displayed will decrease the size of the pixels and increase spatial resolution.

CHAPTER 6: EXPOSURE TECHNIQUE FACTORS

Adjusting Milliamperage (mA) or Exposure Time

$$200 \text{ mA} \times 0.100 \text{ s} = 20 \text{ mAs}$$

To increase the mAs to 40, one could use the following formulas:

$$400 \text{ mA} \times 0.100 \text{ s} = 40 \text{ mAs}$$

$$200 \text{ mA} \times 0.200 \text{ s} = 40 \text{ mAs}$$

Adjusting mA and Exposure Time to Maintain mAs

$$200 \text{ mA} \times 100 \text{ ms} \ (0.100 \text{ s}) = 20 \text{ mAs}$$

To maintain mAs, use the following formulas:

$$400 \text{ mA} \times 50 \text{ ms} \ (0.050 \text{ s}) = 20 \text{ mAs}$$

$$100 \text{ mA} \times 200 \text{ ms} \ (0.200 \text{ s}) = 20 \text{ mAs}$$

Using the 15% Rule

To increase exposure to the image receptor (IR), multiply the kVp by 1.15 (original kVp + 15%):

$$75 \text{ kVp} \times 1.15 = 86 \text{ kVp}.$$

To decrease exposure to the IR, multiply the kVp by 0.85 (original kVp − 15%):

$$75 \text{ kVp} \times 0.85 = 64 \text{ kVp}.$$

To maintain exposure to the IR, when increasing the kVp by 15% (kVp × 1.15), divide the original mAs by 2:

$$75 \text{ kVp} \times 1.15 = 86 \text{ kVp and mAs} / 2.$$

When decreasing the kVp by 15% (kVp × 0.85), multiply the mAs by 2:

$$75 \text{ kVp} \times 0.85 = 64 \text{ and mAs} \times 2.$$

Inverse-Square Law Formula

$$\frac{I_1}{I_2} = \frac{(D_2)^2}{(D_1)^2}$$

If the intensity of radiation at a source-to-image receptor distance (SID) of 40 inches is equal to 400 mR, what is the intensity of radiation when the distance is increased to 72 inches?

$$\frac{400 \text{ mR}}{X} = \frac{(72)^2}{(40)^2} \quad 400 \text{ mR} \times 1600 = 640{,}000$$

$$= 5184X;$$

$$\frac{640{,}000}{5184} = X; 123.5 \text{ mR} = X$$

Direct Square Law or Exposure Maintenance Formula

$$\frac{mAs_1}{mAs_2} \quad \frac{(SID_1)^2}{(SID_2)^2}$$

Optimal exposure to the IR is achieved at an SID of 40 inches using 25 mAs. The SID must be increased to 72 inches. What adjustment of mAs is needed to maintain exposure to the IR?

$$\frac{25}{X} = \frac{(40)^2}{(72)^2}; 1600X = 129{,}600;$$

$$\frac{129{,}600}{1600}; X = 81 \text{ mAs}_2$$

Magnification Factor

An anteroposterior projection (AP) of the knee is produced with an SID of 40 inches and an object-to-image-receptor distance (OID) of 3 inches (source-to-object distance [SOD] is equal to 37 inches). What is the magnification factor (MF)?

$$\text{SOD} = \text{SID} - \text{OID}, \text{MF} = \frac{40}{37}; = 1.081$$

$$37 = 40 - 3$$

Determining Object Size

On an AP image of a knee taken with an SID of 40 inches and an OID of 3 inches (SOD = 37 inches), the size of a lesion measures 0.5 inches in diameter on the radiographic image. The MF has been determined to be 1.081. What is the object size of this lesion?

$$\frac{40}{37} = 1.081\,MF \quad Object\ size = \frac{0.5\ inch}{1.081}$$

The object size is 0.463 inches.

Determining Object % of Magnification

A lesion on the radiographic image measures 1.16 cm, and the lesion's (object's) true size measures 1.06 cm. What is the object % of magnification?

$$Object\ \%\ of\ magnification = \frac{1.16 - 1.06}{1.06\ cm} \times 100$$

$$\frac{0.10}{1.06} = 0.09434 \times 100 =$$
$$9.43\ \%\ Object\ magnification$$

Adjusting mAs for Changes in the Grid

A quality radiographic image is obtained using 5 mAs at 70 kVp without using a grid. What new mAs is needed when adding a 12:1 grid to maintain the same exposure to the IR?

$$\frac{5\ mAs}{X} = \frac{1}{5};\ 1X = 25;\ X = 25\ mAs$$

The new mAs produces an exposure comparable to the IR without the grid.

CHAPTER 7: SCATTER CONTROL

Calculating Grid Ratio

What is the grid ratio when the lead strips are 2.4 mm high and separated by 0.2 mm?

$$Grid\ ratio = h\,/\,D$$
$$Grid\ ratio = \frac{2.4}{0.2} = 12\ or\ 12:1$$

Adding a Grid

If a radiographer produced a shoulder radiograph with nongrid exposure using 3 mAs and then wanted to use a 12:1 ratio grid, what mAs should be used to produce the same exposure to the IR?
Nongrid exposure = 3 mAs
Grid conversion factor (GCF) (for 12:1 grid) = 5 (from Table 7-2)

$$GCF = \frac{mAs\ with\ the\ grid}{mAs\ without\ the\ grid}$$
$$5 = \frac{mAs\ with\ the\ grid}{3}$$
$$15 = mAs\ with\ the\ grid$$

When adding a 12:1 ratio grid, mAs must be increased by a factor of 5 (in this case to 15 mAs).

Removing a Grid

If a radiographer produced a knee radiograph using an 8:1 ratio grid and 10 mAs and on the next exposure wanted to use nongrid exposure, what mAs should be used to produce the same exposure to the IR?
Grid exposure = 10 mAs
GCF (for 8:1 grid) = 4 (from Table 7-2)

$$GCF = \frac{mAs\ with\ the\ grid}{mAs\ without\ the\ grid}$$
$$4 = \frac{10\ mAs}{mAs\ without\ the\ grid}$$
$$2.5 = mAs\ without\ the\ grid$$

When removing an 8:1 ratio grid, mAs must be decreased by a factor of 4 (in this case to 2.5 mAs).

Decreasing the Grid Ratio

If a radiographer used 40 mAs with a 12:1 ratio grid, what mAs should be used with a 6:1 ratio grid to produce the same exposure to the IR?
Exposure 1: 40 mAs, 12:1 grid, GCF = 5
Exposure 2: _____ mAs, 6:1 grid, GCF = 3

$$\frac{mAs_1}{mAs_2} = \frac{GCF_1}{GCF_2}$$
$$\frac{40}{mAs_2} = \frac{5}{3}$$
$$mAs_2 = 24$$

Decreasing the grid ratio requires less mAs.

Increasing the Grid Ratio

If a radiographer performed a routine portable pelvic examination using 40 mAs with an 8:1 ratio grid, what mAs should be used if a 12:1 ratio grid is substituted?

Exposure 1: 40 mAs, 8:1 grid, GCF = 4

Exposure 2: _____ mAs, 12:1 grid, GCF = 5

$$\frac{mAs_1}{mAs_2} = \frac{GCF_1}{GCF_2}$$

$$\frac{40}{mAs_2} = \frac{4}{5}$$

$$mAs_2 = 50$$

Increasing the grid ratio requires additional mAs.

CHAPTER 9: FILM-SCREEN IMAGING

Adjusting mAs for Changes in Film-Screen System Speed

A quality radiograph is obtained using 10 mAs at 65 kVp and a 100-speed film-screen system. What new mAs is used to maintain radiographic density when changing to a 400-speed film-screen system?

$$\frac{10 \, mAs}{X} = \frac{400 \, speed}{100 \, speed}$$

$$10 \, mAs \times 100; 1000 = 400X;$$

$$\frac{1000}{400} = 2.5 \, mAs = X$$

Summary of Radiation Protection Alerts

CHAPTER 1: RADIATION AND ITS DISCOVERY

ALARA Principle

It is the radiographer's responsibility to minimize the radiation dose to the patient, to themselves, and to others in accordance with the **as** **l**ow **as** **r**easonably **a**chievable (ALARA) principle.

Cardinal Principles for Minimizing Radiation Dose

Time: Limit the amount of time exposed to ionizing radiation.

Distance: Maintain a safe distance from the source of ionizing radiation exposure.

Shielding: Maximize the use of shielding from ionizing radiation exposure.

Beam Restriction

Limiting the size of the x-ray exposure field reduces the volume of tissue irradiated and reduces the radiation dose to the patient.

Primary Exposure Factors

The combination of kilovoltage peak (kVp) and milliamperage-seconds (mAs) is selected based on a number of considerations, including the anatomic part being examined, patient age, condition, and pathology, and should be ideally suited to the circumstance to minimize radiation dose while producing optimum exposure to the image receptor (IR).

Avoid Unnecessary Duplicate Exams

The radiographer must recognize and accept his or her role as a patient advocate and do what is necessary to avoid unnecessary duplication of exams.

Screening for Pregnancy

Screening for pregnancy is another important task for minimizing unnecessary exposure to a developing fetus. When it is necessary to perform a radiographic exam on a pregnant patient, shielding materials and precise collimation should be used to minimize the radiation dose administered to the fetus.

CHAPTER 2: THE X-RAY BEAM

Beam Filtration

Low-energy photons, created during x-ray production, are unable to penetrate the patient. Patients are protected from unnecessary exposure to this low-energy radiation by the placement of inherent and added filtration in the path of the x-ray beam.

CHAPTER 4: DIGITAL IMAGE CHARACTERISTICS, RECEPTORS, AND IMAGE ACQUISITION

Digital Detectors and Dynamic Range

Because digital IRs have a wide dynamic range, a quality image can be produced when using more radiation exposure than necessary. Radiographers must take extra precautions to not unnecessarily overexpose patients and select exposure techniques within the exposure latitude established by the department.

CHAPTER 5: DIGITAL IMAGE PROCESSING, DISPLAY, AND DATA MANAGEMENT

Exposure Indicators

The radiographer should strive to select techniques that result in exposure indicator values falling

319

within the indicated optimum range for the corresponding digital imaging system. However, the radiographer also needs to recognize the limitations of exposure indicators for providing accurate information.

CHAPTER 6: EXPOSURE TECHNIQUE FACTORS

Excessive Radiation Exposure and Digital Imaging

Although the computer can adjust image brightness for technique exposure errors, routinely using more radiation than required for the procedure in digital radiography unnecessarily increases patient exposure. Even though the digital system can adjust overexposure, it is an unethical practice to knowingly overexpose a patient.

kVp/mAs

Whenever possible, a higher kilovoltage and lower mAs should be used to reduce patient exposure. Increasing kilovoltage requires a lower mAs to maintain the desired exposure to the IR and decreases the radiation dose to the patient. For example, changing kVp from 75 to 86 when imaging a pelvis is a 15% increase and would require half the mAs needed for the original 75 kVp. Higher kVp increases the beam penetration, and therefore, less radiation is needed to achieve a desired exposure to the IR.

Grid Selection

Decisions regarding the use of a grid and grid ratio should be made by balancing image quality and patient protection. To keep patient exposure as low as reasonable, grids should be used only when appropriate, and the grid ratio should be the lowest that would provide sufficient contrast improvement.

Beam Restriction

In performing a radiographic examination, the radiographer should be aware of the anatomic area of interest and limit the x-ray field size to just beyond this area. Collimating to the appropriate field size is a basic method for protecting patients from unnecessary exposure.

CHAPTER 7: SCATTER CONTROL

Appropriate Beam Restriction

In performing a radiographic examination, the radiographer should be aware of the anatomic area of interest and limit the x-ray field size to just beyond this area. Collimating to the appropriate field size is a basic method for protecting patients from unnecessary exposure.

Post-exposure Electronic Masking or Cropping

Post-exposure electronic masking or cropping the displayed image should never replace pre-exposure collimation because it does not reduce scatter production, reduce patient radiation exposure, or increase image contrast.

Limit Field Size to the Anatomic Area of Interest

The radiographer should always be sure that the size of the x-ray field is restricted to the anatomic area of interest. Digital IRs are typically of a similar size, and, in many instances, larger than the anatomic area of interest. Therefore, it is crucial for the radiographer to appropriately collimate for the imaging procedure so that the patient is not unnecessarily exposed to radiation.

Grid Selection

Decisions regarding the use of a grid and grid ratio should be made by balancing image quality and patient protection. To minimize patient exposure, grids should be used only when appropriate, and the grid ratio selected should be the lowest capable of providing sufficient contrast improvement. In exams in which the anatomic part does not produce excessive scatter, a grid may not be necessary because the computer can vary contrast in the displayed image.

CHAPTER 8: EXPOSURE TECHNIQUE SELECTION

Kilovoltage Selection

Using a higher kVp with automatic exposure control (AEC) decreases the exposure time and the overall mAs needed to produce a diagnostic image, significantly reducing patient exposure. The kVp selected for an examination should produce the desired subject contrast for the part examined while being as high as possible to minimize the patient's radiation exposure.

Monitoring Backup Time

To minimize patient exposure, the backup time should be neither too long nor too short. Backup time that is too short results in the exposure being stopped prematurely, and the image may need to be repeated because of poor quality. Backup time that is too long results in the patient receiving unnecessary radiation if a problem occurs and the exposure does not end until the backup time is reached. In addition, the image may have to be repeated because of poor quality.

Errors in AEC Use

It is important for radiographers to evaluate image quality, the applied mAs, and the exposure indicator when using the AEC device. Errors in selecting the appropriate combination of AEC detectors, detector size, or positioning errors may not be visually apparent because of computer adjustment.

Patient Variability

Factors related to the patient affect the time of exposure reaching the IR and ultimately the image quality; such factors include pathology, contrast media, foreign objects, and pockets of gas. Increases or decreases in patient thickness result in changes in the time of exposure if the AEC system is functioning properly.

Anatomically Programmed Technique and Patient Exposure

When using a preprogrammed set of exposure factors, the radiographer must evaluate the appropriateness of the selected exposure technique factors. Adjustment of the preprogrammed exposure factors may be necessary for that patient or procedure.

Chapter Review Questions Answer Key

CHAPTER 1: RADIATION AND ITS DISCOVERY

1. B	4. A	7. B	10. C	13. A
2. C	5. D	8. D	11. C	14. D
3. D	6. C	9. A	12. B	

CHAPTER 2: THE X-RAY BEAM

1. B	4. A	7. D	10. D	13. D
2. D	5. C	8. A	11. C	14. D
3. B	6. A	9. C	12. B	15. A

CHAPTER 3: IMAGE FORMATION AND RADIOGRAPHIC QUALITY

1. D	4. B	7. A	10. C	13. B
2. D	5. D	8. A	11. B	14. D
3. C	6. B	9. C	12. D	15. A

CHAPTER 4: DIGITAL IMAGE CHARACTERISTICS, RECEPTORS, AND IMAGE ACQUISITION

1. D	5. D	9. A	13. C	17. D
2. C	6. C	10. C	14. A	18. A
3. A	7. D	11. B	15. B	
4. D	8. C	12. A	16. D	

CHAPTER 5: DIGITAL IMAGE PROCESSING, DISPLAY, AND DATA MANAGEMENT

1. C	5. D	9. D	13. B
2. A	6. A	10. D	14. C
3. C	7. D	11. B	15. B
4. D	8. A	12. A	16. A

CHAPTER 6: EXPOSURE TECHNIQUE FACTORS

1. D	4. B	7. C	10. D
2. C	5. D	8. D	11. B
3. A	6. C	9. A	12. B

CHAPTER 7: SCATTER CONTROL

1. C	5. B	9. B	13. C	17. C
2. B	6. A	10. A	14. D	18. D
3. D	7. D	11. D	15. A	
4. B	8. D	12. A	16. B	

CHAPTER 8: EXPOSURE TECHNIQUE SELECTION

1. B	5. B	9. C	13. B
2. C	6. D	10. B	14. C
3. D	7. B	11. D	15. A
4. D	8. A	12. D	16. C

CHAPTER 9: FILM-SCREEN IMAGING

1. D	5. B	9. D	13. C
2. B	6. A	10. C	14. A
3. A	7. A	11. B	15. D
4. D	8. D	12. C	16. A

CHAPTER 10: DYNAMIC IMAGING: FLUOROSCOPY

1. A	4. B	7. B	10. B	13. D	16. A
2. D	5. D	8. B	11. D	14. B	
3. C	6. C	9. B	12. C	15. D	

GLOSSARY

A

15% rule Rule stating that changing the kVp by 15% has the same effect on image receptor exposure as doubling or halving the mAs.

absorbed dose The transfer of radiation energy into matter (e.g., tissue).

absorption As the energy of the primary x-ray beam is deposited within the atoms composing the tissue, some x-ray photons are completely absorbed. Complete absorption of the incoming x-ray photon occurs when it has enough energy to remove (eject) an inner-shell electron.

accelerating anode Attracts and sets the electron stream in motion at a constant velocity inside the image intensifier tube.

active layer The radiation-sensitive and light-sensitive layer of the film.

actual focal spot size The size of the area on the anode target that is exposed to electrons from the tube current. Actual focal spot size depends on the size of the filament producing the electron stream.

added filtration The filtration that is added to the port of the x-ray tube.

air gap technique Based on the simple concept that much of the scatter will miss the image receptor if there is an increased distance between the patient and the image receptor (increased OID).

air kerma (kinetic energy released in matter) Specifies the intensity of x-rays at a given point in air at a known distance from the focal spot or source of x-rays.

ALARA As low as reasonably achievable.

alternative algorithms A mechanism for the radiographer to reprocess the image data by selecting an alternative anatomical region or projection to improve its presentation at the display monitor.

ambient lighting The level of light in the room while viewing images.

anatomically programmed techniques A radiographic system that allows the radiographer to select a particular button on the control panel that represents an anatomic area; a preprogrammed set of exposure factors is displayed and selected for use.

anode A positively charged electrode within the x-ray tube composed of molybdenum, copper, tungsten, and graphite. It consists of a target and, in rotating anode tubes, a stator and rotor.

anode heel effect The x-ray beam has greater intensity (number of x-rays) on the cathode side of the tube, with the intensity diminishing toward the anode side. The heel effect occurs because of the angle of the target.

aperture diaphragm A flat piece of lead (diaphragm) containing a hole (aperture) for beam restriction.

artifact Any unwanted image on a radiograph.

attenuation Reduction in the energy or number of the primary x-ray beam as it passes through anatomic tissue.

automatic brightness control (ABC) A function of the fluoroscopic unit that maintains the overall appearance of the fluoroscopic image (contrast and density) by automatically adjusting the kVp, mA, or both.

automatic collimator/positive beam-limiting device Automatically limits the size and shape of the primary beam to the size and shape of the image receptor.

automatic exposure control (AEC) A system used to consistently control the amount of radiation reaching the image receptor by terminating the length of exposure.

automatic exposure rate control (AERC) Automatically adjusts the tube current (mA), voltage (kVp), filtration, and pulse width to maintain radiation exposure to the flat panel detector.

automatic film processor A device that encompasses chemical tanks, a roller transport system, and a dryer system for the processing of radiographic film.

automatic rescaling Occurs during histogram analysis and is used to maintain consistent image brightness despite overexposure or underexposure of the digital image receptor.

average gradient The slope of the straight-line region of a film's sensitometric curve.

B

backup time The maximum length of time for which the x-ray exposure continues when using an AEC system.

base plus fog (B + F) The lowest amount of density on the radiographic film caused by the tint added to its base and any slight amount of fog added during processing.

beam restriction/collimation Interchangeably used terms that refer to a decrease in the size of the projected radiation field.

beam-restricting device Changes the shape and size of the primary beam, located just below the x-ray tube housing.

bit 0 or 1 that refers to the computer's basic unit of information.

bit depth Number of bits.

body habitus The general form or build of the body, including size. The four types of body habitus are *sthenic, hyposthenic, hypersthenic,* and *asthenic.*

body mass index (BMI) A person's weight in kilograms divided by the square of height in meters. A high BMI (>30) can be an indicator of obesity.

bremsstrahlung interactions Occur when a projectile electron completely avoids the orbital electrons of the tungsten atom and travels very close to its nucleus. The very strong electrostatic force of the nucleus causes the electron suddenly to "slow down." As the electron loses energy, it suddenly changes its direction, and the energy loss reappears as an x-ray photon.

brightness The amount of luminance (light emission) of a display monitor.

brightness gain The product of both flux gain and minification gain; this results in a brighter image on the output phosphor.

Bucky Located directly below the radiographic tabletop, the grid is found just above the tray that holds the image receptor. More accurately called the *Potter-Bucky diaphragm.*

Bucky factor/grid conversion factor Used to determine the adjustment in mAs needed when changing from using a grid to nongrid (or vice versa) or when changing to grids with different grid ratios.

byte 8 bits combined.

C

caliper A device that measures part thickness.

camera tube A device used to convert the light emitted from the output phosphor to an electrical signal sent to the television monitor.

cassette Container for both the intensifying screens and the film.

cathode A negatively charged electrode (within the x-ray tube). It comprises a filament and a focusing cup.

characteristic interactions Produced when a projectile electron interacts with an electron from the inner (K) shell of the tungsten atom and ejects it. An outer-shell electron drops into vacancy and the energy difference is emitted as an x-ray photon.

charge-coupled device (CCD) A light-sensitive semiconducting device that generates an electrical charge when stimulated by light and stores this charge in a capacitor.

coherent scattering An interaction that occurs with low-energy x-rays, typically below the diagnostic range. The incoming photon interacts with the atom, causing it to become excited. The x-ray does not lose energy but changes direction.

collimator Two sets of adjustable lead shutters located 3 to 7 inches below the tube that consist of longitudinal and lateral leaves or blades, each with its own control; this makes the collimator adjustable in terms of its ability to produce projected fields of varying sizes.

comparative anatomy Concept stating that different parts of the same size can be radiographed using the same exposure factors, provided the minimum kVp value needed to penetrate the part is used in each case.

compensating filter Special filters added to the primary beam to alter its intensity. These types of filters are used to image anatomic areas that are non-uniform in makeup and assist in producing more consistent exposure to the image receptor.

complementary metal oxide semiconductor (CMOS) A scintillator device made up of a crystalline silicon matrix. Each detector element has its own amplifier, photodiode, and storage capacitor and is surrounded by transistors. Can be used to convert the light image from the intensifier's output phosphor to an electronic signal that can be reconstructed on the display monitor. Recent advances in CMOS technology, particularly the creation of crystal light tubes that prevent light spread and methods for increasing their size, make them applicable for radiographic imaging.

Compton effect The loss of energy of the incoming photon when it ejects an outer-shell electron from the atom. The remaining lower-energy x-ray photon changes direction and may leave the anatomic part.

Compton electron/secondary electron The ejected electron resulting from the Compton effect interaction.

cone An aperture diaphragm that has an extended flange attached to it. The flange can vary in length and is shaped as a cone. The flange can also be made to telescope, increasing its total length.

continuous fluoroscopy The x-ray exposure continues without interruption while the exposure pedal or button is activated.

contrast enhancement A postprocessing technique that alters the pixel values to increase image contrast.

contrast medium A substance instilled into the body by injection or ingestion that is used when imaging anatomic tissues that have low subject contrast. Also called *contrast agent.*

contrast resolution The ability of the image receptor to distinguish between objects having similar subject contrast.

contrast-to-noise ratio A method of describing the contrast resolution with the amount of noise apparent in a digital image.

convergent line If points were connected along the length of the grid, they would form an imaginary line.

convergent point If imaginary lines were drawn from each of the lead lines in a linear focused grid, these lines would meet to form an imaginary point.

conversion factor An expression of the luminance at the output phosphor divided by the input exposure rate; its unit of measurement is candela per square meter per milliroentgen per second.

CR fading When the imaging plate is not processed in a timely manner, the latent image dissipates over time because some of the signal (released energy) captured in the imaging plate is lost.

crossed/crosshatched grid A grid containing lead lines that are perpendicular to one another. Crossed grids remove more scattered photons than linear grids because they contain more lead strips, oriented in two directions.

cylinder An aperture diaphragm that has an extended flange attached to it. The flange can vary in length and is shaped as a cylinder.

D

data management A complex system-wide effort to ensure that people, equipment, and processes are in place to expand health care communication and improve patient outcomes.

densitometer A device used to numerically determine the amount of blackness on the radiograph.

density The amount of overall blackness of the processed image.

density controls A mechanism that allows the radiographer to adjust the amount of preset radiation detection values.

detective quantum efficiency (DQE) A measurement of the efficiency of an image receptor in converting the x-ray exposure it receives to a quality radiographic image.

detectors The sensors, cells, or chambers within an AEC device that sense how much radiation has reached the imaging plate to terminate the exposure.

developing or reducing agents Agents that reduce exposed silver halide to metallic silver and add electrons to exposed silver halide during film processing.

deviation index (DI) A value that reflects the difference between the desired or target exposure to the image receptor and the actual exposure to the image receptor.

diagnostic densities The appropriate range of optical densities.

differential absorption A process whereby some of the x-ray beam is absorbed in the tissue and some passes through (transmits) the anatomic part.

digital image processing Various computer algorithms (mathematical computations) applied to digital data for the purpose of optimizing the image for display.

digital imaging Constructing an image from numeric data.

digital imaging and communications in medicine (DICOM) A communication standard for information sharing between PACS and imaging modalities.

direct square law A formula that provides a mathematical calculation for adjusting mAs when changing the SID.

disaster recovery A requirement to duplicate all files in a remote location so that recovery is possible in the event of a disaster and the primary files are lost.

display workstation A desktop computer that allows for the retrieval and viewing of medical images from one of the modalities or storage components of the PACS.

distortion Results from the radiographic misrepresentation of either the size (magnification) or the shape of the anatomic part.

D_{max} The point on the sensitometric curve where maximum density has been produced.

D_{min} The point on the sensitometric curve where the minimum amount of radiation exposure produced the minimum amount of optical density.

dose area product (DAP) A measure of exposure in air, followed by a computation to estimate absorbed dose to the patient. It is the same as KAP.

dose equivalent Units of radiation exposure used in measuring occupational exposure in radiation equivalents in man (rem) and sieverts (Sv).

dosimeter A device that measures x-ray exposure.

double-emulsion film Has an emulsion coating on both sides of the base.

dual energy subtraction A technique that can remove superimposed structures so that the anatomic area of interest becomes more visible. Because the image is in a digital format, the computer can subtract selected brightness values to create an image without superimposed structures.

dynamic range The range of exposure intensities an image receptor can accurately detect.

E

edge enhancement A postprocessing technique that improves the visibility of small, high-contrast structures.

effective dose An expression of the *relative risk to humans* (whole-body exposure) of exposure to ionizing radiation and measured in sieverts (Sv).

effective focal spot size Focal spot size as measured directly under the anode target.

electromagnetic radiation Radiation that has both electrical and magnetic properties. All radiations that are electromagnetic make up a spectrum.

electronic health record (EHR) The system for patient health information (PHI) that can be shared outside the facility and among many health care systems.

electronic magnification The selection of a smaller field of view (FOV). When a smaller FOV is selected, an area smaller than the size of the detector is exposed by the x-ray beam, but the area is enlarged to fill the display monitor area magnifying the anatomic structures.

electronic masking Also known as *shuttering*. A postprocessing function that can remove regions of the digital image.

electrostatic focusing lenses Focuses and accelerates the electrons through the image intensifier toward the anode.

elongation Images of objects that appear longer than the true objects.

emulsion layer The radiation- and light-sensitive layers of the film.

equalization A postprocessing function whereby underexposed areas (light areas) are made darker and overexposed areas (dark areas) are made lighter. The effect is an image that appears to have lower contrast so that dense and lucent structures can be better seen within the same image.

exit radiation When the attenuated x-ray beam leaves the patient, the remaining x-ray beam is composed of both transmitted and scattered radiation.

exposure The amount of ionizations or electrical charge in a specified amount of air expressed by Roentgen (R).

exposure adjustment A mechanism that allows the radiographer to adjust the amount of preset radiation detection values.

exposure indicator A numeric value that is displayed on the processed image to indicate the level of x-ray exposure received on the digital image receptor.

exposure intensity The amount and energy of the x-rays reaching an area of the image receptor.

exposure latitude The range of exposures that produce optical densities within the straight-line region of the sensitometric curve.

exposure maintenance formula A formula that provides a mathematical calculation for adjusting the mAs when changing the SID.

exposure technique charts Pre-established guidelines used by the radiographer to select standardized manual or AEC exposure factors for each type of radiographic examination.

exposure time Determines the length of time that the x-ray tube produces x-rays.

extrapolated Mathematically estimated; the mathematical process used to create technique charts.

F

feed tray   A flat metal surface with an edge on either side that permits the film to enter the processor easily and correctly aligned.

filament   A coiled tungsten wire that is the source of electrons during x-ray production.

filament current   Heats the tungsten filament. This heating of the filament causes thermionic emission.

fill factor   The percentage of the x-rays reaching the sensitive area of the detector element (DEL).

film contrast   Controlled by the design and manufacturing of the film components and the effect of processing.

film-screen contact   The contact between the film and intensifying screens. Good film-screen contact exists when the screen or screens are in direct contact with the film.

film speed   The degree to which the emulsion is sensitive to x-rays or light. The greater the speed of a film, the more sensitive it is.

fixed kVp/variable mAs technique chart   A type of exposure technique chart that is based on the concept of selecting an optimal kVp value that is required for the radiographic examination and adjusting the mAs for variations in part thickness.

fixing agent   Clears undeveloped silver halide from the film during processing.

flat-panel detectors (FPDs)   Solid-state image receptors using a large-area active matrix array of electronic components ranging in sizes from 43 × 35 to 43 × 43 cm.

fluorescence   The ability of phosphors to emit visible light only while exposed to x-rays (with little or no afterglow).

fluoro loop save   A feature that saves a fluoro sequence loop to memory (based on the equipment's memory capacity).

fluoroscopy   Allows imaging of the movement of internal structures. It differs from film-screen imaging in that it uses a continuous beam of x-rays to create images of moving internal structures that can be viewed on a television monitor.

flux gain   The increase in light intensities at the output phosphor by accelerating the electrons.

focal distance   The distance between the grid and the convergent line or point, sometimes referred to as *grid radius*.

focal range   The recommended range of SIDs that can be used with a focused grid. The convergent line or point always falls within the focal range.

focused grid   Grid that has lead lines that are angled, or canted, to approximately match the angle of divergence of the primary beam.

focusing cup   Made of nickel and nearly surrounds the filament. It is open at one end to allow electrons to flow freely across the tube from cathode to anode. It has a negative charge, which keeps the cloud of electrons emitted from the filament from spreading apart. Its purpose is to focus the stream of electrons.

fog   Scatter radiation (Compton interactions) that reach the image receptor and creates unwanted exposure on the radiographic image.

foreshortening   Images that appear shorter than the true objects.

frame averaging   An operation that reduces overall patient dose and image noise by averaging multiple image frames together. Because the combining of frames reduces noise, less radiation is needed to maintain image quality; however, spatial resolution will be decreased.

frequency   The number of waves passing a given point per given unit of time. Frequency is represented by a lowercase *f* or by the Greek letter *nu* (ν), and values are given in Hertz (Hz).

G

gradient point   The slope along any portion of the sensitometric curve.

grayscale   The number of different shades of gray that can be stored and displayed by a computer system.

grayscale standard display function (GSDF)   The DICOM recommended standard for consistent display characteristics, such as grayscale appearance and image quality.

grid   A device that has very thin lead strips with radiolucent interspaces, intended to absorb scatter radiation emitted from the patient.

grid cap   Contains a permanently mounted grid and allows the image receptor to slide in behind it.

grid cassette   An image receptor that has a grid permanently mounted to its front surface.

grid cutoff   A decrease in the number of transmitted photons that reach the image receptor because of some misalignment of the grid.

grid focus   The orientation of the lead lines to one another.

grid frequency   Expresses the number of lead lines per unit length inches, or centimeters, or both. Grid frequencies can range from 25 to 45 lines/cm (60 to 110 lines/inch).

grid pattern   The linear pattern of the lead lines of a grid. The two types of grid pattern are linear and crossed or crosshatched.

grid ratio   The ratio of the height of the lead strips to the distance between them.

H

half-value layer (HVL)   The amount of filtration that reduces the intensity of the x-ray beam to half of its original value is considered the best method for describing x-ray quality. The HVL also can be used as an indirect measure of the total filtration in the path of the x-ray beam. It is expressed in millimeters of aluminum (mm-Al).

Health Insurance Portability and Accountability (HIPAA)   National standards for electronic health care transactions and national identifiers for providers, health insurance plans, and employers.

Health Level Seven Standard (HL7)   A communication standard for medical information.

heat unit (HU)   The amount of heat produced from any given exposure.

high contrast   A radiograph with few densities but great differences among them.

histogram   Graphic display of the distribution of pixel values. Each image has its own histogram, and it is evaluated to determine the adequacy of the image receptor exposure to x-rays.

histogram analysis The computer analyzes the histogram using processing algorithms and compares it with a pre-established (reference) histogram specific to the anatomic part being imaged.

hospital information system (HIS) A facility's system to collect and store personal patient information gathered (e.g., demographic data, relevant history, physician orders) that will assist in his or her care.

I

illuminator Device that provides light illumination so that the anatomy, displayed as various shades of optical densities, can be visualized. It is also known as a *viewbox*.

image intensifier An electronic vacuum tube that converts the remnant (exit) x-ray beam to light, then to electrons, then back to light, increasing the light intensity in the process.

image receptor (IR) A device that receives the radiation leaving the patient.

imaging informatics Involves data management for radiology services both within and outside the health care system, also known as radiology informatics.

imaging plate (IP) Located in the CR image receptor, where the photon intensities are absorbed by the phosphor.

immersion heater A heating coil that is immersed in the bottom of the developer and fixer tank. It is thermostatically controlled to heat the developer solution to its proper temperature and maintain that temperature as long as the processor is turned on.

inherent filtration The filtration that is permanently in the path of the x-ray beam. Three components contribute to inherent filtration: (1) the glass envelope of the tube, (2) the oil that surrounds the tube, and (3) the window in the tube housing.

input/output phosphor Phosphors within the image intensifier. The input phosphor converts incoming radiation into visible light energy, and the output phosphor converts the electrons into a brighter image.

integrating the health enterprise (IHE) Initiative by health care professionals and industry to improve the way computer systems in health care share information.

intensifying screen A device in radiographic cassettes that contains phosphors that convert x-ray energy into light, which exposes the radiographic film.

intensity of radiation exposure The amount and energy of the x-rays reaching an area of the image receptor.

interspace material Radiolucent strips between the lead lines of a grid; generally made of aluminum.

inverse-square law The relationship between distance and x-ray beam intensity, which states that the intensity of the x-ray beam is inversely proportional to the square of the distance from the source.

inversion A postprocessing technique that reverses the grayscale from the original image.

invisible image The latent image not visible within the image receptor.

ionization The ability to remove (eject) electrons; a property of x-rays.

ionization/ion chamber A hollow cell that contains air and is connected to the AEC timer circuit via an electrical wire.

irreversible compression Image compression where there is no loss of image data (lossless) at the end user.

K

kerma area product (KAP) The product of the total air kerma (intensity of x-rays at a given point in air) and the area of the x-ray beam at the entrance of the patient. It is the same as dose area product.

kilovoltage (kVp) Potential difference applied across the x-ray tube at the time the exposure is initiated, kVp determines the speed at which the electrons in the tube current move.

L

last image hold (LIH) The last fluoroscopic image displayed without any radiation exposure.

latent image The invisible image within the image receptor.

latent image centers Several sensitivity specks with many silver ions attracted to them.

latent image formation The Gurney–Mott theory used to explain what happens to silver halide crystals when exposed to x-rays and light.

leakage radiation Any x-rays, other than the primary beam, that escape the tube housing.

line focus principle Describes the relationship between the actual and the effective focal spots in the x-ray tube. A smaller target angle produces a smaller effective focal spot.

linear grid Contains lead lines that run in only one direction.

long-dimension linear grid Contains lead strips that run parallel to the long axis of the grid.

long-scale/low contrast A radiograph with a large number of densities but little differences among them.

lookup tables (LUTs) Provide a method of altering the image to change the display of the digital image in a variety of ways.

luminescence The emission of light from the screen when stimulated by radiation.

M

magnification An increase in the image size of the object compared with its true or actual size. Also known as *size distortion*.

magnification factor (MF) Indicates how much size distortion or magnification is shown on a radiograph. MF = SID divided by SOD.

magnification mode Image intensifiers have a multifold function to increase the size of the area of interest displayed on the television monitor. Changing the voltage of the electrostatic focusing lenses tightens the diameter of the electron stream, giving the appearance of magnification.

manifest/visible image The visible image after processing.

mAs readout The actual mAs used for the image is displayed immediately after the AEC exposure, sometimes for only a few seconds.

matrix A digital image is displayed as a combination of rows and columns (array) of small, usually square, "picture elements" called *pixels*.

maximum contrast The greatest difference in optical densities.

milliamperage (mA) The unit used to measure the tube current.

minification gain Increased light intensities as a result of the reduction in size of the output phosphor image compared with that of the input phosphor image.

minimum response time The shortest exposure time that the AEC system can produce.

modulation transfer function (MTF) A measure of the imaging system's ability to display contrast of anatomic objects varying in size.

moiré effect An artifact that can occur when a stationary grid is used during computed radiography imaging if the grid frequency is similar to the scanning frequency. Also known as the *Zebra pattern*.

N

Nyquist frequency A standard formula for converting analog data into discreet digital units to accurately represent the analog signal or imaging data in digital radiography. To accurately reproduce an image from the continuous analog signal, the sampling rate must be at least two times the highest spatial frequency in the exit x-ray intensities (signal).

O

object-to-image-receptor distance (OID) Distance created between the object radiographed and the image receptor.

off-focus radiation Occurs when projectile electrons are reflected and x-rays are produced outside the focal spot.

optical density (OD) A numeric calculation that compares the intensity of light transmitted through an area on the film (I_t) with the amount of light originally striking (incident) the area (I_0).

optimal density Densities that lie within the straight-line region of the sensitometric curve.

optimal kVp The kVp value that is high enough to ensure penetration of the part but not too high to diminish radiographic contrast.

P

parallel/nonfocused grid A grid with lead lines that run parallel to one another.

penetrometer A device comprising uniform absorbers of increasing thicknesses.

phosphor layer Active layer that is the most important screen component because it contains the material that absorbs the transmitted x-rays and converts them to visible light.

photocathode Converts the visible light in the image intensifier into electrons.

photoelectric effect Complete absorption of the incoming x-ray photon occurs when it has enough energy to remove (eject) an inner-shell electron. The ionized atom has a vacancy, or electron hole, in its inner shell, and an electron from an outer shell drops down to fill the vacancy.

photoelectron The ejected electron resulting from ionization during the photoelectric effect.

photoemission A process of emitting electrons in response to light stimulus.

photomultiplier (PM) tube An electronic device that converts visible light energy into electrical energy.

photon A small, discrete bundle of energy.

photostimulable luminescence (PSL) The emission of visible light from the photostimulable phosphor when stimulated by a high-intensity laser beam.

photostimulable phosphor (PSP) The phosphor layer of the imaging plate composed of barium fluorohalide crystals doped with europium.

phototimer Uses a fluorescent (light-producing) screen and a device that converts light to electricity in an AEC device.

picture archival and communication system (PACS) A computer system designed for digital imaging that can receive, store, distribute, and display digital images.

pixel The smallest component of the matrix. Also known as *picture elements*.

pixel density The number of pixels per unit area.

pixel pitch The pixel spacing or distance measured from the center of a pixel to an adjacent pixel.

pulse rate The number of pulses (frames) per second of operation.

pulse width The length of the radiation exposure for each pulse (frame).

pulsed fluoroscopy The x-ray exposure has gaps of exposure between each image frame.

Q

quantum A small, discrete bundle of energy.

quantum noise Visible as brightness or density fluctuations on the image as a result of too few photons reaching the image receptor to form the image. *Quantum mottle* is the term typically used when referring to noise on a film image.

R

radioactivity Unstable atoms spontaneously emitting particles and energy from the nucleus in an effort to attain stability.

radiographic contrast In film-screen imaging it is the degree of difference between adjacent densities and a result of both the subject contrast and the film contrast.

radiographic density The amount of overall blackness produced on the processed film image.

radiology information system (RIS) Similar to the HIS but specific to radiology. If the patient is scheduled for a radiology procedure, patient electronic information (demographics, relevant history, digital images, and interpretations) is stored and becomes a part of the radiology workflow.

rare earth elements Chemical compounds of elements that are relatively difficult and expensive to extract from the earth and range in atomic number from 57 to 71 on the periodic table of elements.

recirculation system Acts to circulate solution in a film processing tank by pumping the solution out of one portion of the tank and returning it to a different location within the same tank from which it was removed.

reducing agents Developing agents that reduce exposed silver halide to metallic silver and add electrons to the exposed silver halide during film processing.

region of interest Postprocessing function that provides calculation of selected pixel values within the area of interest to provide quantitative information about the tissue.

relative speed   Results by comparing film-screen systems on the basis of the amount of light produced for a given exposure.

remnant radiation   When the attenuated x-ray beam leaves the patient, the remaining x-ray beam is composed of both transmitted and scattered radiation. Also known as *exit radiation*.

replenishment   The replacement of fresh chemicals after the loss of chemicals during film processing, specifically, developer solution and fixer solution.

reversible compression   Image compression where there is no loss of image data (lossless) at the end user.

rotor   A device in the x-ray tube that causes the target to rapidly rotate during x-ray production.

S

sampling frequency   How often the analog signal is reproduced in its discrete digitized form.

sampling pitch   The distance between the sampling points.

saturation   The image receptor is extremely over exposed, cannot be properly processed, and the quality is severely degraded.

scale of contrast   The range of densities visible in a film image.

scattering   Some incoming photons are not absorbed; instead they lose energy during interactions with atoms comprising tissue.

scintillator   A phosphor material that converts the exit radiation into visible light.

screen film   Radiographic film sensitive to light emitted by the intensifying screen.

screen speed   The capability of an intensifying screen to produce visible light. The greater the speed, the more sensitive it is.

secondary electron   The ejected electron resulting from the Compton effect interaction. Also known as a *Compton electron*.

sensitometer   A device designed to produce consistent step-wedge densities.

sensitometric curve   A graph of step-wedge optical densities that visually demonstrates the relationship between the intensity of radiation exposure (x-axis) and the resultant optical densities (y-axis).

sensitometric strip   A density step-wedge image.

sensitometry   The study of the relationship between the intensity of radiation exposure to a film and the amount of blackness produced after processing (density).

shape distortion   Images of objects that appear longer or shorter than the true objects.

short-dimension linear grid   Contains lead strips running perpendicular to the long axis of the grid.

short-scale contrast   A film radiograph with few densities but great differences among them is said to have *high contrast*.

shoulder region   A point on the sensitometric curve where changes in exposure intensity no longer affect the optical density.

signal-to-noise ratio (SNR)   A method of describing the strength of the radiation exposure compared with the amount of noise apparent in a digital image.

silver halide   A material sensitive to radiation and light.

silver recovery   The removal of silver from used fixer solution.

size distortion or magnification   An increase in the image size of an object compared with its true, or actual, size.

slope   Steepness of the sensitometric curve indicated by the ratio of the change in y (optical density) for a unit change in x (log relative exposure).

smoothing   A postprocessing technique that suppresses image noise (quantum noise). However, spatial resolution is degraded.

source-to-image-receptor distance (SID)   The distance between the source of the radiation and the image receptor.

source-to-object distance (SOD)   The distance from the x-ray source (focal spot) to the object being radiographed.

space charge   The electrons liberated from the filament during thermionic emission that form a cloud around the filament.

space charge effect   The tendency of the space charge not to allow more electrons to be boiled off the filament.

spatial frequency   Variation in anatomic details imaged as white to black brightness levels that can be defined by the unit of line pairs per millimeter (lp/mm).

spatial resolution   The smallest detail that can be detected in an image; the term typically used in digital imaging.

spectral emission   The color of light produced by a particular intensifying screen.

spectral matching   Correctly matching the color sensitivity of the film to the color emission of the intensifying screen.

spectral sensitivity   The color of light to which a particular film is most sensitive.

speed   A film's sensitivity to radiation exposure.

speed exposure point   The area on the x-axis (log of exposure) that produced the optical density of 1.0 plus B + F.

speed point   The point on a sensitometric curve that corresponds to the optical density of 1.0 plus B + F.

standby control   An electric circuit that shuts off power to the roller assemblies when the film processor is not being used.

stator   An electric motor that turns the rotor at very high speed during x-ray production.

step-wedge densities   A radiograph of uniform densities resembling a step wedge.

stitching   A postprocessing operation to combine multiple images into one image for viewing anatomic areas such as for a scoliosis series.

straight-line region   The area on the sensitometric curve where the diagnostic or most useful range of densities is produced.

subject contrast   A result of the absorption characteristics of the anatomic tissue radiographed along with the quality of the x-ray beam.

T

target   A metal that abruptly decelerates and stops electrons in the tube current, allowing the production of x-rays.

teleradiology   The practice of diagnostic image interpretation outside the facility (offsite) from where the imaging data is acquired.

thermionic emission   The boiling off of electrons from the cathode filament.

tissue density   Matter per unit volume or the compactness of the anatomic particles comprising the anatomic part.

toe region   The area of low density on the sensitometric curve.

total filtration   The sum of the x-ray tube's added and inherent filtration.

transmission   The incoming x-ray photon passes through the anatomic part without any interaction with the atomic structures.

trough filter   A double-wedge compensating filter added to the primary beam to produce more consistent exposure to the image receptor.

tube current   The flow of electrons from cathode to anode, measured in milliamperes (mA).

V

values of interest (VOI)   Determines the range of the histogram data set included in the displayed image.

variable kVp/fixed mAs technique chart   A type of exposure technique chart based on the concept that kVp can be increased as the anatomic part size increases. The baseline kVp is increased by 2 for every 1-cm increase in part thickness, and the mAs is maintained.

vendor neutral archives (VNAs)   Allows for images and data from different systems and in different formats to be stored using a singular system on a common infrastructure.

virtual collimation   Lines on the last image hold indicating the position of the collimator plates that allows for collimation without exposing the patient to additional radiation.

voltage ripple   The amount of consistency in voltage waveforms during x-ray production.

W

wafer grid   A type of stationary grid placed on top of the image receptor.

wavelength   The distance between two successive crests or troughs.

wedge filter   The most common type of compensating filter. The thicker part of the wedge filter is lined up with the thinner portion of the anatomic part that is being imaged, allowing fewer x-ray photons to reach that end of the part.

window level   Sets the midpoint (center) of the range of brightness visible in the digital image.

window width   The range or number of shades of gray visible on the digital image.

X

x-ray emission spectrum   The range and intensity of emitted x-rays.

Page numbers followed by '*f*' indicate figures, '*t*' indicate tables, and '*b*' indicate boxes.